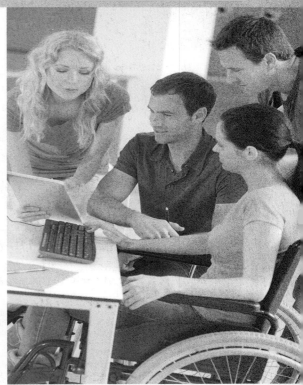

Introduction to Research

Understanding and Applying Multiple Strategies

Fifth Edition

Elizabeth DePoy, PhD, MSW, OTR
Professor, Interdisciplinary Disability Studies and Social Work
Cooperating Professor, Mechanical Engineering, Cooperating Faculty
School of Policy and International Affairs
University of Maine, Orono, Maine
Senior Research Fellow, Ono Academic College
Research Institute for Health and Medical Professions

Laura N. Gitlin, PhD
Professor, School of Nursing and School of Medicine
Director, Center for Innovative Care in Aging
Johns Hopkins University
Baltimore, Maryland

ELSEVIER

ELSEVIER

3251 Riverport Lane
St. Louis, Missouri 63043

INTRODUCTION TO RESEARCH: UNDERSTANDING AND APPLYING
MULTIPLE STRATEGIES, 5TH EDITION

ISBN: 978-0-323261715

Notices

Knowledge and best practice in this field are constantly changing. As new research and experience broaden our understanding, changes in research methods, professional practices, or medical treatment may become necessary.

Practitioners and researchers must always rely on their own experience and knowledge in evaluating and using any information, methods, compounds, or experiments described herein. In using such information or methods they should be mindful of their own safety and the safety of others, including parties for whom they have a professional responsibility.

With respect to any drug or pharmaceutical products identified, readers are advised to check the most current information provided (i) on procedures featured or (ii) by the manufacturer of each product to be administered, to verify the recommended dose or formula, the method and duration of administration, and contraindications. It is the responsibility of practitioners, relying on their own experience and knowledge of their patients, to make diagnoses, to determine dosages and the best treatment for each individual patient, and to take all appropriate safety precautions.

To the fullest extent of the law, neither the Publisher nor the authors, contributors, or editors, assume any liability for any injury and/or damage to persons or property as a matter of products liability, negligence or otherwise, or from any use or operation of any methods, products, instructions, or ideas contained in the material herein.

Library of Congress Cataloging-in-Publication Data-
DePoy, Elizabeth, author.
  Introduction to research : understanding and applying multiple strategies / Elizabeth DePoy, Laura N. Gitlin.—Fifth edition.
    p. ; cm.
  Includes bibliographical references and index.
  ISBN 978-0-323-26171-5 (pbk. : alk. paper)
  I. Gitlin, Laura N., 1952– , author. II. Title.
  [DNLM: 1. Research Design.   2. Biomedical Research.   W 20.5]
  RA440.85
  362.1072—dc23
                                                                        2014038272

Professional Reference Director: Penny Rudolph
Content Development Manager: Jolynn Gower
Associate Content Development Specialist: Katie Guitierrez
Publishing Services Manager: Hemamalini Rajendrababu
Project Manager: Umarani Natarajan
Design Direction: Brian Salisbury

Working together
to grow libraries in
developing countries

www.elsevier.com • www.bookaid.org

Printed in the USA
Last digit is the print number: 9 8 7 6 5 4 3 2 1

To my husband Stephen, who lovingly challenges and thinks with me, and to my family

ED

To my husband Eduardo; my children Keith and Eric; my mom, dad, and brother, all of whom inspire

LNG

And to all of our students, from whom we have learned and continue to learn

ED and LNG

Foreword to Third Edition

This edition of DePoy and Gitlin provides health and human service students and professionals with significantly expanded material for understanding the philosophical foundations of research, the value of systematic inquiry, and the concrete steps for moving through the process of generating and sharing knowledge. What continues to distinguish this text from other research methodological volumes is that readers are exposed to what the authors identify as the 10 essentials of research, which involve the fundamental thinking and action processes required for the conduct of either naturalistic or quantitative approaches to research. The authors walk readers through each of the processes involved in framing a research problem, developing a knowledge base, understanding the role of theory, formulating research questions, and sequencing research. Readers will also learn action steps involved in determining the scope or "boundaries" of a study, data collection and measurement, data analysis, and report writing.

Despite its importance to practice, research method courses are often a required upper-division or graduate-level course that students in health and human service dread—thinking they will need to memorize facts and figures that have little relevance to their career goals and daily practices. DePoy and Gitlin offer an antidote to such fears, making research come alive by the generous use of examples throughout the text, chapters specific to using research in practice, and a final chapter on "stories from the field." Such examples and stories bring life to the essential thinking and action processes of research, enable practitioners to envision the value of research, and zero in on challenges that they may face in their own research endeavors. Of major significance is that the reader will gain a real appreciation of the research enterprise, be able to read and critique literature, and be guided in the conduct of different research approaches to answer practical and clinically relevant research questions. Of added value, this introductory text provides checklists that will help the researcher get started, as well as a list of references for more in-depth examination. Thus the reader gains greater insight into the role of research in improving practice and an increased appreciation of the science and artistry of research.

Whereas most texts emphasize one research tradition over another, the philosophical underpinnings of experimental and naturalistic inquiry are both presented, with the emphasis on the value and importance of each approach. Readers learn about how research questions are framed in each approach and the unique designs and methods appropriate to each research tradition. The take-home message is that both approaches have legitimacy and their own standards of excellence. Rigor is expected whether the approach is experimental or naturalistic, and studies that include both approaches often provide unique insights that go beyond what can be learned from a single approach. This perspective represents an important aspect of this text that contributes as well to the broader debate and discussions about the role and value of different research traditions and design strategies.

This edition contains several new sections and chapters that address topics on the cutting edge of the research venture: information on ethics and evidence-based clinical practices, as well as informed consent documentation. Ethical considerations are paramount these days, and each researcher should be fully aware of requirements for human subject protections and new federal privacy rules that have implications for the type of data that can be collected. This new edition also includes a chapter on seeking financial support for research ideas and practical hints for getting started on writing a research proposal. This is particularly important as health professionals are increasingly expected to seek resources for their programs and related evaluations.

Especially notable is the chapter on practice efficacy. The processes of reviewing and rating existing literature and developing consensus around practice guidelines and best practices are delineated. With tight resources for health and human services, there are increasing demands for accountability to demonstrate the worth of different programs and practices. This chapter provides important information for understanding the pros and cons of the evidence-based movement that is gaining popularity among researchers and funding agencies. Although this approach has strong endorsement in the experimental research field, there are cautions in assuming that randomized clinical trials are the gold standard for research. Although such studies are important for maximizing internal validity, they can be criticized for limited generalizability, are difficult to implement in community-based settings, and do not address the full range of questions relevant to clinical practice. DePoy and Gitlin's Evaluation Practice conceptualization makes a substantial contribution to the literature, providing an easy-to-follow model that incorporates both thinking and action processes, including clarification of the problem, reflexive intervention, and outcome assessment. These concepts are critical to understanding the long-term sustainability of a program or service and offer an innovative approach to integrating research into practice and bridging the research-practice gap.

As in many disciplines, the health and human services field is characterized by a research-to-practice gap. Researchers are generally focused on research theories and designs, data collection, and statistics, which are typically uninformed by practice. On the other hand, practitioners typically rely on clinical practice informed by individual experience independent of a larger theory- and research-driven knowledge base. This gap limits the ability of research to translate into meaningful programs and practices that can make a real difference in people's lives.

This book provides a critical bridge between research and practice by having practitioners understand that their clinical intuition can inform research thinking and action processes and by having researchers learn to appreciate the contexts in which systematic thinking and action processes are implemented. It reflects a significant paradigm shift in thinking about and acting on the essential research elements. Its presentation also represents a fundamental shift in the teaching paradigm from a "talking at" approach to engaging text that emphasizes a "listening to" philosophy.

A major joy of this text is the stories woven by two esteemed researchers who draw on a lifetime of practical experiences that have improved the conceptualization, implementation, and evaluation of different research traditions. The passion of DePoy and Gitlin for their research and practice comes through every page of the book and serves to make this book a truly enjoyable reading and learning experience.

Marcia G. Ory, PhD, MPH
Professor, Social and Behavioral Health
Director, Active for Life National Program Office
School of Rural Public Health
The Texas A & M University System

Preface

Our main purpose in writing this fifth edition is to continue to share with the student, health and human service professional, and beginning researcher our great enthusiasm and passion for conducting research in health and human service using multiple research strategies. Research is an important way of helping to make a difference in the provision of health and human service and the quality of life and well-being of individuals. We have made some substantive changes to this edition that we hope will demystify the research process and provide a foundation from which to critique, understand, and apply multiple research strategies to health and human service concerns. In this fifth edition, we have refined and expanded our framework from which to examine and integrate different research traditions in diverse physical, virtual, and conceptual contexts. In so doing, our goal remains to challenge traditional teaching approaches to research processes, to further narrow the gap between quantitative and qualitative paradigms, and to create a meaningful and useful bridge between research and practice.

Why do health and human service professionals need yet another research text and this new edition? As we stated in the previous editions of this book, health and human service professions continue to stand at the crossroads of significant megatrends in the delivery and financing of services to clients and families, as well as local, global, and virtual communities. These trends continue to change at a rapid pace and include the movement from an acute, medical framework to diverse on-site and virtual models of care; a focus on health promotion, disease self-management, and disease prevention; the development of new paradigms for examining the interplay of behavioral, environmental, economic, political, spiritual, and biological interactions and their impact on health; an increased emphasis on the design and testing of innovative services for under-recognized, underserved, and diverse populations; and recognition of the importance of using systematically derived knowledge to drive care decisions and program development.

These new directions in health and human services require the most current and innovative approaches to research. The traditional research paradigm taught to students of the social sciences and health professions, referred to as quantitative, empiricist, positivist, or rationalist, represents only one approach to scientific inquiry. Historically, the quantitative or experimental-type approach to research has been upheld as the most scientific, valid, and precise methodology. Unfortunately, this belief lingers in the health and human service worlds, is favored in practice models such as evidence-based practice, and significantly limits the efficacious use of other research strategies. This, in turn, continues to restrict knowledge building and use of research knowledge in practice settings. In light of these limitations and the expanded contexts in which research is being conducted, such as the Internet, other research traditions—such as discovery-oriented, interpretive, qualitative, naturalistic, participatory, visual cultural, and mixed methodologies—are rapidly gaining importance and recognition as forms of inquiry with their own rules and systematic approaches to understanding human behavior in context.

The viewpoint we present in this fifth edition reflects an increasingly accepted school of thought that recognizes and values multiple research strategies. This contemporary perspective proposes that naturalistic, experimental-type, and mixed method research strategies have equal value and contribute in complementary and distinct ways to the science of practice. Knowledge of all of these research traditions presents new opportunities for addressing the complex health and human service research questions that are emerging as a consequence of today's diverse health care environments. Students, professionals, and researchers need a research text that prepares them for using the full range of research traditions to meet the scientific challenges posed by changing service systems. For example, to develop effective health promotion programs for global communities composed of individuals from diverse backgrounds requires an understanding of the specific health beliefs and self-care practices of different groups. Traditional survey techniques have not always been successful in identifying different self-care practices, and existing standardized health belief questionnaires do not necessarily represent the varied values of diverse groups across the globe. Different methodologies and approaches that uncover and accurately represent personal beliefs and practices are required for knowledge building in this area.

Since our previous editions were published, many articles and books have discussed and evaluated new methodologies, particularly those from the tradition of naturalistic inquiry and, more recently, mixed methods. However, our approach in this edition continues to differ significantly from other research texts, including these more recent editions to the literature. Most texts for health and human service professionals still identify quantitative research as the most valid approach to scientific inquiry. Some of these research texts include a discussion of other research traditions but most often in comparison to the gold standard of the experiment. Still other texts explain naturalistic and mixed methods inquiry by using the framework or lens of the experimental researcher. In doing so, the authors assume that the three genres differ only with respect to specific procedures. They do not present an approach to understanding each tradition from within its own lens, nor do they discuss the philosophical roots of each tradition and the essential thinking processes that underlie the activity of each. Thus, the research student cannot come to fully understand and accurately implement different design strategies from all three traditions. The student does not obtain a critical understanding of the vast array of research possibilities, or learn strategies by which to purposively select a particular research approach.

In contrast, this text provides a comprehensive understanding of how researchers think and act within and across the research traditions and in diverse contexts. It provides a basic introduction to the essential components of a wide range of research approaches. It offers the researcher and student a framework for understanding the research enterprise overall—one that embraces each of the research traditions and methodologies. The reader learns how to critically evaluate, respect, and implement each research strategy from its own philosophical perspective, thinking process, language, standards of rigor, and specific actions that engage the researcher.

Writing the fifth edition of *Introduction to Research: Understanding and Applying Multiple Strategies* has given us an important opportunity to reflect on and advance our ongoing conceptualization of the three research traditions and their use in expanded health and social service contexts. In this edition we have refined our thinking and present the 10 essential thinking and action processes of research that appeared in previous editions across all three traditions. We show how these highly integrated processes are thought about and solved differently, depending on the particular research tradition being pursued. We have seen from our previous editions that a process approach improves our ability to describe and capture the essence of a range of research strategies and is easily grasped by readers.

Readers of our previous editions will experience the fifth edition as an improvement in several ways. Not only have we updated our major discussion of the research traditions and their philosophical foundations, but we have also added new material on ethics and on global to local contexts in which research is initiated, conducted, and disseminated, as well as discussion about the nature of evidence, its integration within practice settings, and how practice settings can generate evidence systematically. We have updated all examples and expanded our discussion to include new methodologies such as visual culture object analysis. Nevertheless, our underlying assumptions about the purpose and conduct of research and much of our discussions remain intact. We believe all readers will benefit from the clarity that a process approach brings to understanding the fundamentals of conducting research in each of the research traditions.

Readers will also have access to a wealth of resources on our Evolve site. Our Evolve student learning resources offer the following features: crossword puzzles, sample forms, reference lists linked to PubMed, and math tips to accompany Chapter 20. The Evolve instructor teaching resources offer multiple-choice test bank questions with answers, teaching tips, and PowerPoint lecture slides.

The fifth edition reflects an organization similar to that in previous editions. The book is organized into five major sections. The first four sections move the reader from an understanding of the meaning, elements, and importance of research (Part I) to an examination of the specific thinking processes (Part II), design approaches (Part III), and action processes (Part IV) of distinct research traditions. Each chapter in Parts I to IV focuses on one of the 10 essentials of the research process, all of which are discussed using the language of experimental-type, naturalistic, and mixed method researchers. Part V is devoted to using research to improve professional practices and outcomes. Throughout the text, many actual and suggested research examples are provided from diverse bodies of literature and our own research experiences that are relevant to all health and human service providers. As in previous editions, we end with field stories—real-life snapshots of what it is like to participate in different types of research processes based on our own experiences. These brief narrative accounts reveal the hidden side of the research process, how a study unfolds, what it is like to be an investigator, and what really happens after entering the research context. Research, after all, is a human endeavor. Too few researchers dare to discuss the personal ups and downs and common blunders that inform knowledge construction.

In this text, we do not intend to solve the controversy over which tradition (qualitative, quantitative, mixed method) or design approach is best, nor do we think that is the debate to be undertaken. Rather, we urge health and human service professionals to transcend this age-old disagreement and go beyond attempts of the health care and scientific communities to polarize research practices. We propose that knowing the strengths and weaknesses of the full range of approaches to thinking and conducting research provides the basis from which to select, combine, and use multiple strategies to answer research questions.

Who should use this text? This fifth edition, like our previous editions, can be used by undergraduate and advanced students in the health and human service professions. It can also be used by practitioners and beginning researchers who want to broaden their understanding of research traditions to which they have not been previously exposed. Health and human service professionals will continue to experience increasing pressure to initiate research, participate as members of research teams, and use research findings to assess and justify their practice and service programs. This text provides a solid and current foundation from which to pursue these activities. We hope you enjoy and become hooked as we have on the thinking and action processes of research.

Elizabeth DePoy
Laura N. Gitlin

Contents

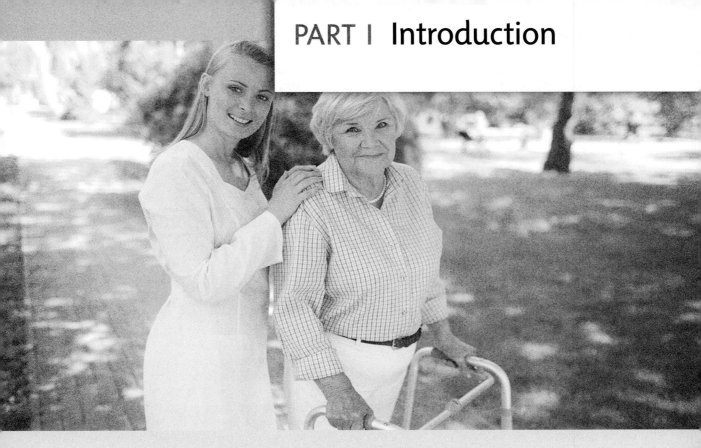

PART I Introduction

Welcome to the world of research!

Conducting research is one of the most challenging, creative, and intellectually satisfying professional activities. Research is an important professional responsibility that develops and advances knowledge from which to base practice. This knowledge is essential if we, as health and human service professionals, are to provide informed quality services that enhance the health, lives, and outcomes of our clients, their families, and their communities.

Part I begins with our definition of research. We identify and discuss the 10 elements of the research process that are essential to the traditions of all research designs.

At this point you may be thinking, "What is research?" "Why is it necessary?" "How does research differ from other ways of learning about things?" "How does one engage in research?" and "What is the process?"

These important questions are examined in the chapters of Part I.

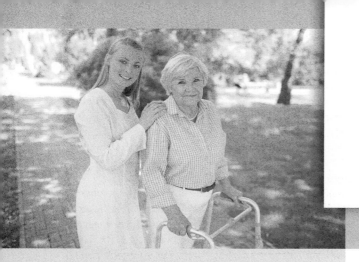

Chapter 1
Research as an Important Way of Knowing

A 74-year-old single African-American woman with a fractured hip will be discharged shortly from rehabilitation to her home. She appears reluctant to use the self-care techniques you taught her. You wonder whether rehabilitation has been effective in meeting its specified goals and what her future capabilities will be after she returns home.

You have learned how to use a new tool to assess the environmental barriers encountered by children with intellectual impairments. You wonder whether this instrument is more accurate and useful than previous ones you have tried.

A research article describes a progressive approach to promoting physical fitness for adults with intellectual impairments. You wonder whether you should implement these planning procedures in your own practice and whether they will be effective in meeting their goal in diverse geographic locations.

You need to initiate a new program to prevent low back injury in migrant farmworkers. Existing prevention strategies have not been effective in reducing the incidence of low back injury in this population. You wonder why traditional approaches have failed and how to develop an appropriate knowledge base from which to develop an efficacious program.

You notice in your home care practice that some clients need more visits than others to achieve the same health outcomes. You wonder what factors influence service need. You wonder how to increase health literacy and access to health information for people who cannot see.

You are interested in how the outcomes of Internet counseling for minor depression compare to on-site counseling outcomes.

What Is Research?

Research is not "owned" by any one profession or discipline. It is a systematic set of ways of thinking and acting and has distinct vocabularies that can be learned and used by anyone.

Many definitions of research can be found in texts, ranging from a very broad to a very restrictive understanding of the research endeavor. A very broad definition suggests that research includes any type of investigation that uncovers knowledge. In contrast, a formal and more restrictive definition of research implies that only one type of strategy, such as a quantitative orientation, is valid. Many researchers use the classic (but we believe restricted) definition offered by Kerlinger, who defined scientific research as "systematic, controlled, empirical, and critical investigation of natural phenomena guided by theory and hypotheses about the presumed relations among such phenomena."[1] Whereas a broad definition includes any type of activity as research, a restrictive definition, such as Kerlinger's viewpoint, implies that the only legitimate approach to scientific inquiry is hypothesis testing.

In contrast, we define research to reflect and allow for a wide range of systematic and logical ways of knowing or approaches to knowledge building. As such, our definition of research is as follows:

> *Research is defined as multiple, systematic strategies to generate knowledge about human behavior, human experience, and human environments in which the thinking and action processes of the researcher are clearly specified so that they are logical, understandable, confirmable, and useful.*

Our definition has three important components (Box 1-1). First, we state that research is more than one type of investigative strategy; that is, research is not just hypothesis testing, as suggested by Kerlinger, but rather is represented by a broad range of strategies that are systematically implemented. In contrast

---

BOX 1-1 *What Is Research?*

Multiple Systematic Strategies
- Experimental-type design
- Naturalistic inquiry

Thought and Action Processes
- Inductive
- Abductive
- Deductive

Four Criteria
- Logical
- Understandable
- Confirmable
- Useful

---

to the definition offered by the restrictive view, we recognize the legitimacy and value of many distinct types of investigative strategies. Second, our definition emphasizes that research is composed of thinking processes and specific actions (action processes) that must be clearly delineated and articulated. We believe that the beauty and efficacy of the research process lie in the explication of how and on what basis a knowledge claim is made. Third, we characterize thinking and action processes as logical, understandable, confirmable, and useful to meet the criteria of research. That is, in contrast to the broad inclusive definition of research, our approach clearly distinguishes the boundary between research and other forms of knowing (e.g., through trial and error) by establishing these important criteria. Let us examine the three major components of our definition in greater detail.

Research as Multiple Systematic Strategies

The first component of our research definition emphasizes the value of varied systematic strategies to understand the depth and range of research questions and queries posed by health and human service professionals. These multiple research strategies can be categorized as representing *naturalistic inquiry*, *experimental-type research*, or *mixed methods that contain parts of both classical traditions*. The two classical categories of research, experimental-type and naturalistic, are based in distinct philosophical traditions, follow different forms of human reasoning, and define and obtain knowledge differently. Naturalistic inquiry refers to a wide range of research approaches characterized by a focus on understanding and interpreting human experience within the context in which experience occurs. Experimental-type research refers to a range of designs characterized by a focus on prediction and hypothesis testing. Naturalistic inquiry tends to be *idiographic;* that is, it focuses on specific phenomena in a context and seeks to highlight the complexity of these phenomena. Experimental-type approaches examine and characterize what is typical about one or more groups; this approach is referred to as *nomothetic.* Mixed methods are anchored in philosophical pragmatism and thus employ strategies from both experimental-type and naturalistic methods to account for the limitations of each classical approach. Chapter 4 examines the differences between these three research traditions, their philosophical roots, and their implications for health and human service research.

Our viewpoint, however, reflects a school of thought that has been expressed in numerous professional and academic disciplines. This school of thought proposes that naturalistic inquiry, experimental-type research, and mixed methods hold equal importance in establishing a knowledge base of health and human service practice and in adequately examining the diversity of human experiences and behaviors. Idiographic and nomothetic understandings each reveal different, valuable, and necessary knowledge.

This viewpoint also firmly asserts that it is not reasonable to critique naturalistic research using experimental language because each approach represents a distinct *epistemology*, or way of knowing and obtaining knowledge.[2] As Gareth Morgan, cited by Patton in one of his classic works, eloquently claimed:

> *It is not possible to judge the validity or contribution of different research perspectives in terms of the ground assumptions of any one set of perspectives, since the process is self-justifying. Hence the attempts in much social science debate to judge the utility of different research strategies in terms of universal criteria based on the importance of generalizability, predictability and control, explanation of variance, meaningful understanding, or whatever are inevitably flawed: These criteria inevitably favor research strategies consistent with the assumptions that generate such criteria as meaningful guidelines for the evaluation of research.... Different research perspectives make different kinds of knowledge claims, and the criteria as to what counts as significant knowledge vary from one to another.*[2]

Another implication of our perspective is that combining or mixing methods is an important and purposive approach to the study of many of the complex issues of current concern to health and human service professionals. As Bonilla-Silva asserts with regard to the study of contemporary racism, "The research strategy that seems more appropriate for our times is mixed research designs because it allows researchers to cross-examine their results."[3]

Research as Thinking and Action Processes

The second important component of our definition of research refers to *thinking* and *action processes*. Thinking processes and action processes represent the different ways of reasoning and the specific series of actions that distinguish naturalistic and experimental-type investigators in the conduct of their research. Experimental-type research uses primarily a deductive form of logical reasoning. Naturalistic inquiry primarily uses inductive and abductive forms of logic. Each leads to different types of research actions and generates different information or knowledge. Table 1-1 summarizes the major characteristics of these approaches to logical reasoning.

Deductive Reasoning and Actions

Experimental-type researchers primarily use *deductive logic*. This type of reasoning involves moving from a general principle to understanding a specific case. On the basis of a theory and its propositions, hypotheses are derived and then formally tested. Health and human service professionals use deductive reasoning every day in their practices.[4,5] As an example, a professional proceeding from the theory that clinical depression is a mood state that manifests in flat affect, sleep disturbance, change in appetite, and dysphoria would ascertain the

TABLE 1-1	Major Characteristics of Inductive/Abductive and Deductive Thinking	
Inductive/Abductive		**Deductive**
No a priori acceptance of truth exists		A priori acceptance of truth exists
Alternative conclusions can be drawn from data		One set of conclusions is accepted as true
Theory is developed		Theory is tested
Relationships are examined among unrelated pieces of data		Relationships are tested among discrete phenomena
Concepts are developed based on repetition of patterns		Concepts are tested based on application to discrete phenomena
Perspective is holistic		Perspective is atomistic
Multiple realities exist		Single, separate reality exists

degree to which a client had these symptoms. If each of these symptoms were found to be sufficiently present, the provider would deduce, on the basis of the general theory, that the client was clinically depressed. The provider would then use theory deductively to determine how best to treat the depression, to define outcomes, and then to test treatment efficacy by assessing the theorized outcomes. Thus the theory accepted as accurate is applied as a guide for intervention and expected outcomes. Clinical assessment would examine the achievement of desired outcomes as defined within the theory and clinical context.

A similar process occurs in research. Using a deductive type of reasoning, the researcher begins with the acceptance of a general principle or belief based on a particular theoretical framework. This principle is then applied or used to explain a specific case or phenomenon. This approach involves "drawing out" or verifying what is already accepted as accurate.[6]

> For example, a researcher is interested in testing an intervention to improve the health of caregivers of people with dementia. In this case, the researcher may begin from a framework of caregiver-burden theory that assumes the characteristics or behaviors of the person with dementia negatively affect the health and well-being of and therefore place a burden on caregivers. Accepting this principle as accurate, the deductive researcher will be interested in testing the effectiveness of interventions that are designed to reduce burden by providing education, teaching behavioral skills management, or providing respite. •

Inductive Reasoning and Actions

Researchers who work within a naturalistic framework primarily use *inductive reasoning*. This type of reasoning involves moving from specific cases to a broader generalization about the phenomenon under study.[9] In some forms of naturalistic inquiry, inductive reasoning involves fitting data, such as a set of observations or propositions, into existing theory. Health and human service professionals also use this form of reasoning in everyday practice.

> For example, assume you need to determine the discharge plans for a woman with dementia. You have concerns about her ability to live alone, based on your knowledge of dementia as a progressively deteriorating condition. However, you do not know anything about the circumstances of this particular woman, her personal goals and those of her family, or her specific living arrangements. By observing her in a clinical context, as well as conducting in-depth interviews with the patient and her family members, you discover that an adequate plan for monitoring and caring for this woman has been put into place. Thus, you make a discharge decision based on systematic information you uncovered inductively. •

A similar reasoning process occurs in research. Reflecting the inductive logical thinking process, the researcher seeks general rules or patterns emerging from specific observations. In pure inductive thinking, there is no "truth" or general principle that is accepted *a priori* ("from the former") or before the study begins. Consider the example of caregiving previously discussed. To derive an understanding of the nature and scope of caregiver burden, one type of inductive research approach could involve examining the daily life experiences of caregivers and their own perceptions of their activities. Using a variety of data collection techniques, such as observation and in-depth interviewing, the researcher might reason inductively by searching for patterns across observations of different caregivers. From this approach, the researcher would be able to develop an understanding of the specific situations that cause stress and burden, or perhaps their absence, as well as the types of interventions that would be most useful in promoting caregiver health. The researcher, proceeding inductively, might seek to reveal or uncover knowledge based on the perceptions of caregivers. Intervention principles would then be developed based on the researcher's interpretations of the perceptions of caregivers. In this example, the researcher might use the principles learned from those who do not experience stress to inform intervention for those who do.[7]

Abductive Reasoning and Actions

As we just discussed, the two research traditions are typically characterized as using deductive and inductive reasoning processes; experimental-type research uses deductive reasoning, and naturalistic inquiry uses inductive reasoning. However, according to Flick, von Kardorff, and Steinke,[10] this representation is not complete. Some approaches in naturalistic inquiry are best characterized as "abductive."[2,9,10] Abduction is a term introduced by Charles Peirce[6] and currently used by researchers and logicians to refer to an iterative process in naturalistic inquiry. This process involves the development of new theoretical propositions that can best account for a set of observations, which cannot be accounted for or explained by a previous proposition or theoretical framework. The new theoretical proposition becomes validated and modified as part of the research process. In this way, ethnography and some other forms of naturalistic inquiry, such as grounded theory,[16] are considered to be "theory generating." In deductive reasoning the data are contained and controlled by the hypotheses. In inductive reasoning, an attempt is made to fit the data to a theoretical framework or to generate a set of identified and well-defined concepts that emerge form the data. In *abductive reasoning*, the data are analyzed for their own patterns and concepts, which in some cases may relate to available theories and in other cases may not relate.

As we discuss in depth throughout the book and in Chapter 12, mixing methods may involve all three logical structures or just two of the three. As an example, returning to the caregiver burden inquiry, the researcher may accept existing theory as accurate in some instances but not in others. Thus, a deductive process may be used to test the presence of caregiver burden using a survey deductively developed from caregiver burden theory and then followed with open-ended interviews to seek new theoretical insights.

Differences in Knowledge

Each type of reasoning will result in the generation or production of a different form of knowledge. An inductive or abductive reasoning approach in research is used to "uncover" or "reveal" theory, rules, and processes.[2] A deductive reasoning approach is used to describe, test, or predict the application of theory and rules to a specific phenomenon. Both approaches can be used to describe, explain, and predict phenomena. The acceptance of mixed methods is becoming increasingly widespread, as complex phenomena often require a combination of logical approaches to both test and revise theory and its application to health and human service concerns.

Let us examine the type of knowledge that is generated by each reasoning approach. The researcher working deductively will assume a theoretical truth before engaging in the research process and will apply that truth to the investigation. In the caregiver example, the researcher would assume that all caregivers will experience a form of burden in which they experience stress. The researcher therefore hypothesizes that caregivers will benefit from a stress-reduction intervention that may take the form of group psychoeducational counseling sessions and would be based on existing caregiver burden theory. Research that tested this intervention approach has found it to be only mildly effective in reducing caregiver stress and only for some caregiver study participants.[7] Thus, the question remains as to why all caregivers do not benefit at the level at which researchers expect.

In a study proceeding inductively or abductively, the researcher might be looking for an intervention approach to emerge from what is learned from those who will receive the intervention or those who do not need it. Caregiver research that uses an inductive process may therefore find that caregiver experience cannot be completely understood or explained by caregiver burden theory or addressed by stress-oriented interventions alone. New interventions would be suggested by inductively oriented inquiry, such as a broader array of services, based on the specific needs and care issues identified by the study participants and the strategies used by those who do not experience stress.

The deductive approach could show that a stress-reduction intervention benefits some caregivers. The inductive approach could reveal that burden theory is too limited to describe comprehensively the multiple strengths and needs of this group and that other theories and types of interventions would be helpful to consider.

As you can see, each type of reasoning and research approach produces important information from which to advance services to caregivers. It is also possible to use both types of reasoning to address a research problem. For example, you can use an inductive or abductive approach to identify specific areas of caregiver needs and then use a deductive strategy to test systematically the outcome of an intervention that addresses the identified needs. This inductive-abductive-deductive approach has been successfully used to develop and test community-based health and human service programs for underserved and culturally diverse populations. First, investigators used inductive strategies to uncover the health and wellness beliefs and needs of the target group. On the basis of the findings and theoretical frameworks that were refined, intervention strategies were developed, implemented, and systematically evaluated.

The integration of different forms of reasoning makes intuitive sense. In our daily lives, we naturally engage in all forms of reasoning. Likewise, health and human service professionals combine knowledge gained from both deductive and inductive reasoning to derive appropriate treatment plans. For this reason, if possible, mixing methods is desirable.[13] As we discuss throughout, integrating logic and the methods based on diverse structures provides the opportunity for both building and testing knowledge.

Research as Four Basic Characteristics

The third important component of our research definition refers to the criteria we use to characterize the research activity and differentiate it from other ways of knowing about a phenomenon. We have stated that scientific knowledge may be generated by multiple research strategies using inductive or abductive or deductive reasoning. Any research strategy, whether based on inductive or abductive or deductive reasoning, must conform to the four criteria of being logical, understandable, confirmable, and useful.

Logical

In research, there is a unique way of thinking and acting that distinguishes it from other ways we use to know, understand, and make sense of our experiences. Charles Peirce,[6] one of the founders of the scientific research process, identified other ways of "knowing" as the following: (1) authority—being told by a respected or trusted source; (2) hearsay—secondhand information that is not verified; (3) trial and error—knowledge gained through incremental doing, evaluating, and modifying actions to achieve a desired outcome; (4) history—knowing indirectly through collective past experiences (also referred to as memory); (5) belief—knowing without verification; (6) spiritual understanding—knowing through divine belief; and (7) intuition—explanations of human experience based on previous unique and personal organization of one's own experience. More recent theorists of knowledge espouse a range of ways of knowing from skepticism (doubt) to the inability to come to know anything at all suggested by some postmodernists.[14]

In these other forms, knowledge is gained unsystematically or even doubted as possible, and it is not necessary to clarify the evidentiary basis or the logical thinking and action processes by which the information is obtained and asserted. Think about how an individual gains knowledge about parenting or providing care to a person who requires assistance. Informal caregivers tend to learn how to provide care through trial and error. Information as to what works and what does not work to achieve a desired goal is gained incrementally, over time, by trying different techniques and informally evaluating their outcome. Many caregivers also use intuition and hearsay or information from other caregivers, family, and friends who may make suggestions based on their own history and experience. In contrast to this informal set of thinking and action processes, research must be based on systematic thought processes and methical investigative activities that include documentation, analysis, and drawing conclusions.

By "logical," we mean that the thinking and action processes of a research study are clear, rational, and conform to accepted norms of deductive, inductive, or abductive reasoning. Logic is a set of reasoning methods that involves defined ways of thinking and methodically relates ideas to develop an understanding of phenomena and their relationships.[2] The systematic nature of research requires that the investigator proceed logically and articulate each thought and action throughout the research process.

Understandable

Using our definition, it is not sufficient for a researcher to articulate a logical process. This process, the study outcomes, and conclusions need to be explicit, make sense, be precise, be intelligible, and be credible to the reader or research consumer. If you cannot understand the research process, it cannot be used, confirmed, or replicated and thus does not meet the criteria for research specified in our definition.

Historically, researchers using naturalistic inquiry did not typically identify the specific steps involved in their investigative process. Currently, however, a significant body of literature describes and makes explicit the thinking and action processes of different forms of naturalistic inquiry.[15-17] Investigators who work out of the naturalistic tradition are advancing the standards of quality by which to judge such research. How are we to distinguish a casual observation from a scholarly interpretation of underlying patterns in that setting? Researchers have actively addressed this critical issue.[15-18]

Confirmable

By "confirmable," we mean that the researcher clearly and logically identifies the evidence and strategies used in the study so that others can reasonably follow the path of analysis and arrive at similar outcomes and conclusions. The claims made by the researcher should be supported by the evidence and research strategy and should be accurate and credible within the stated boundaries of the study.

Useful

Research generates, verifies, or tests theory and knowledge for use. In other words, the knowledge derived from a study should be purposive[19] and should inform and potentially improve professional practice and client outcome. Each researcher, consumer, or professional judges the utility of a study on the basis of his or her own needs and purposes. Usefulness is a subjective criterion in that it is based on the judgment about the value of the knowledge produced by a study. However, the value of a study and the usefulness of knowledge become more widely accepted as the new knowledge increasingly stimulates further research and promotes the testing or verification of new or existing theory and practice.

What Research Is Not

We have just discussed what research is and defined it as four major criteria. You may have noticed that we did not say that research is a way to prove a theory, to come to a single truth, or to create static knowledge.[20] Research cannot tell us what is true or correct. Research cannot prove a point of view.[2] Rather, research is a set of logical reasoning processes in which theory is supported or developed, not proven. Given the essential place of theory within the research enterprise, you may now begin to see why there may be multiple perspectives, each accurately supported by research. Consider the example of depression. Suppose two researchers are seeking to evaluate the outcomes of interventions designed to alleviate depressive symptoms. The researcher proceeding from psychoanalytic theory would define depression as anger turned inward and thus the intervention would be designed to assist a client to express anger and place it external to the self. In this example, the researcher would likely test success by measuring or assessing the extent to which anger is displaced outward, referred to as a catharsis.[19] However, the researcher proceeding from the theory that anger is a chemical imbalance would be likely to examine the behavioral and physiological outcomes of antidepressant medications.

Which approach is correct or truth? Both and neither. As you can see, research cannot tell us what the one truth is. What if a researcher is not satisfied with any of the theories that currently are published to explain depression? This researcher might use inductive naturalistic inquiry to develop yet another theory.

Setting the Stage by Example

To illustrate the points discussed earlier and revisited throughout the book, consider this example. As a professional in a public health agency, you are focusing on smoking cessation and prevention. Given the increasing use of the Internet for disseminating health information, you decide to use this venue as a major part of your work. However, the literature reveals that there are significant disparities in access to Web-based health information due to literacy and visual access barriers. You decide to verify this theory with research and proceed to test your solutions systematically.

To inform your work, you conduct your first research project to answer the following questions:

1. What is the literacy level of smoking cessation and prevention websites?
2. How accessible are these websites to screen readers?

To conduct this initial project, you systematically measure two variables for smoking on selected websites: literacy level and ability for a text reader to convert text to oral presentation. To measure these variables, you select instruments that match the definitions of reading level and access and provide numeric ratings of each. Your results reveal that only one of the 50 randomly selected websites that you tested could be translated from text to oral presentation by a text reader and that the average website was written at an 11th-grade literacy level.

Now that you have verified the accuracy of the theory, you once again return to the literature. On the basis of research demonstrating that few web designers address visual access and literacy level, you develop an innovation that uses automated software to translate existing websites into fourth-grade literacy (the average reading level of the American public) and to accessible formatting. To test the efficacy of your innovation, you formulate the following research questions:

1. To what extent did users improve in their comprehension when using the translated websites?
2. To what extent do diverse web users feel comfortable in using, navigating, and interacting on the new websites?

3. What changes need to be made to improve Web use and comprehension?

To answer these questions, you design a mixed method study relying on the three logic structures. You recruit individuals with diverse visual abilities (full vision to no vision) and with low literacy levels. After screening them for inclusion into the study and testing their comprehension of the original site, you then ask them to access and read or hear the information on the experimental site. To answer question 1, you compute statistics to determine the differences in comprehension of the original and of the experimental website.

Questions 2 and 3 are answered in a focus group (a group interview in which a facilitator poses questions, and group members respond in an open-ended fashion).

Your finding indicates that comprehension and access improved when using the new website. Moreover, even many subjects who had typical vision preferred the oral version of the text. Subjects provided multiple recommendations for improving navigation and ease of use, as well as appearance preferences for the websites.

From this research agenda, you have learned important principles and knowledge to guide practice. First, you have verified the magnitude of literacy and visual access barriers to health information on the Web. Second, you have identified that these barriers could be remediated and selected software innovation as the method to do so. Third, you tested the intervention and found that it met your goals of comprehension and accessibility. Finally, you have Web user recommendations to further improve the website. You are now ready to expand this pilot to decrease disparities in Web-based health information.

When and Why Is Research Necessary and Useful?

The preceding discussion has alluded to the "when" and "why" of research. Here we explicate its necessity. Health and human service professionals routinely have questions about their daily practice and seek guidance from legitimate professional knowledge.[21] Many of these questions, such as those just listed, are answered best through systematic investigation, or the research process. Moreover, professionals should be able to articulate a body of knowledge that guides their decision making and activity in all phases of their professional interactions. It is therefore unfortunate that many practitioners do not engage in research both to master the precision of the thinking and action processes and to generate knowledge to advance their professions. This reluctance may be caused in part by unfamiliarity with and misconceptions about the research process.

Research is challenging, exhilarating, and stimulating. As with other professional activities, research can also be time-consuming, tedious, and frustrating. The challenges and frustrations of conducting research occur because it is not a simple activity—particularly health and human service research, in which conducting research in service environments and understanding human behavior are often complex matters. Implementing a research study in the home, community, school, outpatient clinic, or medical facility can be much more challenging than conducting research in a laboratory or a setting that the investigator can control. Throughout this book, we discuss the specific dilemmas and design implications posed by research that is implemented in the health and human service practice.

There are many important reasons why you should understand the research process and participate in research activities (Box 1-2).

BOX 1-2   *Seven Reasons to Learn About the Research Process*

1. Systematically build knowledge and test treatment efficacy
2. Have an impact on health policy and service delivery
3. Participate in research activities
4. Enhance understanding of daily practice
5. Become a critical consumer of research literature
6. Understand the method of clinical trials and apply this knowledge to professional practice
7. Apply the precision of research to all professional thinking and action

---

First, research is a systematic process to obtain scientific knowledge about specific problems encountered in daily life and professional practice.[5,12,22] Thus it is an important way of finding answers to questions about needed interventions, practice outcomes, and clinical puzzles. The fundamental goal of research for health and human services is to develop and advance a body of knowledge to guide professional activity. Research contributes to the development of a systematic body of knowledge in several ways. It generates relevant theory and knowledge about human appearance, experience, and behavior; it develops and tests theories that form the basis of specific practices and treatment approaches; and it examines, validates, or determines the effectiveness of different practices in attaining their intended and sometimes unintended outcomes.[12]

The second important reason to understand and participate in research is its overall impact on health definitions and theories, health care policy, and service delivery. The knowledge obtained through research is often used directly or indirectly to set standards for population health—to inform legislators and regulatory bodies about issues necessary to develop the most efficacious health and human service policies and service delivery models. Federal regulatory agencies and other fiscal intermediaries base many of their decisions and practice guidelines on empirical evidence or knowledge generated through the research process. Evidence from research has become increasingly used to identify "best" or evidence-based practices, as described in Chapter 24. Consider managed care; its very foundation uses systematic cost measures and specific outcome measures to yield data that then form the basis for policy, practice decisions, and implementation of treatment guidelines. In addition, research provides the tools by which to compare diverse health definitions and needs, practices, health outcomes, and costs across practice settings. Using systematic, standard approaches allows professionals to make comparisons among different populations and diverse health and human service contexts to determine their level of efficiency and effectiveness.

The third reason to learn about research is to enable you to participate in research activities in your own practice setting. In many health and human service settings, practitioners establish or maintain a database of health information and derive statistical reports on client outcomes. In some settings, particularly in an academic health science center or teaching hospital, you or other members of your agency will participate in research to advance the research goals of the institution. You may have many diverse roles as a member of a research project. You may initially want to participate in the process as a data collector, chart extractor, interviewer, provider of an experimental intervention, or recruiter of participants into a study. These are all excellent, time-limited roles to learn firsthand the art and science of the research process. When you feel more comfortable and gain some experience with the process, you may want to serve as a project coordinator and become responsible for the coordination of the detailed tasks and daily activities of a research endeavor, or you may choose the role of the co-investigator and assist in the conceptual development, design, implementation, and analytical components of a study. If you really become hooked on research, you may want to be a principal investigator and assume responsibility for initiating and overseeing the scientific integrity of the entire research effort.

The fourth reason to know about research is that it provides the tools by which you can learn about and be responsive to the experiences and needs of the individuals and groups you help in your professional practice.

The fifth reason to learn about and participate in research is to become a critical consumer of the growing body of research literature that is published in professional journals and other venues. Research not only yields a body of knowledge but also provides the evidence and reasoning strategies on which the investigator bases knowledge claims. Thus, research provides the foundation for informed professional decision making and action. By understanding the research enterprise when you read a research study, you will learn specific findings and also how the knowledge was generated and whether it can be applied to various settings, persons, or areas of practice. Understanding the thinking and action processes of research will provide you with the necessary skills to determine the adequacy of research

outcomes and their implications for daily practice.[5] Most important, the knowledge you gain about research findings has the potential to improve your practice and thus improve the health and quality of life of the people you serve (patients, clients, families) and the health of your community.

Sixth, within health and human service research is the method of clinical trials. Clinical trials are research studies that use human subjects to test and verify the efficacy and safety of new health and human service interventions. This type of research is critical for the development of a sound knowledge base to guide practitioner clinical reasoning and outcome expectations.[22]

Finally, because research is precise, systematic, and logical, understanding and mastering the thinking and action processes of research will enhance, focus, and sharpen your thinking and action in all parts of your professional (and personal) life.

As you can see, there are many reasons to learn about the research process. Most important, whether conducting a formal study or just using systematic techniques in your professional activity, the procedures and methodologies used in research can improve how you think and act in your daily practice. They answer two fundamental questions: "How do you know?" and "So what?" "How do you know" is answered by explicating the evidence to support claims and the ways in which the evidence was obtained and interpreted. The ability to articulate a sound rationale for decisions and activity is an obligation for all professionals. The "so what" question refers to use of knowledge. Now that you have the knowledge, how can you best and most ethically put it to use? This text offers a range of methodologies and techniques, including case study, analysis of audio or video recordings, single-case design, observation, and in-depth interviewing. As a health care or human service professional, you can use each to gain better insight into a particularly difficult practice situation or, in general, to advance all aspects of your professional practice. For example, if you are experiencing difficulty effectively interacting with and thus treating a child with a developmental disability, borrowing a technique from research (e.g., recording a session and systematically analyzing verbal and nonverbal interactions frame by frame) may provide important insights to better approach this particular individual.

> 🔍 Consider another example:
> Let us assume you have been asked to assess the functional ability of residents who live in an assisted living facility in the community to improve self-care skills and participation in daily activity. You may want to set up a single-subject design to monitor your program and its effectiveness in attaining its outcome and then share findings with staff and administrators. First, you would take several baseline assessments of the resident's functioning over several days using a standardized functional measure. Second, you would introduce your strategies to improve self-care and participation in activity. Then you would reassess the residents over several days using the same functional assessments. This simple and easy approach allows you to obtain systematic information about your treatment and its outcome. The point is that many aspects of the research process can be easily incorporated into your daily practice to improve your own as well as professional knowledge about methods to achieve practice outcomes. ●

One final point should be made regarding the importance of participating in research. As health and human service professionals engage in the research process, they contribute to the development of knowledge and theory and help to identify new practice approaches, validate existing strategies, and improve practice. Through this research activity, health and human service professionals are participating in the advancement and refinement of the research process itself and its application to professional issues and service settings. Health and human service professionals who are involved in research today will make significant contributions to the evolution of research methodologies.[21]

Summary

Our definition of research represents our conceptual framework and guides our subsequent discussions in this book. It is based on a philosophical position that the multiple realities that shape health and human services require an approach to research that is informed by multiple research traditions and design strategies. Our approach to research is practical; that is, the purpose and question of an investigator guide the selection of appropriate methodologies, and in turn the questions asked and the knowledge gained must be useful to the clinical, professional, and consumer communities.

Research is critical to health and human service professionals to advance the knowledge base by which clinical decisions are made. Research informs knowledge development and daily practice, and professionals can participate in this activity in many ways.

EXERCISES

1. Select a research article in a peer-reviewed health and human service journal. Identify the source from which the investigator obtained the research question. Decide whether the study fits the four characteristics of research as being logical, confirmable, understandable, and useful, and give the reasons for your opinions.

2. Record three issues that are within the scope of your profession or that have emerged from your daily practice. Determine whether each issue reflects a topic that can and should be researched. How do you currently address these issues? What knowledge is needed that does not exist or that is not complete or compelling? Provide the rationale for your thinking.

References

1. Kerlinger FN: *Foundations of behavioral research*, ed 3, New York, 1986, Holt, Rinehart, & Winston.
2. Patton M: *Qualitative evaluation and research methods*, ed 3, Newbury Park, Calif, 2001, Sage.
3. Bonilla-Silva E: *Racism without racists: color-blind racism and the persistence of racial inequality in the United States*, New York, 2003, Rowman & Littlefield.
4. Kreuger L, Neuman L: *Social work research methods*, Boston, 2006, Allyn & Bacon.
5. Westerfelt A, Deitz TJ: *Planning and conducting agency-based research*, ed 4, Boston, 2009, Allyn & Bacon.
6. Peirce CS: *Essays in the philosophy of science*, Indianapolis, 1957, Bobbs-Merrill.
7. Gitlin LN, Hauck WW, Dennis MP, et al: Maintenance of effects of the home environmental skill-building program for family caregivers and individuals with Alzheimer's

disease and related disorders. *J Gerontol Med Sci* 60A(3): 368–374, 2005. Available at: http://www.rosalynncarter.org/evidence_based_resources.

8. Flick U, Von Kardorff E, Steinke I, editors: *A companion to qualitative research*, London, 2004, Sage.

9. Hoover KR: *The elements of social scientific thinking*, ed 2, New York, 1980, St Martin's Press.

10. Agar M: *An ethnography by any other name*. 2006. Available at: http://www.qualitative-research.net/index.php/fqs/article/view/177/395.

11. Glaser B, Strauss AL: *The discovery of grounded theory: strategies for qualitative research*, Chicago, 1967, Aldine de Gruyter.

12. Audi R: *Epistemology*, New York, 2011, Routledge.

13. Creswell J: *Qualitative inquiry and research design: choosing among five approaches*, ed 3, Los Angeles, 2013, Sage.

14. Sim S: *The Routledge companion to postmodernism*, ed 3, Abington, UK, 2011, Routledge.

15. Silverman D: *Doing qualitative research: a practical handbook*, ed 4, Los Angeles, 2013, Sage.

16. Berg B, Lune H: *Qualitative research methods for the social sciences*, ed 8, Long Beach, Calif, 2014, Longman.

17. Denzin N, Lincoln YS: *Sage handbook of qualitative research*, Thousand Oaks, Calif, 2011, Sage.

18. Swedberg R: *Theorizing in social science: the context of discovery*, Stanford, Calif, 2014, Stanford University Press.

19. Tashakorri A, Teddlie C: *Handbook of mixed methods in social and behavioral research*, ed 2, Thousand Oaks, Calif, 2010, Sage.

20. Safran J: *Psychoanalysis and psychoanalytic therapies*, Washington, DC, 2012, American Psychological Association.

21. DePoy E, Gilson SF: *Human behavior theory and applications: a critical thinking approach*, Thousand Oaks, Calif, 2012, Sage.

22. Wodarski J, Hopson L: *Research methods for evidence-based practice*, Los Angeles, 2012, Sage.

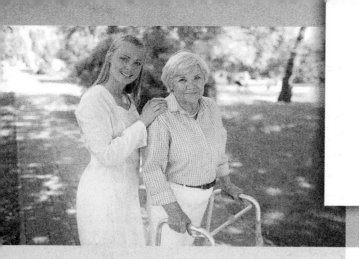

Chapter 2
Essentials of Research

What are the essential characteristics of the research enterprise? This chapter addresses this fundamental question. You will learn in this chapter that any type of research endeavor, whether it be naturalistic, experimental, or a mixed type of inquiry, confronts similar challenges and requirements. We categorize these challenges and requirements into what we refer to as the *10 essentials* of the research process (Box 2-1). How these 10 essentials are interpreted and acted on differs depending on the type of inquiry (naturalistic, experimental-type, or mixed) that is being pursued.

This chapter provides an overview of the 10 essentials and serves as a summary for the entire book. Subsequent chapters in this book examine each of these research essentials from the perspectives of naturalistic inquiry, experimental-type, and mixed methods research. We recommend that you consider this chapter as a guide to the entire text and refer to it as you read each chapter as a way to summarize and reinforce the meaning of these 10 essentials. Also, you can refer to Table 2-1 as a quick guide as you move through this text as well.

Ten Essentials of Research

The 10 essentials of research should be addressed in any type of research that is conducted. These essentials appear as the critical elements of a research proposal and also when reporting findings from a completed inquiry. The first important point to know about the 10 essentials is that the order in which each is addressed will depend on the research tradition and the research design that is chosen. Each essential is highly interrelated with the others, but the essentials may not necessarily occur in the order presented in Box 2-1 and this text. Thus, their order of presentation in this text should not be construed as representing a step-by-step, procedural, or "recipe"-type formula for the research process.

Let's examine briefly how each research essential is addressed in each of the research traditions.

BOX 2-1 *Ten Essentials of Research*

1. Identify philosophical foundation
2. Frame a research problem
3. Determine supporting knowledge
4. Identify a theory base
5. Develop a specific question or query
6. Select a design strategy
7. Set study boundaries
8. Obtain information
9. Analyze information and draw conclusions
10. Share and use research knowledge

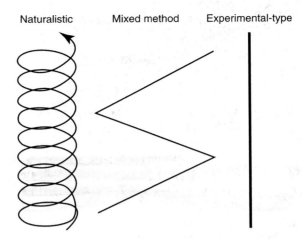

Figure 2-1 **Sequence of the Essentials in Each Tradition.**

TABLE 2-1 *Ten Essentials of Research*

Essential	Explanation
Identify a philosophical foundation	Reveal underlying assumptions of ontology and epistemology
Frame a research problem	Identify broad topic or problem area
Determine supporting knowledge	Review and synthesize existing literature to examine knowledge development in identified problem area
Identify a theory base	Use existing theory to frame research problem and interpret result, or construct theory as part of research process
Develop a specific question or query	Identify specific focus for research, based on knowledge development, theoretical perspective, and research purpose
Select a design strategy	Develop standard procedures or broad strategic approach to answer research question or query
Set study boundaries	Establish scope of study and methods for accessing research participants
Obtain information	Determine strategies for collecting information that is numerical, visual, auditory, or narrative
Analyze information and draw conclusions	Employ systematic processes to examine different types of data and derive interpretative scheme
Share and use research knowledge	Write and disseminate research conclusions

Experimental-type research is hierarchical in its sequence and approach to addressing the 10 essentials. It tends to follow the 10 essentials in a precise, ordered, and highly structured manner such that each essential purposely builds on the other in a linear,

systematic, and stepwise manner. The line in Figure 2-1 depicts this sequential trajectory, and the graphic is used throughout this book to describe the enactment of the 10 essentials. However, it is important to note that even within experimental-type research, the 10 essentials are not mutually exclusive. As one moves along stepwise, previous steps may be revised as a consequence of new methodological decisions. Naturalistic inquiry, in contrast, embodies the 10 essentials using more diverse and complex processes, in which each essential is related to the other and revisited at different points throughout the research process. We use a spiral image throughout this book to depict this type of iterative form of inquiry (Figure 2-1), which links the 10 essentials in different orders, depending on the specific philosophical foundation in which the research is based and the design that is adopted. The sequences of the 10 essentials will differ for each of the research traditions in naturalistic inquiry. This will become clearer to you as you make your way through this book.

Similarly, a mixed methods approach will sequence the 10 essentials differently depending on the way in which the different research traditions and methods are integrated in the particular study. As in naturalistic inquiry, there are numerous approaches to mixing methods, and hence the 10 essentials will be addressed accordingly (Figure

2-1). This point will become clearer as you move through this text.

Let us now examine the meaning of each essential.

Identify a Philosophical Foundation

Identifying a *philosophical foundation* is an important essential that occurs first or in the early stages of the research process. By philosophical foundation, we mean an individual's particular orientation to how a person learns about human behavior, health, and personal abilities and experiences or other phenomena of importance in health and human services. In Chapter 4, we classify these orientations into three overarching philosophical categories through which knowledge is viewed and built, each of which gives rise to one of the primary research traditions. Thus, the researcher's particular philosophical orientation toward learning about phenomena determines the specific research tradition that is selected and the nature of the knowledge generated[1]: experimental-type, naturalistic inquiry, or an integration of the two. In naturalistic inquiry, articulating a philosophical tradition is especially important because of the many distinct philosophical schools of thought that inform the various research approaches subsumed within this form of inquiry (see Chapter 4). When using naturalistic inquiry, it is expected that the researcher will discuss his or her philosophical perspective in a research proposal or in writing a report to provide an understanding of the thinking context in which the research is being conducted.

For example, researchers who identify their philosophical perspective as symbolic interaction tend to use highly interpretative forms of naturalistic inquiry that focus on the meanings and behaviors of individuals in social interaction.[2] Examples of studies may be examining client-health provider exchanges, family dynamics, or even virtual interactions as they concern defining and responding to serious illness. Researchers working out of this tradition may pursue ethnographic research methodology. In contrast, researchers who identify with the philosophical foundation of phenomenology will focus on how individuals perceive their own particular personal experiences. Examples of studies may be how people living with acquired immunodeficiency syndrome (AIDS), renal dysfunction, or spinal cord injury experience their illness or injuries and construct their daily lives, or how diverse groups experience their encounters with health care providers. Researchers working in this tradition tend to pursue methodologies that elicit the telling of a person's personal story or narrative and draw on sources such as direct observations of personal interactions, in-depth interviews, diary or social networking reviews, and other relevant materials such as historical documents, blogs, photos, or narratives.

In contrast, experimental-type research is based on one unifying philosophical foundation—logical positivism.[1] Positivism is a broad term that refers to the belief that there is one truth independent of the investigator and that this truth can be discovered by following strict procedures (see Chapter 4). It is not necessary for an experimental-type researcher to identify the philosophical root of his or her research when submitting a research proposal or a published report, because all experimental-type inquiry is based on a single philosophical base. For example, a researcher trained in survey techniques will naturally assume a positivist or empiricist approach to describe a particular phenomenon. Therefore, it is not necessary for this researcher to state formally the epistemological assumption embedded in the study. Although the philosophical foundation is implicit in the researcher's orientation, it is still important to understand the assumptions about human behavior on which this form of inquiry is based.

You might be thinking that both of these approaches—experimental and naturalistic—would be informative to use in a study in order to advance an effective pregnancy prevention program. You are correct! It is possible to pursue a research study that integrates both approaches; this is referred to as a mixed methods approach. As we discuss in Chapter 4 in more detail, although it may seem that the philosophical foundations of experimental-type and naturalistic traditions are mutually exclusive and thus incompatible, the purposive aim of mixing methods places this third tradition within the philosophical home of pragmatism.[3] For example, to inform the development and then assessment of a pregnancy prevention program, a researcher might start with a naturalistic approach to identify beliefs, values, and preferences of this group. The researcher might then test the program using experimental methodologies and further evaluate who benefited and why, using both naturalistic and experimental strategies to achieve a programmatic purpose.

A philosophical foundation provides the backdrop from which specific methodological decisions in research are made. This does not mean that you must first become a philosopher to participate in research. However, you do need to know that research methodologies reflect different assumptions about human behavior, experience, meaning, and knowledge and about how we learn about these phenomena. By selecting a particular research strategy, you will automatically adopt a particular worldview and philosophical foundation. We believe that, at the very least, you should be aware that you are adopting a specific set of assumptions about human behavior, contexts, and how people come to understand them. Understanding this philosophical foundation is particularly critical because assumptions about knowledge and their use have major implications for how health and human service professionals understand and respond to the diversity of human characteristics.

How does one's philosophical foundation shape research decisions? Consider the example of a health care provider who is hired to design and examine a pregnancy prevention program for Asian-American teenagers. From a logical positive tradition, one approach would be to select an existing and previously validated program, or what is referred to as an evidence-based program,[4] and then implement and test it to ascertain its effectiveness in achieving pregnancy prevention for this particular group. In contrast, a naturalistic researcher would begin by discovering the cultural norms and values of Asian-American teenagers that might be important to informing a prevention program and then, based on this knowledge, construct an intervention tailored to that group.

Each research approach including mixed methods has its distinct advantages as well as limitations that you will learn about in this book. It is important to recognize the assumptions and tradeoffs in your selection of any approach.

You probably already have a particular philosophical foundation or preferred way of knowing, perhaps without fully labeling or recognizing it as such. Sometimes personality, or how one naturally views the world, influences the particular research direction that is adopted. If you prefer to make and follow detailed plans, if you feel uncomfortable with the view that values and biases shape one's worldview, or if you do not like "hanging out" in someone else's world and trying to uncover his or her perspectives or experiences, you may have difficulty with naturalistic inquiry. In contrast, if you are uncomfortable working with and understanding numerical values or feel that numbers do not capture the complexity of the human experience, you may have difficulty with experimental-type inquiries. Many articles have been written about the personality types of individuals who pursue naturalistic inquiry versus those who pursue experimental-type research. However, there is nothing definitive about this literature. Certainly, all types of personalities are capable of learning the practices of multiple research paradigms. Also, as you will learn, it is viable for one researcher to work out of both research paradigms or to use an approach that integrates the two.

Frame a Research Problem

To engage in the research process, the investigator identifies in advance a particular problem area or broad issue that necessitates systematic investigation. Not every problem may need to be addressed through systematic investigation. Research, regardless of the form of inquiry used, is a focused, systematic endeavor that addresses a social problem or issue, theoretically derived prediction, practice question, or personal concern. One of the first thinking processes in which you must engage is to identify the problem area and the specific purpose for your research, and to understand why and how research can address the area of concern. Research topics should come from personal, professional, theoretical, scholarly, political, or societal concerns. To engage in research, it is important that you identify an area that holds personal interest and meaning to you. The research process is challenging and requires time and commitment. You cold lose momentum if you do not pursue a topic that intrigues you personally. Some researchers study areas that have been problematic in their own lives. For example, some investigators who pursue studies on chronic illness have had a personal encounter with chronicity, such as growing up with a sibling or parent with a serious chronic illness or having a chronic condition themselves. Research in an area that has personal significance provides a scholarly forum from which to examine and then personally understand the issues. This is not to say that you have to be an individual with chronic illness to want to study this area, or that you need to have experienced child abuse to study the phenomenon. However, something about a topic should "grab" you. It has to have personal meaning or some level of importance to your life—intellectually, emotionally, or professionally—for the research endeavor to be personally worthwhile. Because research is a long and engaging process, being passionate about a particular topic area or problem is important and is likely to facilitate and solidify your commitment to the research process.

Once you have identified a topic (e.g., coping strategies of diverse caregivers of individuals with dementia; impact of maternal alcohol abuse on early childhood development; quality of life and individuals with multiple sclerosis; end of life decision-making among individuals with cognitive impairment; use of virtual interaction in clinical counseling practice), you can begin to think about your particular purpose in exploring the topic. What do you want to know about the topic? What will be the purpose of your particular research, and how will the knowledge gained be used? Recall our discussion of ethical use of knowledge in Chapter 1. To determine the direction, purpose, and uses of a study, the researcher critically reads what is already known about the topic.

Determine and Evaluate Supporting Knowledge

Another research essential involves conducting a critical review of existing theory and research that concerns your topic or area of inquiry.

Let us assume, on the basis of your practice with individuals hospitalized with spinal cord injury, that to improve their care you need to know more about their self-care practices and social and technological supports after they return home. This information would help determine the types of knowledge, skills, and equipment training that would be important to introduce in the hospital and how best to prepare your patients for the challenges they will confront at home. Or let's say you are concerned about home safety of older adults after they are hospitalized and have reduced functional capacity returning to their home. What would be your first task for either of these concerns? It will be to determine what is already known in the published literature about the population and particular topic. If there is little or no knowledge about the topic, for examples the use of smart home technology in older people's homes, then you would likely want to design a study that obtains foundational knowledge and that initially describes self-care practices and the role of social networks. If there is some relevant descriptive knowledge of daily practices of individuals with spinal cord injuries or the safety issues of older adults post-hospitalization but little information about differences across diverse populations or the role of social supports and technology, you may want to conduct a study that investigates these aspects of either of these topics. Alternatively, suppose there is a body of well-constructed knowledge about gender and ethnic differences in practices of caregivers. This information may lead you to examine the impact of these practices on the general well-being and self-care of individuals who will be discharged to their homes after spinal cord injury or other reason for hospitalization. Existing literature should be consulted to help identify and guide the direction of the research you plan to pursue to build knowledge in your area of interest. •

A critical review of the literature initially helps the investigator frame a specific research direction so that the study will systematically contribute to the building of knowledge in the topic or area of concern that is meaningful, systematic, and purposeful.

A critical literature review is also used for other purposes throughout the research process. In some forms of naturalistic inquiry, a literature review is used as an additional source of data or as a data set. Literature review may also be used to help the investigator further explore his or her emerging interpretations of observations. In experimental-type research, a critical review of a body of published studies using the methodology of meta-analysis is a type of research study in its own right (see Chapter 6). Within any research tradition, the researcher draws on and places his or her new findings within the context of previous studies when reporting the knowledge developed in a study. The findings of a particular study are always interpreted through or added to other studies to add incrementally to a body of knowledge in the topic area.

Identify a Theory Base and Evaluate Its Adequacy

Theory is formally defined as a set of interrelated propositions that provide a framework for understanding or explaining phenomena.[5] (Theory and its relationship with research are described in greater detail in Chapter 7.) The purpose of research is to construct theory and/or to test theory. Research that does not contribute to the building of theory or that is not based on theory produces findings that contribute nothing to the knowledge canon that professionals use. Findings from a study that are not based in or related to a theoretical context cannot be adequately interpreted or understood. Atheoretical collection of data (enumeration) therefore does not contribute to the systematic building of knowledge. Experimental-type researchers tend to test different aspects of a theory; that is, the research begins with a theoretical framework from which specific hypotheses (hunches about what should occur) are generated and tested using various design strategies. Even in a descriptive or correlational study that is not designed to test a specific theory, theory is essential in guiding the research process, such as which constructs and their associated variables to examine, as well as in interpreting study results.

Naturalistic inquiry primarily is designed to generate new theories, expand existing theories, or relates research findings to existing theoretical frameworks. In actual research practice, theory is used by both research traditions for multiple purposes and in many ways. Similarly, a research study that mixes methodologies from experimental-type

and naturalistic traditions also draws on theories at different junctures and in different ways. Thus, the use of theory is interjected at various points in the research process, in the beginning of the experimental-type and throughout the process in naturalistic inquiry and mixed methodological approaches.

Develop a Specific Question or Query

After a problem area is identified, the researcher specifies a particular research direction. In experimental-type research, this direction takes the form of a highly specified *question* that details the exact factors and the characteristics or phenomena that will be examined.

> Consider the issue of well-being for adults with new spinal-cord injuries. An experimental-type researcher who is interested in this topic would pose a question such as, "What is the relationship between robotic technology availability and use and psychological well-being in individuals with spinal-cord injury?" With this question, the researcher identifies three concepts that will be studied—robotic technology availability and use, and psychological well-being—in a targeted population, adults with new spinal-cord injury. The researcher will then carefully define conceptually each of these terms and determine how each will be operationalized or measured. A study design would then be selected that will enable an analysis of the relationship between these three concepts or how they are associated for this particular population. The design would be set a priori or up front and serve as a blueprint for the conduct of the study. The design would remain fixed throughout the course of the study.

In naturalistic inquiry, the research direction is broadly represented and becomes highly specified only through the process of conducting the study itself. In this type of research, the investigator develops a broad working question, or what we call a *query,* that initially identifies the "who, what, and where" of the boundaries of the study, but no other procedural or design details are decided on up front or before engaging in the research process.

The naturalistic-type researcher may pose a different type of query such as, "What are the attitudes about and experiences with robotic technology use of adults with new spinal-cord injuries?" With this broad question, the researcher has identified who will participate in the study (adults with new spinal-cord injuries), where the study will be initiated (at home), and what the focus of the query will be (attitudes and experiences with robotic technology use). Other concerns may emerge in the course of the study that will lead the researcher to redefine the initial query, to broaden or narrow the working definition of attitudes and experiences with robotic technology use, or to consider more specific questions, such as the relationship between attitudes and experiences with robotic technology use and personal well-being. For example, the researcher may learn in the course of the study that it is important to understand attitudes about robotic technology use by evaluating a broader range of attitudes and underlying values about technology in general. The researcher may learn that attitudes are defined differently by participants. The decision to expand the inquiry to other technologies is based on the initial analyses and formative information that have been gathered by the researcher conducting the study. The design is fluid and emerges in the course of conducting the study. •

question within this topic area? The first step would be for the investigator to identify and evaluate the published literature on this topic. This step would shape all other subsequent decisions concerning the research essentials (e.g., development of a specific question or query, setting boundaries, and so forth). •

Thus, in naturalistic inquiry, the research question is framed broadly and represents a query from which more specific research questions and investigative approaches emerge in the course of learning about a particular phenomenon. The specific questions that arise in the course of being in the context of the study cannot be anticipated before entering the research setting.

In any type of research approach, however, a broad topic or area of concern is framed or specified in such a way as to facilitate its exploration.

Consider the broad topic of aging in place with a physical impairment. What are some of the specific questions you might have about this topic? Within this topic, many subtopics and specific research questions or queries can be formulated. What is the first essential that would need to be pursued to address a

The level of knowledge development and theoretical understanding of the topic will direct the researcher to the specific research question or query that represents the next logical step to build knowledge in the chosen area.

Select a Design Strategy

Design is perhaps the most fundamental aspect of the research process. On the basis of one's philosophical position, research purpose, theory, and specific research question or query, the researcher will select a set of action processes by which to explore or answer the query. In naturalistic inquiry, research design is fluid and evolves as the investigator gains access to a natural setting and explores the phenomenon of interest. Further, terms that refer to designs can represent both the process and the end product. For example, "ethnography" is a term that refers to the process of performing fieldwork to understand the cultural patterns of a specified group. Ethnography also refers to the end product: the published report or book about the particular cultural group. Design in naturalistic inquiry means a set of strategies that are employed by the investigator to gain access to a natural setting (e.g., homes of adults with new spinal-cord injuries) and to collect and analyze information using a combination of procedures that unfold in the course of conducting the study (e.g., video recording, participant observation, interviewing, email exchanges, or robotic technology sensors).

In experimental-type research, design is highly structured with a specified set of procedures that are decided on before conducting the study, and then implemented uniformly and systematically by the investigator. In this tradition, a design is similar to a "blueprint" that details each procedure or action process.

Let's say you are interested in understanding safe sexual practices of teenagers in the United States. Given the scope of your interest and perhaps limited knowledge of the current cohort of teenagers, you might want to conduct a survey of high school students in different geographic regions (North, South, East, and West) to determine their level of knowledge about safe sexual practices. Before conducting the study, the investigator will develop a sampling plan (how study participants will be recruited and selected), frame a set of survey questions with a fixed response set (e.g., agree a lot, agree a little, disagree a little, disagree a lot), and identify specific statistical analyses that will be conducted. All these essential decisions are made before beginning the study and then strictly followed according to the plan. •

It is impossible to discuss the vast array of research design strategies in each of the research traditions in one text. We present the most fundamental, commonly used, and useful approaches for health and human service professionals, with a particular emphasis on designs that are amenable to or that can be integrated within professional practices and varied settings.

Set Study Boundaries

Another essential is what we refer to as boundary setting. In conducting this essential a researcher limits the boundaries or scope of a study. Boundaries are established for a number of reasons, the most important of which is to delimit the study so that it is "doable" or feasible to conduct. Ways of setting boundaries include determining the length or duration of the study, who can participate in what part of the study, the conceptual dimensions to be examined, and the type and range of questions that will be asked. Establishing and implementing the boundaries of a study are different for experimental-type, naturalistic inquiry, and mixed method studies. In experimental-type designs, the boundaries of the study are clearly and precisely defined before entering the investigation or starting the study. The researcher establishes a concise plan for identifying and enrolling subjects into the research, determines which instruments or data collection strategies to

use, and identifies, before (or a priori) conducting the study, the specific conceptual dimensions and analytic strategies that are to be included. In naturalistic-type studies, setting boundaries is more fluid. It is an evolving process that occurs once the investigator enters the field or research setting. After gaining access to the context, the investigator continually makes boundary-type decisions such as whom to interview, how and which data to collect, and what conceptual issues to explore. Mixed methods are diverse in boundary setting strategies.

In setting boundaries, a major action process is the protection of those boundaries, particularly if the study involves human subjects and/or informants. Protection can take various forms. For example, in an experimental-type study, boundaries such as who can and who cannot participate must be carefully followed and protected; procedures for ensuring that eligibility rules are followed or protected are part of the study design. The engagement of human subjects in studies requires specific ethical and legal protections as discussed in Chapter 3.

Obtain Information

Obtaining information is the eighth essential of the research process. A researcher can choose from a wide variety of techniques for obtaining information or data. Later in this text, we examine these techniques along a continuum, from unstructured looking and listening techniques to structured, fixed-choice observation and ways of asking questions. Also, a wide range of sources can be used to obtain information from historical documents to Internet-based information to personal diaries.

Analyze Information and Draw Conclusions

Analyzing information, the ninth essential of the research process, involves a series of planned activities that differ depending on the specific research tradition in which one works. One of the initial analytical tasks of experimental-type researchers is to aggregate each individual datum and reduce this large volume of numerical data into meaningful and manageable indicators, such as means, mode, and median. Other statistical techniques are then employed depending on the characteristics of the measures, the size of the sample, and the specific research questions to be answered. The analytical task typically occurs once all the data have been collected and is used to answer the initial research questions that were posed.

In naturalistic inquiry, other analytical approaches are used that are appropriate for the analysis of narrative and other numerical and nonnumerical types of data. The analytical task has several purposes in naturalistic inquiry. First, it is an ongoing process that occurs throughout the study and is used to inform decisions on next directions while the study is in process, to specify additional questions, and to reset boundaries. Second, the analysis systematically applies techniques that can lead to an interpretation of the information that has been obtained (when interpretation is indicated).

Mixed method studies may use multiple forms of analysis depending on purpose, questions and queries, and the nature of design integration.

Share and Use Research Knowledge

The 10th essential, sharing and using research knowledge, completes the research process, at least to the extent that the resulting knowledge is a starting point for new research. Reporting conclusions involves preparing a report and disseminating the knowledge gained from the research. Each research tradition approaches the reporting of newfound knowledge somewhat differently. However, in reporting research-derived knowledge, researchers usually describe the purpose of their study; how it contributes to a particular field or topic; the specific procedures that were followed by the researcher, including analytical strategies; and the findings and interpretations of the information obtained. Research conclusions may take different forms, including providing an understanding of the clinical relevance of the findings—how the knowledge gained can be translated for use in specific clinic or service settings or to guide professional practice, or as a step from which other research questions are posed.

Ethical Considerations

We have identified 10 essentials or characteristics of any type of research study. Researchers address each essential, although this may occur at different points in the research process. The application of these essentials, particularly as it concerns health and human service settings, raises special issues and ethical dilemmas that we discuss and illustrate throughout the book. Underlying each research essential are ethical considerations. Ethical concerns focus on (1) the rights of human research participants to full knowledge of the purpose of the study and the nature and scope of their involvement; (2) the specific behaviors or conduct of the investigator; (3) the *ethics* underlying the research question or query, boundary-setting strategies, and design procedures that will be implemented; (4) the ethics of reporting; and (5) the ethics of selecting and using knowledge to inform professional action. Ethical considerations are explored in each chapter, with specific reference to how these considerations influence and shape each essential.

So now it is your turn. Identify a social or health problem, clinical challenge, puzzle, or personal query that intrigues you and warrants systematic investigation. Think through how you might apply the 10 essentials of the research process to that problem. Also, be sure to consider the ethical issues related to each essential when applied to your area of concern. Think about how your research activities will affect the community in which it will be conducted, about how your actions may affect participants, and about how your data collection efforts will protect confidentiality and ensure respect for participants and their rights to agree or not agree to participate in your study and its procedures. Also consider the strengths and weaknesses or limitations of each of your decisions along these 10 essentials.

Summary

All research, regardless of the topic, approach, and use, consists of 10 essentials. In experimental-type research, these essentials are ordered, linear, and performed in a stepwise manner. In naturalistic inquiry as well as mixed methods, the essentials are carried out in different sequences depending on the particular research tradition/s and the design/s used. Ethical considerations intersect with each of these essentials.

Figure 2-1 is used throughout this text to signify the specific tradition and essential that we are discussing. As you proceed through the world of research with us, you will note that the graphic also depicts the integration of experimental-type and naturalistic research into a third tradition, mixed methods. Research integrating experimental-type and naturalistic traditions can occur in any of the thinking processes or action processes that constitute the 10 essentials, as discussed throughout this book.

EXERCISES

1. Select two research articles and identify the 10 essentials in each.
2. Using both articles, compare and contrast how the essentials are sequenced and described by the investigators.

3. For each article, identify up to three ethical considerations.

References

1. Audi R: *Epistemology*, New York, 2011, Routledge.
2. Hewitt J, Shulman D: *Self and society: a symbolic interactionist social psychology*, ed 11, New York, 2011, Pearson.
3. Tashakorri A, Teddlie C: *Handbook of mixed methods in social and behavioral research*, ed 2, Thousand Oaks, Calif, 2010, Sage.
4. Rubin A, Bellamy J: *Practitioner's guide to using evidence-based practice*, ed 2, Hoboken, NJ, 2012, Wiley.
5. DePoy E, Gilson SF: *Human behavior theory and applications: A critical thinking approach*, Thousand Oaks, Calif, 2012, Sage.

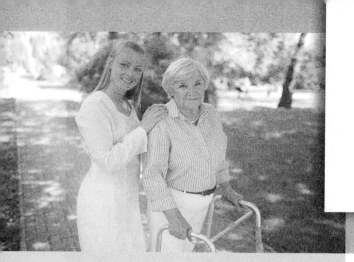

Chapter 3
Research Ethics

Ethics of Knowledge Generation and Use in Professional and Personal Lives

Ethics of Conduct Throughout the Research Process

Research ethics is a term most typically applied to rules for "proper" behavior during the thinking and action processes of research and particularly to the protection of human subjects. In this chapter we address critically important ethical issues including ethical decision making, knowledge generation and use of knowledge in professional practice.

Consider this example as we begin this important topic. Suppose you are interested in examining the outcomes on family of a trauma-focused clinical intervention for adult women of child-bearing age. In your research, you find that as the therapy proceeds two outcomes occur: the alliance between the clinician and the client is improved, but positive interactions between parents and their adult children decreases, negatively affecting parental mental health and leading to family of origin estrangement.[1] As you continue your research agenda, you find that clinical assessment is based on recall of how children were treated by their parents over the course of their development. Issues such as working parents not spending sufficient time with their children were interpreted by the clinician as traumatizing and articulated as such.

Many ethical dilemmas present themselves in such a scenario, including, but not limited to, whom

> **BOX 3-1** *Ethical Decision-Making Models*
> ....
> Principlism: based on five principles: autonomy,
>   beneficence, non-malfeasance, autonomy, justice
> Consequentialism: the outcome or consequences of
>   action form the basis for value judgment
> Non-consequentialism: inherent qualities of goodness
>   or badness
> Casuistry: idiographic (individualized) approach to
>   ethical decision making

the intervention is benefitting and harming, how theory is being applied to clinical practice, and who oversees the use of knowledge in professional practice. How do you proceed to think about and articulate these dilemmas, not only in your research, but also in the way in which you intend your research to be used?

Ethical Frameworks and Reasoning

There are numerous ethical decision-making models to guide your reasoning. Ethics forms a major division of philosophy, axiology, and thus is far beyond the scope of this book. Models have been categorized and analyzed in numerous formats. The models that we briefly present and illustrate are only one organizational method.[2] Look at Box 3-1 for descriptions of each model. The ethical generation and use of knowledge is a critical concern not only for researchers but for all who use knowledge to guide professional practice.

Principlism is the basis for ethics that protect human subjects. We discuss this model and its application to research methods later. Principlism refers to a set of four rules that guide ethical behavior. Autonomy proposes that one should respect an individual's right to choose. Beneficence refers to optimal intent for an action to do good work; non-malfeasance guides one to do no harm. Finally, justice refers to fairness of an act. Considering the example from earlier, it is unclear in judging the therapist's use of trauma-informed therapy whether any of the principles are violated. Those who would suggest that the greatest benefit for the client would be for the whole family to work together as a unit would not see the therapist's use of trauma theory as

ethical. Yet, others who espouse client autonomy and beneficence for the client only might judge the therapist's intervention as ethical. Still others might see the therapist as unethical in placing the alliance above all, creating harm for the parents and possibly the adult child. Fairness is just as complicated. To whom is this intervention fair or not fair?

The *consequentialist* would look at the outcome of the knowledge use to judge its goodness. However, once again, outcome for whom and over what period of time are in question. If, for example, the outcome for the client is estrangement from her family, for the short term this consequence may be useful in light of harm that she perceives as resulting from parenting behavior. Over the long run, however, some might argue that such isolation is harmful for the client as well as the family.

From a *non-consequentialist* perspective, if the therapist is deemed as a good and well-intended individual (of course, who is sitting in judgment determines the extent to which the therapist meets this criterion), then goodness is affirmed. However, if the therapist's concern with the alliance as the basis for prolonging intervention supersedes concern for the welfare of the client and family, then this behavior is not a virtue.

Casuistry would require that ethical knowledge use be judged for its relevance to this particular situation, and thus the ethics of evidence-based practice might be violated under this structure. However, for those who resonate with relativism and the primacy of individuality, casuistry would be a sound ethical decision-making framework to apply to knowledge generation and use in this example.

Although not all of the ethical dilemmas just illustrated are specific to the conduct of research, we started the ethics chapter with this introduction to bring your attention to both the complexity and critical importance of considering ethics in all parts of knowledge generation and use.

We had an experience several years ago when the outcome of a study was used to do the opposite of what was intended. As the basis for informing the development of community-based social opportunities for individuals living in group homes, we conducted an inquiry to answer the following questions:

1. What degree of socialization is available for cognitively impaired adults residing in congregate, community-based homes in the northwestern region of the United States?
2. How does living environment relate to level of socialization for this population?

To obtain data, we tested the social opportunities and level of socialization in two groups, individuals in congregate community-based homes and individuals in long-term care facilities. We also looked at community-based opportunities for socialization. The results indicated that adults in long-term care socialized more than those in community settings, and that the opportunity for socialization was greater in long-term care environments. Although our purpose was to inform efforts to "deinstitutionalize" adults and develop social opportunities, the governor of the state in which we conducted the study used the results to suggest that long-term care should be expanded because it provided social opportunity for residents. The consequences of this research could have increased institutionalization. What, then, were the duties of the researchers, the users of the knowledge, the residents and their families, the long-term care facilities managers and owners, and so forth? We relate this story to demonstrate the critical importance of ethical decision making in all aspects of knowledge generation and use.

With this brief introduction to ethical models, we now move to research ethics that are specifically focused on protecting humans participating in research studies.

As we discuss in Chapter 13, health and human service professionals frequently delimit or, as we refer to it, set boundaries by engaging humans through sampling plans or other participant recruitment strategies. Involving human subjects in research requires important considerations that not only uphold ethics but also are legally binding.[3] The basic ethical model that underpins human subject protection is principlism. In each of the research traditions, the researcher is obligated to ensure the protection of human subjects through principlist decision making.

What do we mean by "the protection of human subjects"? All research in which people are directly involved has potential risks to its participants, even if such risks are minimal or simply involve momentary discomfort with a personal question on a survey. According to federal law,[2-4] investigators must submit a plan (proposal) for the ethical conduct of any inquiry involving human subjects to a board or group composed of both lay and scientific representatives. This board is mandated to examine proposals with regard to critical considerations that include: (1) the level of risk posed to study participants and relationship of risk to potential benefits to society; (2) the adequacy of the plan to provide participants with necessary knowledge about study procedures, risks, and benefits, referred to as "full disclosure"; (3) the plan for ensuring that study participation and all procedures are voluntary; and (4) the plan for ensuring confidentiality.

Large institutions such as hospitals and universities have formal committees, usually called institutional review boards (IRBs). In smaller agencies, review boards may be ad hoc committees (with a particular purpose). Regardless of where you are conducting an inquiry, however, you are required both ethically and legally to seek human subjects review to protect those who are devoting time and effort to serve as participants in your study. Also, if you obtain funding for your research, you will not be allowed to conduct the study until such a review has been conducted and formal approval obtained. Even if you are conducting a small or pilot-level research study, such as for a research class, you are obligated to seek IRB approval. IRBs are the main mechanisms through which protection strategies are reviewed and monitored in the conduct of any type of research study.

Principles for Protecting Human Subjects[2]

Human subject protection is based on three primary principles: full disclosure, confidentiality, and voluntary participation (Box 3-2). All investigators, regardless of the scope or type of research, must follow these principles.

Full Disclosure

Any person who participates in a study, whether participatory action research, single-subject design, or randomized trial, has the absolute right to full disclosure of the purpose and procedures of the study. *Full disclosure* means that the investigator must clearly share with the informant, subject, or research participant the types and content of interviews, length of time of participation, types and length of observations, and other data-collection procedures that will occur, as well as the scope and nature of the person's involvement. Full disclosure also means that any risk to a subject, even if the potential is rare or minimal, must be clearly identified and a plan for remediation offered for each risk to every subject.

Identifying and sharing specific study procedures tend to be straightforward in experimental-type research. However, such disclosure can create difficulties for certain forms of naturalistic and mixed method inquiry. In an experimental-type study, all the procedures are clearly articulated and determined before the researcher enters the field. Therefore, the researcher can identify in layperson's terms the purpose and scope of the study and the types of data collection efforts that will occur. In naturalistic and some mixed methods designs, most bounding-type decisions are made in the field and change or evolve over time as knowledge about the context emerges. Researchers who work in this tradition must solve this dilemma in creative, thoughtful, and ongoing ways. In some studies, it may be necessary to introduce a consenting process for each data-collection effort.

Discussion in the research literature is ongoing about effective approaches that investigators can use to remain ethical while preserving the integrity of their methodology. All researchers, regardless of tradition, will no doubt struggle over the best way to describe the study truthfully without revealing specific aims or hypotheses or introducing factors that may shape and/or influence the informant's responses during the study. For example, within the experimental-type tradition, although it is necessary to state the overall research objective, it is not appropriate to indicate a directional hypothesis that could influence how an informant responds during an interview. Some designs present unique challenges when explaining study procedures. For example, when employing a randomized trial design (see Chapter 10), care must be taken to explain all procedures and activities associated with both the treatment and control groups. However, one group must not be portrayed and perceived as being better or more preferred than the other. In experimental-type approaches, the researcher must maintain a neutral stance and does not suggest that one group is being hypothesized to have a better outcome than the other. Although the researcher may firmly believe that treatment is better than its absence, the point of a randomized trial is to determine whether that claim can be supported. Maintaining a stance of neutrality in the way in which all study procedures are explained and implemented is referred to as assuring *equipoise* in the conduct of the study.

Full disclosure of study intent and procedures is usually provided when initially enrolling and recruiting participants into a study and when obtaining informed consent. In addition to consent forms, some investigators also provide an informational sheet, brochure, or Web description to participants as a handy reference that outlines the study purpose and the procedures used. In studies that involve multiple testing occasions, the investigator may restate the study purpose and procedures at each follow-up to ensure that study participants understand what to expect next and at which stage they are in the research study.[5]

Although full disclosure is mandatory in all studies and with all human subjects, it is important to recognize the importance of disclosure, particularly as it concerns vulnerable populations (e.g., children, individuals with cognitive impairments, prisoners) and minority groups, for which there has been a long history of unethical research practices. Take, for example, the Tuskegee syphilis experiment conducted between 1932 and 1972 in Tuskegee, Alabama, by the U.S. Public Health Service. The study recruited 399 poor African-American share-croppers with syphilis to evaluate the natural course of the disease. Even though by 1947, penicillin had become the standard of treatment for syphilis, this information and access to drug treatment were not offered to study participants. The failure to treat study participants resulted in unnecessary suffering and death of participants and their family members.[5] The unethical practices in this and other studies have led to major regulatory changes to protect partici-pants of studies, including full disclosure through the informed consent process and accurate and timely reporting of study results, including informing par-ticipants of changes in risk or treatment discoveries. Disclosure is particularly challenging when involv-ing individuals with cognitive and sensory impair-ments.[3] Ensuring that persons with compromised cognition and/or poor hearing and vision can fully and clearly understand study procedures is critical.

Confidentiality

The investigator is required to ensure that all infor-mation shared by a respondent in the course of a study is kept confidential. *Confidentiality* means that (1) no person other than specified members of the research team can have access to the respondent's information, unless those who have access to the data are identified to the participants before their participation (usually stated in informed consent); and (2) the information provided by a respondent cannot be linked to the person's identity.[3] This second consideration, although relevant to all research involving human subjects, is especially important in studies that focus on sensitive and potentially stig-matizing topics, such as acquired immunodeficiency syndrome (AIDS), teenage pregnancy and birth control use, mental health issues, crime, and drug abuse.

An investigator can ensure confidentiality in several ways. The name of the respondent can be removed from the actual information that is obtained. This procedure ensures that the identity of respon-dents in your study is protected and that the informa-tion they provide will not be linked to their names in the future. One typical way to protect a study participant's identity is the assignment of identifica-tion numbers. However, this action presents some

difficulty for studies that primarily use observation as the principal data-collection effort. Also, ensuring confidentiality can be difficult when using audio and video recordings as data-collection sources. In these instances, the investigator does not usually transcribe names that are recorded. The researcher would more likely establish procedures for coding and storing digital data in locked filing cabinets or offices with restricted access, as well as destroying electronic copies at the conclusion of the study.

Confidentiality of research participants must also be protected when results are reported. In reporting findings from a case study or naturalistic design, the names of individuals and key identifying informa-tion are modified (de-identified) so that there is no direct link between the person's identity and the information the person provides. Most experimental-type studies report findings that reflect summative scores or outcomes of an aggregate of individuals, which makes ensuring confidentiality less challeng-ing in this research tradition than in naturalistic inquiry.

Researchers who investigate controversial topics carefully plan how information will be stored and reported. Studies about human immunodeficiency virus (HIV), sexual activity, drug trafficking, or sexual, physical, or substance abuse may contain information of interest to the legal system. While investigators can refuse to turn over documentation, they may still risk being called into court to testify.

Federal regulations such as the *Health Insurance Portability and Accountability Act (HIPAA)* also impose confidentiality rules and restrictions on research activity. HIPAA requires that all health-related information obtained in the course of a study be "de-identified" so that it is not possible to link a person's name to the health information provided. HIPAA also requires that any health information that is shared in the course of a study be documented in the informed consent form that is signed by a par-ticipant before entering a study. Furthermore, under HIPAA, researchers are not legally permitted to contact individuals about a study unless that person has given prior permission for such contact to be made.[6] To abide by this regulation, many clinical sites ask patients or clients to sign a form that indi-cates their willingness to be contacted and informed about a study of potential interest. Researchers also use similar procedures and create password-protected human subject registries of individuals who have agreed to be contacted in the future about further studies by the research team.

Ensuring confidentiality necessitates that certain office procedures be established. First, written personal identifying information concerning study participants is kept to a minimum. A master list of study participants that includes the assigned identification number (ID#), first and last names, and necessary group designations (e.g., control vs. experimental group) is maintained for tracking purposes on computers and is password protected; hard copies are kept in locked filing cabinets separate from the actual information obtained. In many studies, screening forms and interview cover sheets that include identifying information are used. All this information is considered strictly confidential and is also kept in locked file cabinets separate from study data. Any information with subject identification that is not needed is shredded.

Second, confidentiality should also be maintained when making telephone contact with study participants or potentially eligible persons. Conversations with or about study participants require common-sense discretion. Attempts to schedule appointments with study participants or telephone conversations discussing issues related to a participant should be conducted in a manner that ensures confidentiality. When talking on the telephone or other mobile device, researchers should keep voices low and should not use last names except as necessary, to keep others in the office from hearing. When possible, they should conduct conversations in private. If this is not possible, calls can be made when fewer people are in the office or when only persons directly involved with the research project are present.

Third, computer files used for tracking study participants can be set up with password protection. Access to such files should be restricted to defined key personnel, and any backup disks or cloud sites should be secure and encrypted.

Fourth, interviewers should be trained and certified in "protection of human subject" procedures before any phone, mobile device, or face-to-face interviews with study participants. For face-to-face

contact, interviewers introduce themselves, explain the study's purpose and procedures, and review the informed consent. Informed consent is obtained before collecting any study-related information. For screen or phone-mediated interviews, interviewers frequently read a script approved by the IRB and obtain verbal assent, which is recorded on an institutionally approved form.

Voluntary Participation

When humans are involved in studies, their participation is strictly voluntary. Individuals have the right to choose to participate or not. Also, an individual who initially agrees to participate in a study has the right to withdraw from the study at any point and the right to refuse to answer any particular question(s) or participate in a particular set of procedures. Thus, the voluntary quality of participation is protected at three points in a study: initial enrollment, continuation in the study, and right to refuse to answer specific questions or participate in a study procedure. To ensure *voluntary participation* at each of these points, investigators develop approaches to recruiting participants that are not coercive and that provide full disclosure of all study procedures.

It is important for the investigator to understand why refusals occur. Is withdrawal caused by the nature of the procedures or by excessive demands placed on participants? Is the research team offensive in any way? Is withdrawal based on a change in the health status of the participants or their relocation to another geographic region? Reasons for refusal to participate in a study, withdrawal from a study as a participant, or refusal to answer a particular question may have implications for the ethical conduct of the study, interpretation of results, and ability to generalize outcomes to other groups, as well as planning future studies. Therefore, it is important to keep track of and evaluate the reasons study participants withdraw from a study or refuse participation in a study component. This information enables the investigator to refine ethical plans, evaluate whether differences exist between those who participate and those who do not, and prepare for future research.

Refusal to answer a particular question (e.g., "What is your yearly income?") or to engage in a particular study component (e.g., allow observation of home interactions) presents a methodological challenge that the investigator should be prepared to meet. Missing information can be a greater problem in experimental-type research than in naturalistic inquiry because missing data limit the types of statistical analysis that can be used and the inferences that can be derived from the data. For example, a common question on survey studies is level of income as one indicator of socioeconomic status. However, participants may refuse to disclose this information. Missing information can be handled in numerous ways, including using the mean value of the group or using a statistical program to assign a value randomly.

Missing information is less problematic in naturalistic and some mixed method studies. The refusal to answer a question may be an indicator of the salience (or importance) of that particular topic or area, and its "missingness" becomes, in essence, a type of meaning that enters into an interpretive scheme. For the naturalistic inquirer, however, missing an observation, such as an important community event, may be problematic. To overcome this issue, adjustments in collecting information may need to be made, such as prolonging engagement in a particular context or obtaining information about the event from newspaper reports, community meetings, and personal interviews.

Belmont Report

The ethical issues of conducting research have only recently been a focus of national concern. In 1974, the National Research Act created a commission to delineate the ethical issues and guidelines for the involvement of humans in behavioral and biomedical research in the United States.[7] This act and its subsequent activities arose from revelations of the Nuremberg war crime trials about the devastating human experiments conducted by medical scientists during the Holocaust. Other tragic abuses of human subjects involved in research had occurred in the United States as well—most notably, the Tuskegee experiments discussed earlier, which involved poor rural black men diagnosed with syphilis from whom investigators withheld known curative treatment to observe the natural course of the disease process.[5]

The resulting Belmont Commission issued a report in 1979 that outlined three basic ethical principles to guide all research activity in order to protect human subjects.[7] The Belmont Report is a brief document that is required reading for all those involved in human subject research. Because abuses continue to occur and make national headlines, the Belmont report is a live document, and researchers should refer to it frequently. It is of utmost importance to understand and follow the three principles of this document in the conduct of research involving human subjects.

Based on principlist ethics, the first principle is the importance of distinguishing the boundaries between research and practice. This differentiation may be more complex in health and human service research than in other types of science research. However, it is important to distinguish between daily, traditional practice and systematic efforts to evaluate new approaches and service interventions. This distinction can be challenging. For example, suppose you want to develop a new set of items to assess delirium in dementia patients who are hospitalized. You have a sense of what these items should be, as some have been derived from your own practice when conducting clinical interviews with and examinations of hospitalized elderly patients. However, now you want to formalize those items and determine if they differentiate patients with and without delirium. Using the items in your practice and collecting information to evaluate the sensitivity of items for distinguishing delirium and dementia would require human subject consent. Alternatively, let's say your practice setting determines that use of these items enhances an understanding of the clinical profile of patients and decides that they should be used on a consistent basis. You could then evaluate post-hoc the outcomes of using these items (whether they predict delirium or not) through chart review. In this case, you could seek "exempt" status from the IRB, which means that on being notified of your research plans, they have granted you an exemption from further reporting to them about this study as it is no-risk and involves a post-hoc evaluation of existing clinical data. However, you also need to obtain an IRB waiver for obtaining consents, because the chart review will expose you to protected patient health information such as name, address, age, and other identifying information.

The second ethical principle in the Belmont Report describes three areas to be addressed: respect for persons, beneficence, and justice. The first area, respect, states that individuals should be treated as autonomous individuals who are capable of personal choice and self-determination. A related mandate is that individuals who are not autonomous or who are vulnerable, such as the person with reduced cognitive capacity, must be protected. The second ethical area, beneficence, specifies that research will "do no harm" and will "maximize" benefits and "minimize possible harm" to individuals. The third ethical area, justice, specifies that people should be treated fairly; that is, research should provide full opportunity to include all relevant groups and individuals who could potentially benefit from the knowledge generated. For example, if a study may provide knowledge beneficial to all genders, then the sample or set of informants should seek to include the full range of gender diversity.

The third principle described in the Belmont report concerns the application of these general principles to research activities including the informed consent process, specifying a risk-benefit assessment and how human subjects are selected for participation in a study. Let's examine the elements of this third principle.

Institutional Review Board

On the basis of the Belmont Report, the involvement of humans in research is overseen by a government-mandated board of experts established at each institution that is engaged in the research process. These boards, referred to as *institutional review boards (IRBs)*, are charged with monitoring the ethical conduct of research as outlined by the Belmont Report. Most academic settings have an IRB, but only a few health and human service settings have established research committees or IRBs. If you are located in a setting that does not have an established board, you may need to form a partnership with a university or hospital that can review your protocol. Some universities have arrangements with community-based agencies and organizations in which they agree to review protocols for a fee or

gratis. This linkage is particularly important when seeking funding to support your research effort. All federally funded research studies must be approved by an official IRB. In most institutions, however, any research study—funded or not funded, small scale or large scale—must be reviewed by a committee to examine the nature of human involvement.

Before implementing a study, a researcher writes a proposal describing in detail the plans for involving humans, the procedures of the study, and analytic strategies. This proposal is submitted for review to a designated office of research or to an IRB (see Chapter 22). One of the initial determinations made is whether a particular activity is or is not classified as research. This is not as straightforward as it may sound, particularly in clinical settings, as the earlier example suggests: Some clinical activities can become a form of research. This is also the case in health and educational settings, in which some evaluative activities may become a form of research. Numerous methodologists and scholars differentiate evaluation from research. Some suggest that because of its purposive, political aims, evaluation is distinct from inquiry. Others such as Trochim[8] suggest that evaluation is a specialized brand of the research enterprise. He states:

> *Evaluation is a methodological area that is closely related to, but distinguishable from more traditional social research. Evaluation utilizes many of the same methodologies used in traditional social research, but because evaluation takes place within a political and organizational context, it requires group skills, management ability, political dexterity, sensitivity to multiple stakeholders and other skills that social research in general does not rely on as much.*[8]

We see this distinction between research and evaluation as limiting to health and human service knowledge development and use. Professional inquiry is designed to generate knowledge to guide practice and to determine the extent to which and how interventions met their goals within complex contexts. Health and human service research thus is evaluative of and informing to practice. Thus, we would urge you to seek review whenever human subjects are involved in systematic study, even if the

IRB proposes the distinction between evaluation and research.

Assume you are a health professional working in a rehabilitation setting, and (1) you read about a new therapeutic technique in the literature and want to evaluate its benefits for your clients, or (2) you want to examine case records to see whether you can identify a set of factors that predict rehabilitation improvement. Are these research studies? Would you need to submit these plans to the IRB for review and their approval? It is always best to discuss and seek advice from an IRB to ensure that you uphold the highest degree of ethical principles in your systematic inquiry.

Let's assume your clinical department decides to implement a new technique to track patient outcomes. However, the purpose of this activity is clinical and is designed to improve clinical services. Previous research has shown that this new technique has benefits and is of low risk to patients. As the purpose is clinical, it would not be considered research and hence would not require IRB approval. Suppose, however, that you want to compare outcomes from this new therapeutic approach systematically to traditional care and assign patients to receive the new or typical treatment, aggregate the data, and report the results formally. In this case, the activity should be considered research, even if evaluative, and fall under the purview of the IRB. Alternatively, if the technique were of high risk to patients and the clinic wanted to determine which patients would fare better by this approach, then a research query and IRB review would be necessary.

In the case involving a chart extraction activity, given that you plan to review case records systematically and aggregate the data for reporting purposes, you should seek IRB approval. Because your methodology involves extracting information from the charts of patients but does not require patient contact or disclosure of patient names, you most likely will receive what is referred to as "exempt" status (as discussed earlier and also later); this means your study has minimal risks and thus is exempt from continued reporting requirements. Once again, however, because you will be viewing and collecting patient health information that is considered protected under HIPAA, you need to request from the IRB a waiver for human subject consent. Although you are initially obligated to inform the IRB of any study you plan to conduct, if it is designated as exempt by that board, there will be no further legal or ethical requirements for annual IRB reports and updates.

After the IRB determines that the proposal is research and requires a review, its main goal is to evaluate whether the research protocol will adversely affect study participants, whether study procedures are too burdensome, whether benefits outweigh risks, whether the design is appropriate to address the research questions, and whether the research itself justifies the involvement of humans. Also, the IRB evaluates the procedures that will be used to identify and enroll or engage humans in the study to make certain that participation is voluntary, that confidentiality will be ensured, and that there is full disclosure of study procedures.

Assume you are a rehabilitation clinician and plan to evaluate the relationship between client self-report of functional ability and observation of actual performance. You plan to evaluate the clients you see in the rehabilitation setting. Although this idea does not necessarily present ethical challenges, you carefully consider how you will introduce the study to your clients. Also, you establish clear boundaries between your clinical efforts and the information you need to proceed clinically, and the information you need and will gather for research purposes. You set up procedures to ensure that clients understand three points. First, their participation in the study is strictly voluntary; in other words, it is their decision whether or not to participate in all or part of the study. You establish procedures to enroll clients that ensure that they do not feel coerced into participating because you are working with them clinically. Second, clients must understand that their decision not to participate will not affect the type and quality of service intervention they will receive. Third, if clients decide to participate, they can choose to discontinue participation at any point in the study with no consequences to them or their ability to receive other medical and social services for which they are eligible. In this case, it is usually necessary to involve others in the consenting process so that clients do not feel any pressure or coercion to participate in the study.

Moreover, the IRB will review all study procedures to make certain that they are ethical and not coercive. You will not be able to begin your study until you have received approval from the IRB. IRB approval is provided through a letter to the investigator that is maintained in the study file drawer or electronic file and readily available for any future audits. Also, consents and other study-related materials that are used for recruitment, such as brochures, website announcements, or flyers announcing the study and surveys, will be approved by the IRB. Only forms with an up-to-date approval by the IRB can be used in the study. If you seek a change in protocol or if forms change in any substantive way, then a revision to your protocol and forms is required for re-review and re-approval.

Three Levels of Review

Most IRBs have three levels of review: full, expedited, and exempt. A full board review involves a formal examination of an investigator's research protocol by members who have been officially appointed by an institution. The composition of board members is mandated to include a consumer representative and a member with scientific expertise in the protocols being reviewed. The board can be composed of as many as 20 individuals or as few as 5, depending on how the institution has set up its IRB. A study that involves a vulnerable population must receive a full review. *Vulnerable populations* refer to individuals who may not be able to represent themselves or participate in decision making or who may be at particular risk when participating in a research study (see later discussion). Examples of vulnerable populations are infants, children, pregnant women, prisoners, mentally incompetent individuals, or persons addicted to substances. In addition, research studies involving HIV testing, AIDS, investigational drugs, or medical devices also require a full board review. In a full board review, all members read the research protocol, discuss its merits and weaknesses, and vote to either approve (with changes or no changes to recruitment and consent procedures) or disapprove it. If your protocol is disapproved, you may receive guidance for revision.

An expedited review involves an evaluation of a research protocol by a subcommittee selected from the full IRB membership. Studies that receive an expedited review may not involve vulnerable populations, may not test invasive techniques, and must represent minimal risk to individual participants. Studies that can receive an expedited review may include those that collect data from individuals who are 18 years of age or older using noninvasive procedures routinely used in practice, studies that use existing data, and research on group behavior in which the investigator is not manipulating behavior. The previous example of the study in rehabilitation would be appropriate for an expedited review.

Exempt status means that a study protocol is exempt from formal review from either the full board or its subcommittee. Although it is necessary to inform the IRB of the intent to conduct the research, the IRB will send a letter of approval of its exempt status and indicate that no future or annual review is necessary. Studies that are exempt from formal review procedures may include research involving and assessing normal educational practices or the use of educational tests, as well as research involving the collection or study of existing data, documents, and records, provided these sources are publicly available or the information is recorded so that the individuals cannot be identified. An example of the latter situation is a retrospective study involving chart review or hospital census data from the previous 10 years of individuals who experienced strokes and their level of functional status at discharge.

In submitting a proposal to an IRB, you address each of six considerations (Box 3-3). Although the actual format of a proposal submission to an IRB may differ across institutions, these six points are standard.

Informed Consent Process

The principles outlined in the Belmont Report are applied to the conduct of research through the informed consent process. *Informed consent* is the process through which potential study participants are informed of the study and its participation

---

BOX 3-3 *Six Areas That Must Be Addressed in an Internal Review Board Proposal*

1. Describe the number and characteristics of the persons who will participate in the study.
2. Describe any potential risks and benefits of study participation.
3. Describe procedures to ensure confidentiality.
4. Describe data-collection sources and procedures.
5. Describe plans for recruitment and procedures for obtaining informed consent.
6. Describe procedures for protecting against or minimizing potential risks.

BOX 3-4 *Typical Elements of Informed Consent*

Statement of purpose of study in layperson's terms
Description of study procedures (e.g., number and length of interviews)
Disclosure of any risks or discomforts from study participation
Statement describing how confidentiality will be ensured
Health Insurance Portability and Accountability Act disclosures
Statement describing right of refusal and voluntary consent
Description of benefits of participation
Signatures of study participant, interviewer, and researcher
Name of institute and telephone number of investigator
Disclosure of any monetary support if person requires medical attention because of a study procedure

---

requirements. It usually takes the form of an official written document developed by the researcher that informs study participants of the purpose and scope of the study. Although the specific wording and format of informed consent forms vary widely across institutions, they must contain the basic elements listed in Box 3-4.

Important elements of informed consent include a description of the procedures in which you are asking the person to participate and your assurance that participation is voluntary. Also, you need to specify whether participation in the study carries any known risks, and if so, what these risks are and what measures should be taken if they occur. In proposing a study, you need to consider the elements to include in your informed consent and the procedures you will use to introduce it to study participants. A consent form must be read before collecting any information from a person. Usually the participant, the interviewer, and the principal investigator sign the form, and a copy is made for the participant to keep.

A written consent is not required for every type of study. For example, in conducting an online survey, the act of completing the survey is considered an indication of the respondent's consent to participate. Likewise, in a telephone survey, the act of agreeing to answer questions over the telephone is a sign of volunteering or assenting to the study.

Obtaining consent from participants, whether written or *assent* through verbal acknowledgment, is somewhat straightforward in experimental-type research that involves individuals who are not cognitively impaired. The researcher knows exactly who is eligible to participate in the study and can review informed consent before asking a set of standardized questions. In obtaining consent, the individual and researcher review each section of the consent. Some individuals may wish to review the consent before meeting with the researcher, in which case a copy of the consent can be mailed, emailed, or otherwise delivered to the person. Some individuals may want to share the consent with other family members before signing it. Obtaining written consent can take time. The amount of time may vary depending upon the complexity of the study and the different types of procedures. Also, individuals who have had limited to no exposure to research may find the process intimidating. Every effort should be made to be clear and thorough in reviewing consents and not to rush through this process. Individuals must feel comfortable about asking questions and must have the time they need to understand and process all study procedures.

It can be more difficult to obtain consent in naturalistic inquiry than in experimental-type approaches, especially when data collection involves observing various events in which you cannot predict who will be attending or involved in the setting. Researchers using a naturalistic approach must be creative and thoughtful as to the best and most ethical way of handling consent.

The research of Johansen and Kohli[9] provides an excellent exemplar. This work illustrates the different approaches naturalistic and mixed method researchers consider in addressing ethical dilemmas. Johansen and Kohli studied rural residents diagnosed with AIDS to ascertain their challenges and needs, particularly in small areas where their conditions were known in their communities. The study posed several challenges. First, it involved a vulnerable, protected population—people with AIDS. Second, it involved data collection over time at the informant's home. Third, it involved people who were stigmatized not because of AIDS but because they were perceived by community members as disabled and poor. Consent was first obtained by approaching the staff of the service center where these individuals obtained support and treatment. As the author describes, this population was particularly vulnerable: "The first reactions/emotions included being scared, shocked, angry, delirious, depressed, worried, uncertain, crying uncontrollably, fearful, and lacking hope for the future."[9]

Second, the informants worried about confidentiality because of the stigma attached to AIDS. "Interestingly, more participants related initial concerns about rejection by significant others or employers than those who verbalized fear of death."[9]

As stated by the Office of Human Subjects Research (OHSR) of the National Institutes of Health, informed consent is best conceptualized as a process:

Informed consent is a process, not just a form. Information must be presented to enable persons to voluntarily decide whether or not to participate as a research subject. It is a fundamental mechanism to ensure respect for persons through provision of thoughtful consent for a voluntary act. The procedures used in obtaining informed consent should be designed to educate the subject population in terms that they can understand. Therefore, informed consent language and its documentation (especially explanation of the study's purpose, duration, experimental procedures, alternatives, risks, and benefits) must be written in "lay language" (i.e., understandable to the people being asked to participate). The written presentation of information is used to document the basis for consent and for the subjects' future reference. The consent document should be revised when deficiencies are noted or when additional information will improve the consent process. Use of the first person (e.g., "I understand that...") can be interpreted as suggestive, may be relied upon as a substitute for sufficient factual information, and can constitute coercive influence over a subject. Use of scientific jargon and legalese is not appropriate. Think of the document primarily as a teaching tool, not as a legal instrument.[3]

To more fully understand the significance of informed consent and its pivotal role in the bounding processes of research, access the OHSR website. Although written consents basically contain similar elements, each institution requires slightly different wording and approaches, so be sure to check with your setting. Most IRBs provide scripts and templates from which to develop your consent. See Figure 3-1 for an example.[3]

Study Approval and Monitoring

After you have submitted a proposal and a sample consent form and obtained IRB review, you will receive a letter indicating that your research protocol has been approved as submitted, conditionally approved, or not approved. Conditional approval indicates that the IRB will provide final approval after specific issues are clarified and elements of the consent are modified. However, an investigator cannot begin a study until final approval is obtained. If your study is not approved, you should carefully consider why and what types of changes are necessary and then resubmit your protocol detailing how it was modified to address the concerns that were raised.

In addition to receiving an approval letter, you will also be provided with your original informed

---

Sample Informed Consent Form

You are invited to participate in a research project being conducted by *(name)*, a *(faculty member, staff member, graduate student, undergraduate student)* in the Department of *(name)* at the University of Maine. *(If the principal investigator is a student, also name the faculty sponsor.)* The purpose of the research is _____. You must be at least 18 years of age to participate. *(This statement is not always required. An example of when it is required is if the study involves the UMaine undergraduate student population. If there is a chance that someone in the population you are studying could be under 18, include this statement.)*

What Will You Be Asked to Do?

If you decide to participate, you will be asked to *(describe procedures, give examples of sample questions if applicable. If the study is a survey and the survey is attached, sample questions are not required). If the study involves a focus group, indicate how many people will be in the group.* It may take approximately *(amount of time)* to participate. *(If the procedures are numerous, we suggest you use bullets to make the form easier to read.)*

Risks *(Listed below are examples)*

- There is the possibility that you may become uncomfortable answering the questions.
- There is the possibility that you may have bruising after the blood draw.
- Except for your time and inconvenience, there are no risks to you from participating in this study.

Benefits (Two *benefit statements are required – benefit to participant and potential benefit of the research)*

(Examples of benefits to participants)

- You may learn how your energy level changes your mood.
- You will have a cholesterol screening at no charge.
- While this study will have no direct benefit to you, this research may help us learn more about…

Compensation: *(Listed below are examples; if you are not offering compensation, leave this section out.* **NOTE: See Item #7 on checklist for additional guidance if compensation exceeds $75.)**

- You will receive $X for participating in this study.
- You will receive $X for completing the first part of this study and $X for the remaining part.
- You will receive 1 hour of research credit for participating in this study.

Confidentiality

Your name will not be on any of the documents. A code number will be used to protect your identity. Data will be kept in the investigator's locked office. (List others who may have access to data, such as faculty advisor and/or others working on the project.) Your name or other identifying information will not be reported in any publications. The key linking your name to the data will be destroyed after data analysis is complete (list approximately when), and all data will be destroyed after X years (or the investigator will keep the data indefinitely). If a key will be kept electronically, explain that it will be encrypted (know your audience, you may need to explain, e.g., "the key will be stored using software that provides additional security." Specifically address the retention of any audio, video, or film recordings. Do not state that data will be kept until the study is completed, as that is too vague. If the study involves an online survey, include a description what will be done to protect their information, e.g., encryption, etc.

Figure 3-1 Sample Informed Consent Form.

consent document with a stamped date, indicating when IRB approval was granted and the date that approval will expire. You should use only current, dated consent forms. Each year, a report must be submitted to the IRB indicating the number of study participants who have been enrolled, and general study progress. Each year, the IRB will re-stamp a consent form with the current date. The dated consent document ensures that only the current, IRB-approved informed consent documents are

NOTE: the above is a sample; it may not fit your study. The important aspect is to tell people how the data will be kept to ensure confidentiality – or to inform that that it won't be kept confidential, as in the case of oral histories.

For an anonymous survey, use:

This study is anonymous. Please do not write your name on the questionnaire. There will be no records linking you to the data. *State where and for how long data will be kept.*

For Focus Groups, also include this statement: Due to the focus group format, confidentiality of responses cannot be guaranteed.

Voluntary

Participation is voluntary. If you choose to take part in this study, you may stop at any time *(explain whether stopping will alter the benefit/compensation to be received).* You may skip any questions you do not wish to answer.

(For a mail/internet survey): Return of the survey implies consent to participate.

Contact Information

If you have any questions about this study, please contact me at *(phone, address, e-mail).* You may also reach the faculty advisor on this study at *(phone, address, e-mail).* If you have any questions about your rights as a research participant, please contact Gayle Jones, Assistant to the University of Maine's Protection of Human Subjects Review Board, at 581-1498 (or e-mail gayle.jones@umit.maine.edu).

*(If the study is **not** exempt from further review, continue with the following statement.)*

Your signature below indicates that you have read the above information and agree to participate. You will receive a copy of this form.

_____   _____
Signature   Date

NOTE: If your study involves children (<18 years old), the consent letter is written to Dear Parent/Guardian, and reference to "your child" or "your son/daughter" is used.

For studies involving children, an assent script is required. Children with permission to participate in a research study also have the right to be informed about the study and choose whether they wish to participate. Create a script that describes the study, what they'll be asked to do, confidentiality issues, etc. Use age-appropriate language! Children do not sign any documents.

Figure 3-1 cont'd

presented to study participants. It also serves as a reminder to investigators of the need for continuing review of their protocols. In addition, adverse events and whether they can be attributed to study participation must be reported to the IRB within 24 hours of their occurrence, and then summarized at the annual reporting period. Adverse events may include but are not limited to participant hospitalization, nursing home placement, a life-threatening event (suicide or suicidal ideation), or death. For each event, the researcher must have in place a set of procedures to ethically and appropriately manage the event.

Let's say a study participant becomes ill and needs to go to the hospital during an interview. The research staff must be properly trained and prepared for this type of occurrence, particularly if the study involves sick or frail individuals. If the participant is alone with the researcher, then it is the obligation of the researcher to stay with the person until he or she is safe. Calling 911, another family member, or a neighbor would be appropriate. If the person is with a family member, the researcher is obligated to ensure that the family member can manage the situation, and the family should not be left alone until the situation is resolved—that is, until the person is successfully taken to the hospital by ambulance or other means.

Any adverse events such as in this example must be submitted to the IRB for review. In submitting the event, the researcher indicates date of occurrence, briefly describes the event and how it was resolved, and then provides an evaluation of the probability that the event occurred as a result of a study procedure (not at all probable, somewhat probable, or highly probable). If the event is due to the study, a determination will be made about whether the study needs to be terminated because it poses too high a risk to participants. If the potential benefits outweigh the risk or the event was not life threatening, then the IRB may determine that the study can continue but that the consent needs to be modified to reflect the new potential risk that was uncovered in the research process. If the adverse event is not related to the study (e.g., the interviewer discovers that the person is in need of medical attention before engaging in any study-related procedures), then no changes to the study protocol or consent forms will be required and the study can continue as proposed, although tracking and reporting of such events would continue.

Developing an Informed Consent Document

Guidelines for developing the informed consent document reflect the principlist ethical framework established by the Belmont Report. First, the consent should be written at a sixth-grade to eighth-grade level to ensure that persons with diverse levels of literacy can fully understand the research process in which they are being asked to participate. Achieving this literacy level can be very challenging, as typically IRBs require that certain legal language appears in consents. It is helpful to submit your consent to a literacy check to determine the grade level at which it is written. Second, familiar words should be used throughout the consent. Jargon, including medical and legal terms, should be avoided; for example, the term "cholesterol" is preferable to "blood lipids," and when indicating random assignment, explain that assignment will be determined "by chance." If a scientific or medical term must be used, be sure to define it. Avoid the use of abbreviations and acronyms. If they need to be used, you must be sure to clearly define them first.

It is critical that all persons be given the opportunity to participate in the research process (the principle of justice). You need to consider different strategies for involving persons with low literacy or sensory impairments (e.g., vision or hearing) so that they can understand your study procedures and participate in an informed way. For persons with low cognitive capacity, approaches can be used to ensure their understanding of the research process. One approach is to use a more simplified version of the consent and to check in with the person to be sure they understand the intent of each paragraph. For example, following the paragraph describing the study, a person could be asked, "Can you tell me in your own words what this study is about?" If the person is unable to follow or does not feel comfortable, then consent must be obtained from a proxy such as a responsible party or legally authorized person (e.g., spouse). In some cases, you may be aware of a person's cognitive status through a preexisting assessment that you are authorized to view before administering the consenting process. In this case, a protocol could be established that persons with a certain score on the assessment would require proxy consent.

Different approaches may be needed to ensure inclusiveness for different study populations. Involving children, for example, may require use of pictures to explain aspects of the study in addition to also obtaining parental consent. You might develop an explanation of your study, with its risks, benefits, and confidentiality procedures, that can be translated into pictures, languages other than English, or Braille, if necessary, depending on the target group. The point is that you are obliged to consider the characteristics of your target study population and how best to ensure informed participation. Keep in mind that whatever procedures for consenting that you develop, the IRB must review and approve them.

Involving Vulnerable Populations

The involvement of vulnerable persons remains a widely discussed and debated issue in research. As noted earlier, the term "vulnerable populations" refers to a wide range of persons who may be at risk in a research setting not only because of their intrinsic characteristics but also as a result of their life situation or circumstances. For example, persons may be vulnerable because of a medical condition (e.g., terminal illness), a particular setting (e.g., emergency room of hospital, homeless shelter, prison), a baseline limitation of intellectual function (e.g., developmental disability), a psychosocial stressor (e.g., posttraumatic stress disorder), stigma (AIDS or HIV), or an illness that compromises comprehension and decision-making abilities (e.g., dementia, frailty).

The concern with involving vulnerable persons is twofold. First, no ethical justification exists for excluding vulnerable populations. In fact, it is unethical to exclude such populations from research in that their exclusion restricts knowledge development in areas that would ultimately benefit that group.[3] Vulnerable populations are typically underrepresented in studies, and it is usually not possible to generalize research findings to the group. A second concern is determining the best way to involve vulnerable populations. Here the investigator must strike a balance between not excluding a particular study group that is vulnerable and avoiding inducement.

Consider how pharmacological studies that use monetary inducements for participation may be particularly attractive to individuals rendered vulnerable because of their life circumstances, such as persons

who are homeless or live in prison.[10] Participating in a study based on a hefty monetary inducement, however, may not be in the best interest of these groups.

A related issue is how best to apprise persons with compromised decision-making abilities about the procedures of a study so that they can make an informed decision to participate or not, as discussed earlier. Remember that an essential principle established in the Belmont Report and overseen by IRBs is that persons must be fully informed before agreeing to participate in a study. For persons with dementia and other populations with impaired comprehension and judgment, how can we be assured that these groups willingly and knowingly agree to participate in a study?

The research community addresses this important issue and has developed tools that can reliably and validly distinguish between persons who can make a judgment regarding their participation and those for whom proxy consent is necessary.[11] For example, persons at the early stages of dementia may be capable of comprehending a typical informed consent written document, whereas persons at the moderate stage may not fully understand what they are committing to in the study if the document is written at a high literacy level. In persons unable to provide their own consent, consent from a legal guardian or family caregiver can be obtained. Even when proxy consent is obtained, however, before administering a test, interview, or any type of procedure, the person with dementia or compromised cognition should be provided a brief explanation, and assent should be obtained (e.g., "Hello, Mr. Smith. I would like to ask you a few questions about how you are doing; is that okay? You can let me know at any time if you want to stop.").

Although simplifying the language of an informed consent may be helpful for some groups with compromised intellect or decision making, use of pictorial or other visual representations of study procedures may be useful for other populations. Knowing exactly the most effective way to present informed consent can be difficult and is only now becoming the focus of research.

Suppose you want to conduct a study of the quality of life of persons with developmental disabilities living in the community. You want to include persons who have a wide range of capabilities. In this case, your presentation of informed consent may need to be tailored to match persons at different levels of intellectual and cognitive abilities. However, there is no standardized approach to do this, or even to determine how to identify what type of approach a person may need to become fully informed.

Despite the difficulties and challenges of involving vulnerable populations, the research community is committed to developing meaningful approaches that can appropriately involve those who had historically been omitted from research that is critical to their health and well-being. Remember that these populations are vulnerable in large part because of our lack of knowledge and expertise about their involvement in research and their prior exploitation in the research enterprise. Given the challenges in developing informed consent documents for different populations and, in particular, for individuals with low literacy or cognitive impairments, the Agency for Healthcare Research and Quality has developed a helpful toolkit that is available on the Web: "Informed Consent and Authorization Toolkit for Minimal Risk Research" (http://www.ahrq.gov/funding/policies/informedconsent/ictoolkit.pdf). It provides templates for informed consents and strategies to evaluate the literacy level and appropriateness of the documents you develop.

Specialized Oversight of Experimental-Type Designs

The true-experimental design, often referred to as a "randomized controlled trial," requires a specialized level of human subject oversight in addition to IRB review. Given that such trials test the efficacy of a new technology, behavioral intervention, device, or therapeutic program, there is heightened concern for the safety of study participants in this type of design strategy. Thus, in addition to the IRB, another level of oversight is required to monitor the safety of study participants in randomized trials.

Assume you plan to test an intervention that involves introducing balance and strength exercises

to older adults to reduce fear of falling. A potential harmful outcome of the intervention might be muscle strain, back injury, or possibly a fall as a result of increased movement and activity. Thus, the study must be monitored for the occurrence of these possible events. The investigator tracks the occurrence of such events and determines whether a given event is a direct consequence of the intervention.

To monitor the safety of participants in randomized trials, the investigator is responsible for establishing an independent group of experts as a *data and safety monitoring board (DSMB)*.[12] The extent of involvement of a DSMB in oversight of a study depends on the level of risk associated with the treatment and study procedures. Studies that place participants at high risk require greater monitoring, whereas studies with minimal risk require less oversight.

Regardless of risk level, the primary responsibilities of a DSMB in addition to the IRB are to (1) review and approve all study procedures; (2) provide oversight for procedures regarding the safety of human subjects and ethical research practices, including reviewing the investigator's approach to recruitment and the informed consent process; (3) determine whether and when a study should be terminated because of adverse events that can be attributed to study procedures; and (4) determine if interim analyses should be conducted to evaluate study outcomes and if the study should be stopped midstream because it is either overwhelmingly beneficial or harmful.

The requirement for DSMB monitoring recently has expanded beyond pharmaceutical research to include behavioral treatments. Some institutions have created a DSMB to serve as a monitoring group for all clinical trials conducted at that setting. In most institutions, however, the investigator is responsible for establishing a committee composed of persons who have expertise in randomized trials and in the specific content of the treatment and who are not involved with members of the research team so that the potential exists for a conflict of interest.

It is important to recognize that even a controlled trial with minimal risk, such as testing a telephone information service for individuals who are unable to leave their homes, necessitates careful oversight to ensure human subject protection and ethical research practices. The DSMB can be a helpful mechanism for providing feedback and recommendations to the investigative team to enhance study rigor. Search the Internet for DSMBs to see how they function at different institutions. You will find a wide range of approaches, although all cover the essentials of safety monitoring and human subject protection oversight.[12]

Summary

Research ethics are expansive, from generating to using and applying knowledge. We presented several ethical-decision models at the beginning of the chapter and then focused on protection of human subjects as a major obligation, both ethically and legally, that all researchers must incorporate into their investigations irregardless of the type of inquiry that is pursued. Researchers are ethically obligated to design protection strategies so that all populations, regardless of literacy level or physical or cognitive capacity, can engage in the research process in a fully informed and ethical way. Before engaging in any type of research, you are required to submit a proposal to the IRB for review and approval. If a written consent is necessary, it must contain critical elements describing study procedures, voluntary capacity, risk-to-benefit ratio, and confidentiality procedures. A current, dated, and stamped consent precedes the enrollment or recruitment of study participants. The process of obtaining consent is an essential aspect of bounding one's study and ensuring ethical research behavior on the part of the researcher.

As in all other thinking and action processes of research, the construction of protection strategies requires careful and thoughtful consideration. Unethical or inappropriate research harms not only study participants but also the target population, society, and the overall research enterprise.

EXERCISES

1. Contact the office of research of your institution and obtain consent templates. Propose a study and develop a corresponding consent form. What aspects of the consent form were particularly challenging to develop? What literacy level is the actual template?

2. Role-play the introduction of a consent to a peer. What types of questions does the person ask about the study and informed consent process? How did the informed consent process flow? Do you think the person understood the purpose of the study and the nature of his or her participation? What could you have done to improve the clarity and flow of the process?

3. Identify a published study and develop an informed consent document based on the description of the procedures in the article.

4. Identify a particular vulnerable group that you think is important to study. Design a strategy for informing this group about a study.

....

References

1. Goh EC: *De-pathologising children as "victims" in social work practice*. Childhood, 3rd Global Conference, 2013. Available at: http://www.inter-disciplinary.net/probing-the-boundaries/wp-content/uploads/2013/05/gohchildpaper.pdf.

2. Corey G, Corey MS, Callanan P: *Issues and ethics in the helping professions*, Belmont, Calif, 2011, Cenage. National Research Act (Public Law 93-348).

3. Research Compliance—Institutional Review Board for the Protection of Human Subjects (IRB), 2012. Available at: http://umaine.edu/research/research-compliance/institutional -review-board-for-the-protection-of-human-subjects-irb.

4. Office for Protection from Research Risks: *2011 ANPRM for revision to Common Rule*. Available at: http://www.hhs.gov/ohrp/humansubjects/anprm2011page.html.

5. Centers for Disease Control and Prevention: *U.S. Public Health Service syphilis study at Tuskegee*, 2013. Available at: http://www.cdc.gov/tuskegee/timeline.htm.

6. *Summary of the HIPAA Privacy Rule: Health information privacy*, n.d. Available at: http://www.hhs.gov/ocr/privacy/hipaa/understanding/summary.

7. National Commission for the Protection of Human Subjects of Biomedical and Behavioral Research: *The Belmont Report: ethical principles and guidelines for the protection of human subjects of research*, Washington, DC, 1979, The Commission.

8. Trochim W: *Introduction to evaluation*, 2008. Available at Evaluation Research: http://www.socialresearchmethods.net/kb/intreval.php.

9. Johansen PS, Kohli H: Long-term HIV/AIDS survivors: coping strategies and challenges. *J HIV/AIDS Soc Services* 11(1):6–22, 2012.

10. Beauchamp L, Jennings B, Kinney ED, et al: Pharmaceutical research involving the homeless. *J Med Philos* 27:547–564, 2002.

11. Kim SYH, Caine ED, Currier GW, et al: Assessing the competence of persons with Alzheimer's disease in providing informed consent for participation in research. *Am J Psychiatry* 158:712–717, 2001.

12. Ellenberg SS, Fleming TR, DeMets DL: *Data monitoring committees in clinical trials: a practical perspective*, Chichester, UK, 2003, Wiley.

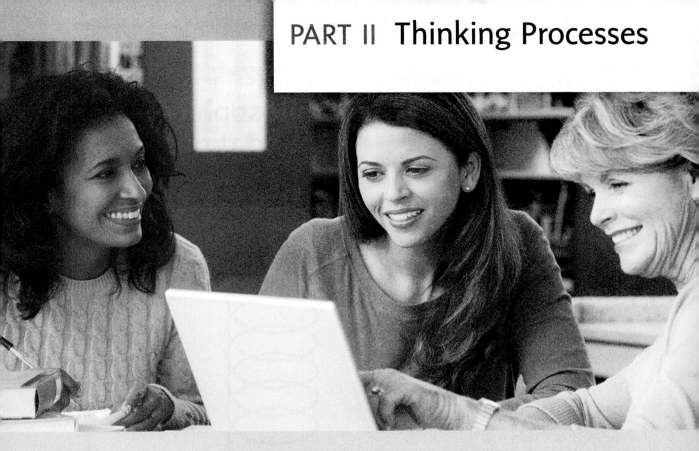

PART II Thinking Processes

In Part I of this text, we introduced the definition, purposes, and essentials of research.

We now delve into Part II, the thinking processes in which all researchers engage to make sound decisions about how to frame, conduct, and use research. These efforts include understanding the philosophical foundations that underpin diverse research traditions, framing the research problem, critically reviewing the literature, linking theory and research, developing a research question or query, and using the appropriate research language to understand and explicate the research process, findings, and interpretations.

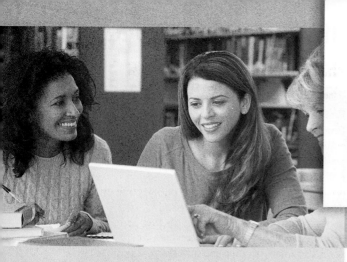

Chapter 4
Philosophical Foundations

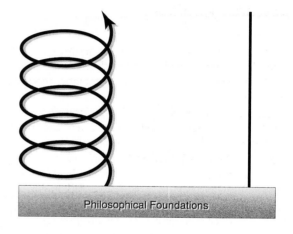

Philosophical Foundations

Although you do not have to be a philosopher to engage in the research process, it is important to understand the philosophical foundations and assumptions about human experience and knowledge on which experimental-type, naturalistic, and, more recently, mixed methods research traditions are based. By being aware of these assumptions, you will be more skilled in directing the research process and in selecting specific methods to use and combine. Also, an understanding of these philosophical foundations will help you recognize that "knowledge" is shaped by the way you frame a research problem and the strategies that are used to obtain, analyze, and interpret information.

The questions, "What is reality?" (*ontology*) and "How do we come to know it?" (*epistemology*) have been posed by philosophers and scholars from many academic and professional disciplines throughout history. As we have suggested, in Western cultures, until recently, there have been two primary but often competing views of reality and how to obtain knowledge. These two perspectives reflect the basic differences between naturalistic inquiry and experimental-type research. *Logical positivism* is the foundation for deductive, predictive designs that we refer to as "experimental-type research." In contrast, a number of *holistic* and humanistic philosophical perspectives use inductive and abductive reasoning, which form the foundation for the research tradition that we refer to as "naturalistic inquiry." The third view, which transcends the seeming incompatibility of these philosophical positions and provides a sound rationale for using mixed methods, is pragmatism.[1] Before exploring these philosophical approaches in more detail, we begin with a brief overview of each tradition. We return to them in more detail following the discussion of philosophical foundations.

Research Traditions

As introduced previously, there are three major traditions into which research falls: experimental-type, naturalistic inquiry, and mixed methods. Within each of these categories are many systematic research strategies.

Studies within experimental-type inquiry share a single philosophical foundation and are characterized by a prescribed sequence of linear processes and rules (as discussed in detail in subsequent chapters).[2,3] In contrast, strategies that share the principles of a holistic pluralistic perspective fall under the category of naturalistic inquiry. Although diverse, these approaches for the most part follow a nonlinear, iterative, and flexible[4] sequence of processes.

The mixed method tradition integrates strategies from both experimental-type and naturalistic traditions but does not share the philosophical foundation of either. Because experimental-type and naturalistic inquiry form the basis for what strategies are used in mixed methods, we suggest that one must become conversant in each of the primary traditions to understand and efficaciously use mixed methods. As we discuss later, this tradition is underpinned by pragmatism, a philosophical school of thought that foregrounds purpose as primary.

Each design tradition has its own language, its own thinking and action processes, and specific design issues and concerns. We use the concept of the three traditions throughout this text as a basis from which to discuss and compare design essentials and research processes within the same philosophical perspective and across philosophical traditions.

Philosophical Foundations of Experimental-Type Research

Experimental-type researchers share a common frame of reference or epistemology that has been called rationalistic, positivist, reductionist, or logical positivism. Although theoretical differences exist between these terms, we use the term "logical positivism" to name the overall perspective on which deductive research design is based.

Descartes, a 17th-century philosopher, is often considered the father of Western philosophy. He proposed dualism, an idea that divided the mind and the body into distinct entities. Building on Cartesian thinking, David Hume, an 18th-century philosopher, was most influential in developing this traditional theory of science,[5] which posited a separation between individual thoughts and what is real in the universe outside ourselves. That is, traditional theorists of science define "knowledge" as part of a reality that is separate and independent from individual perspective and experience. Within this philosophical school of thought, legitimate knowledge is therefore only that which is verifiable through the scientific method. Logical positivists believe that a world apart from our ideas and a single truth, referred to as monism, constitute reality, are objectively knowable, and can be discovered through observation and measurement. If properly conducted, coming to know can be considered free of human bias. This epistemological view is based on the fundamental assumption that it is possible to know and understand phenomena that reside outside ourselves, separate from the realm of our subjective ideas. Only through observation and sense data, defined as information obtained through our senses, can we come to know truth and reality. This type of knowing is named empiricism.

Philosophers in subsequent centuries further developed, modified, and clarified Hume's basic notion of empiricism to yield what today is known as logical positivism. Essentially, logical positivists believe that there is a single reality that can be discovered by reducing it into its parts, a concept known as reductionism.[6] The relationship among these parts and the logical, structural principles that guide them can also be discovered and known through the systematic collection and analysis of sense data, finally leading to the ability to predict phenomena from what is already known. Bertrand Russell, a 20th-century mathematician and philosopher, was instrumental in promoting the synthesis of mathematical logic with sense data.[7]

Statisticians, such as Quetelet, Fischer, and Pearson, developed theories to reveal "fact" (elements of knowledge considered to be real) logically and objectively through mathematical analysis.[8] The logical positivist school of thought therefore provided the foundation for what most laypersons have come to know as "experimental research." In this approach, a theory or set of principles is held as true. Specific areas of inquiry are isolated within that theoretical perspective, and clearly defined hypotheses (expected outcomes of an inquiry that investigate only those phenomena) are posed and tested under carefully controlled conditions. Sense data are then collected and mathematically analyzed to support or refute hypotheses. Through incremental deductive reasoning, which involves theory verification and testing, "reality" can become predictable.

Another major tenet of logical positivism is that objective inquiry and analysis are possible; that is, the investigator, through the use of accepted and standard research techniques, can eliminate bias and achieve results through objective, quantitative measurement.[9,10]

Philosophical Foundations of Naturalistic Inquiry

Another school of theorists has argued an alternative position: Individuals create their own subjective realities, and thus the knower and knowledge are interrelated and interdependent.[4,11-14] In general, these theorists believe that ideas and individual interpretations are the lenses through which each individual knows the universe and that we come to understand and define the world through these ideas and our unique interpretation of symbols. Furthermore, within these traditions, there is a range of beliefs about the stability of ideas, symbols, and the role of language in communicating or even creating ideas and experiences. These epistemological viewpoints are based on the fundamental assumption that it is not possible to separate the outside world from an individual's ideas, language, symbols, and perceptions of that world. Knowledge is based on how the individual perceives experiences and how he or she understands his or her world.

Listen to Byers[15]:

It seems strange to call science a mythology since the story that science tells about itself is precisely that it, an activity pursued by human beings, is objective and empirical; that it concerns itself with the facts and nothing but the facts. . . . And yet science is a human activity. This is an obvious statement but it bears repeating since part of the mythology of science is precisely that it is independent of human beings; independent of mind and intelligence. . . . How do human beings create a system of thought that produces results that are independent of human thought?

A number of research strategies share this basic holistic, epistemological view, although each is rooted in a different philosophical tradition.

Although research based on the understanding that there are pluralistic perspectives has gained acceptance more recently than the espousal of logical positivist approaches, *pluralism* is not new. Ancient Greek philosophers struggled with the separation of idea and object, and philosophers throughout history continue this debate.[16] The essential characteristics of what we refer to as pluralistic philosophies are as follows:

1. Human experience is complex and holistic, and it cannot be understood exclusively by reductionism, that is, only by identifying and examining its parts.
2. Meaning in human experience is derived from an understanding of individuals in their social, economic, political, cultural, linguistic, physical, expressive, emotive, and virtual contexts.
3. Multiple realities exist, and one's view of reality is determined by events viewed through individual lenses or biases.
4. Those who have the experiences are the most intimately knowledgeable about them.

In addition to these common characteristics, pluralistic philosophies encompass a number of princi-

Paradigm ⊃ a model; pattern, example

ples that guide the selection of particular designs in this category. For example, *phenomenologists* believe that human meaning can be understood only through experience.[12] Thus, a phenomenological understanding is limited to knowing experience without an outsider interpreting that experience. In contrast, interpretive and social "semiotic" *interactionists* assume that human meaning evolves from the context of social interaction.[13] Human phenomena can therefore be understood through interpreting the meanings in social discourse, exchange, objects, spaces, and other symbols. Deconstructionists focus on the primacy and fleeting stability of language, and thus research based on that philosophical thought examines how language both forms and undermines what we know.[8,17] Although disparate, these philosophies therefore share a pluralistic, holistic view of knowledge; multiple realities can be identified and understood to a greater or lesser extent only within the natural context in which human experience and behavior occur. To the extent possible, coming to know these realities requires research designs that investigate phenomena in their natural contexts and seek to discover complexity and meaning. Furthermore, those who "own" or have the experience are considered the "intimate knowers," and they transmit their unique knowledge through doing and telling.[16]

Philosophical Foundations of Mixed Methods

Transcending the apparent contradiction between monism and pluralism, Tashakkori and Teddlie[1] have suggested several philosophical foundations that underpin and support mixing experimental-type and naturalistic methods of inquiry. In their classic work,[1] they focused their philosophical lens on the single perspective of pragmatism. Briefly, *pragmatism* is a school of thought characterized as an "unparadigm" (p. 15). That is to say, rather than taking a position on the nature of knowledge itself, pragmatism is turned to the selection of methodological tools that are most purposive in solving a knowledge problem. Thus concepts such as "truth" and "reality" are relative and purposive. Given this philosophical

"unparadigm," the purposive choice of methodology, including mixed methods, is most desirable. However, more recently, Tashakkori and Teddlie have added alternative philosophical thoughts to support mixed methods or what they call paradigm pluralism. Furthermore, these authors distinguish multiple methods as bottom-up, or choosing research strategies that best answer a question without being constrained by one philosophy.

Equipped with this brief philosophical background, we now turn to the discussion of the nature of the traditions themselves.[1]

Experimental-Type Research

Now, let us review the nature of experimental-type designs in more depth. Remember that logical positivists are monistic in that they believe there is a single reality that can be known through reductionism. This deductive process involves theorizing to explain the part of reality about which the investigator is concerned, reducing theory to observable parts, examining the parts through measurement, and determining the degree to which the analysis verifies or falsifies part or all of the theory. Second, a central principle of logical positivism is that it is possible and desirable to understand the world through systematic objectivity that can only occur by eliminating bias in our observations. Given these two critical elements of logical positivism, let us examine how each research essential, as it occurs in a linear sequence, supports the tenets of logical positivist inquiry.[2]

After identifying a philosophical foundation, the researcher begins by articulating a topic of inquiry. Suppose, for example, Web-based health information was your topic of interest. We name this step "framing the problem," which identifies and delimits the part of the "real world" that an investigator will examine. After a research problem is identified, supporting knowledge is obtained by conducting a review of scholarly literature and resources. This research essential discerns how the problem has already been theoretically approached and explained. It examines the extent to which the theory has been objectively and rigorously investigated.[2] The scholarly review of literature and other sources of knowledge therefore provide the researcher with legitimate knowledge for developing a theoretical foundation for the inquiry. With this information, the investigator is now ready to propose a specific research question. This question is derived from and builds on previous inquiry, isolates the theoretical material to be scrutinized, and incrementally advances knowledge about the subject under study. The ultimate goal of experimental-type inquiry is to predict a part of reality from knowing about other parts. To answer the research question objectively, the investigator selects a research design that addresses the level of knowledge sought (e.g., descriptive, predictive) and enacts specific, accepted techniques that control for factors that introduce bias into a study. The design clearly and succinctly specifies all action processes for collecting and analyzing information so that the study may be replicated by other investigators. To ensure that the goals of objectivity and the elimination of bias are met, action processes within the inquiry must proceed exactly as designed. Through data analysis, the investigator examines the extent to which the findings have objectively confirmed or raised doubts about the "truth value" of the theoretical tenets tested and their capacity to explain and ultimately predict the slice of reality under investigation.

Many designs are anchored in the philosophical foundation of logical positivism. Box 4-1 lists the four major categories of design that form the experimental-type tradition, each of which is discussed in this text.

Naturalistic Inquiry

There is great diversity in the strategies that are categorized as naturalistic inquiry. As indicated in this chapter, designs that fit with this tradition are rooted in different philosophical and theoretical perspectives. The language and thinking processes used by naturalistic researchers vary within the tradition and are significantly different from the language and thinking processes found in the experimental-type tradition. However, all naturalistic approaches have seminal characteristics in common and rely primarily on qualitative methodologies, although often for different purposes and to answer distinct types of inquiries.

Designs in the naturalistic tradition vary according to (1) the extent to which inquiry involves the personal "essence," language, experiences, and insights of the investigator; (2) the extent to which individual "experience" and meaning versus patterns of human experience is sought; (3) the extent to which the investigator imposes structure in the data collection and analytical processes; and (4) the sequence of the research process.

Neither the point of entry into the spiral of inquiry nor the sequence of the thinking and action processes is prescribed a priori. Thus an investigator may begin with any of the essential thinking and action processes, change the design or specific action strategies in response to findings throughout the research process, and revisit steps that have already been conducted. Many methodologists use the term "iterative" to describe the repetitive, flexible, and progressively building process of naturalistic inquiry.[14]

Although there are many design variations, Box 4-2 lists the major categories of design that make up the tradition of naturalistic inquiry, as discussed in detail in Part III.

BOX 4-1 *Major Categories of Design in Experimental-Type Research*

- Nonexperimental
- Pre-experimental
- Quasi-experimental
- True experimental

BOX 4-2 *Major Categories of Design in Naturalistic Inquiry*

- Endogenous
- Participatory action research
- Critical theory
- Phenomenology
- Heuristic design
- Ethnography (classic and new)
- Narrative
- Life history
- Meta-analysis
- Grounded theory
- Semiotics

Integrating the Two Research Traditions—Mixed Methods

As we briefly discussed, there has been significant and heated debate over which research tradition is best for advancing our understanding of human experience. Because experimental-type researchers believe that reality can only become known incrementally through implementing objective thinking and action processes, they may not value the naturalistic foundations of pluralism and subjectivity. Conversely, many naturalistic researchers question the extent to which human experience can be reduced to a single, observable, measurable, and predictive reality. Moreover, because of the philosophical incompatibility of monism and pluralism, many scholars and researchers have opposed integrating experimental-type and naturalistic traditions.

As we discussed earlier, there is a growing and now well-accepted usage of mixed methods, as scholars and researchers recognize that the limitations of both traditions can be mediated by the strengths of alternative approaches.[1,18] Moreover, experimental-type methodologists now recognize that naturalistic inquiry represents a legitimate and logical research strategy alternative to experimental-type inquiry, and naturalistic researchers are giving greater attention to the standardization of analysis and procedures and to the complementary role of experimental-type designs. Consistent with a growing number of methodologists, we believe that the following eight points of tension in the health and human service research world have led many investigators to espouse strategies that overcome or transcend the limitations of each research tradition:

1. The focus on the experimental-type tradition as the only viable research option has been brought into question by findings that repeatedly indicate few or no measurable effects of experimental treatments in health and human service research.
2. Many explanatory theories can enrich knowledge, and thus strategies that rely on a single truth can limit rather than expand knowledge.[8]

3. There is growing recognition that many of the persistent and unanswered issues that are critical to health and human services cannot be addressed by the experimental paradigm alone.
4. There is an increasing realization that quantitative information, in and of itself, does not necessarily provide insight into the contexts and processes that influence empirical findings reflected in a numerical report.[18]
5. There are often great discrepancies in knowledge generated from qualitative and quantitative studies.
6. The increasing emphasis placed on the empirical demonstration of the need for outcomes of health and human service has led naturalistic researchers to consider using replicable strategies.
7. Understanding and eliminating disparities in health and wellness among diverse population groups require the use of multiple discovery and verification strategies.
8. Within naturalistic design, the limits of relativism in predicting outcomes can be redressed and improved by purposive addition of experimental-type measurement to qualitative strategies.

Both traditions have strengths and limitations; both have value in investigating the depth and breadth of research topics that inform us about human experience; and both can be integrated in a single study or throughout all or some of the parts of a research agenda involving multiple studies.[1,18] We suggest that an integrated approach can strengthen health and human service inquiry. An integrated approach involves purposively selecting and combining designs and methods from both traditions so that one complements the other to benefit or contribute to an understanding of the whole.

However, as discussed throughout this text, well-conducted integration depends on an investigator's firm understanding of the attributes of thinking and action processes, the design strategies, and the particular methodological approaches of each tradition. Given this understanding, the researcher can mix and combine strategies to strengthen the research effort and to strive for comprehensive and complex understanding of the phenomenon under consideration. In their classic work, Brewer and Hunter used the term *multimethod research* and explain the premise of this approach to inquiry in this way:

> Our individual methods may be flawed, but fortunately the flaws in each are not identical. A diversity of imperfection allows us to combine methods not only to gain their individual strengths but also to compensate for their particular faults and limitations. Its [multimethod research] fundamental strategy is to attack a research problem with an arsenal of methods that have nonoverlapping weaknesses in addition to their complementary strengths.[18]

The use of mixed methods as "the mediator or point of integration" to strengthen and advance scientific inquiry has a 35-year history in sociology, anthropology, and education. Only more recently, however, has the integration of the traditions become acceptable and even popular in health and human service research. Many researchers implicitly use one or more forms of integration discussed throughout this text. For example, there is a long history of the use of simple descriptive statistics, such as frequencies and means, in ethnographic research; quantitative studies frequently use an exploratory, open-ended series of questions before establishing closed-ended and numerically based interview questions; and it is not uncommon for sampling techniques to be mixed with unstructured interviews.

Several points are important here. First, a multimethod approach enables you to generate more in-depth, nuanced, or complex knowledge about phenomena. Consider the example in Chapter 1 in which the investigators used measurement to examine improvement in comprehension and then proceeded, through naturalistic methods, to investigate the "experience" of using the health information website that they developed. Second, although mixed method approaches are complex, like all forms of inquiry they require purposeful and logical development that combines elements of the thinking and action processes from both the naturalistic and the experimental-type traditions for each research essential.

A third important point is that mixed method studies transcend the classic and unresolved philosophical and methodological "monism-pluralism" debates, thereby bring both to bear on enhancing inquiry. Integration is based on philosophical "unparadigms"[1] that propose thinking of and approaching research strategies as a purposive set of knowledge-generating tools. As suggested first by Brewer and Hunter[18] and more recently by Tashakkori and Teddlie,[1] contemporary researchers who adopt integrated or mixed methods are not necessarily proceeding from mixed philosophical bases but from perspectives that can achieve purpose, emancipation, and illumination not possible with single-tradition approaches.

Table 4-1 summarizes the essential characteristics of experimental-type, naturalistic, and mixed method inquiries. Examining the differences will help you understand the foundations of each tradition and its integration with the other.

We suggest five distinct ways in which the research traditions can be integrated. Figure 4-1, *A*, shows a study design that initially involves a form of naturalistic inquiry, followed by an experimental-type approach. Usually in this sequence, the purpose of the naturalistic inquiry is to gain an understanding of the boundaries or dimensions of a particular construct or to generate a theory or set of propositions. If the purpose is to define a particular construct or concept, the investigator uses the naturalistic process

TABLE 4-1   *Four Distinguishing Characteristics of the Research Traditions*

	Experimental-Type	Naturalistic	Mixed Method
Epistemology	Logical positivism	Humanistic or holistic	Multiple
Approach to reasoning	Deductive	Inductive and abductive	All
Theoretical aim	To reduce complexity; test theory	To reveal complexity; develop theory	All
Context	Arranged by researcher	Natural context	Multiple

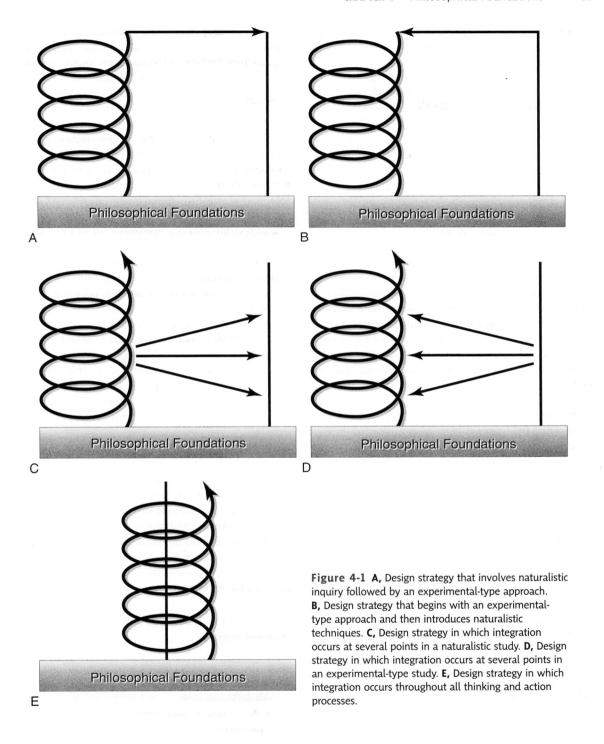

Figure 4-1 A, Design strategy that involves naturalistic inquiry followed by an experimental-type approach. **B,** Design strategy that begins with an experimental-type approach and then introduces naturalistic techniques. **C,** Design strategy in which integration occurs at several points in a naturalistic study. **D,** Design strategy in which integration occurs at several points in an experimental-type study. **E,** Design strategy in which integration occurs throughout all thinking and action processes.

to inform the development of an instrument or set of measures for use in a quantitative study. If the purpose is to generate or modify a theory using the naturalistic process, this study phase is followed by an experimental-type design, which formally tests an aspect of the theory that has been developed.

Figure 4-1, *B,* presents a strategy for integrating the research traditions that involves the opposite sequence of *A.* In this integration scheme, the researcher begins with an experimental-type approach and then introduces naturalistic techniques. Usually in this structure, the quantitative findings suggest the need for more in-depth and complex exploration of a particular phenomenon. In Figure 4-1, *C,* integration occurs at several points throughout the research process. As a naturalistic study unfolds, elements of emerging theory are tested with experimental-type strategies. Similarly, Figure 4-1, *D,* depicts a mixed method design in which experimental-type inquiry reveals the need to develop alternative insights using naturalistic techniques. In their work on the meaning and value of wheeled mobility for persons with mobility impairments, Hoenig, Giacobbi, and Levy[19] suggested mixed methods as one of the most comprehensive and useful ways to conduct research that will improve practice and use of devices. Finally, Figure 4-1, *E,* depicts the most fully *integrated design.* In this scheme, the investigator integrates a study from the beginning and throughout all thinking and action processes.

Implications of Philosophical Differences for Design

The previous discussion provided the basic elements of different philosophical positions concerning how we think about and develop an understanding or knowledge about human life. Although you do not have to take a position on the ongoing debate between different philosophical positions, it is important to recognize that by adopting a particular methodology, you are implicitly adhering to a particular way or multiple ways of viewing the world and knowledge development. You may also find yourself gravitating to a particular research approach because you feel more comfortable with it or because it may resonate with how you see the world. How

full & clearly expressed

you explicitly or implicitly define and generate knowledge and how you define the relationship between the knower (researcher) and the known (research outcomes or phenomena of the study) will direct your entire research effort, from framing your research question or query to reporting your findings. Let us consider some examples of these important philosophical concepts and their implications for research design.

Suppose that four researchers want to know what happens to participants in group therapy who have joined the group to improve their self-confidence. The researcher who suggests that knowing can be objective may choose a strategy in which he or she defines "self-confidence" as a score on a preexisting, standardized scale and then measures participants' scores at specified intervals to ascertain changes. Changes in the scores suggest what changes the group has experienced.

A second investigator, who believes that the world can be known only subjectively, may choose a research strategy in which the group is observed and the members are interviewed to obtain their perspective on their own progress within the group.

A third investigator, who believes that language shapes individual perception of reality, will focus on analysis of language communication and its multiple uses, contexts, and meanings within the group setting.

A fourth researcher, who believes in the emancipatory value of many ways of knowing, may integrate the previous three strategies. This researcher tries to understand and inform change from the communication patterns as well as individual perspectives of the participants and from the perspective of existing theory as measured by a standardized self-confidence scale.

Selecting a Research Tradition and Design Strategy

How does one decide which tradition to choose and which particular design strategy to use? The adoption of a design strategy is based on four considerations: (1) what you want to accomplish, or your purpose in conducting the research; (2) the way in which you think or reason about phenomena; (3) the level of knowledge development in the area to be investigated; and (4) practical considerations.

Purpose of Research

Research is a purposive, "intentional goal directed" activity. That is, research is conducted for a specific reason—to answer a specific question or query, to solve a problem, or to examine a particular controversy or issue. This point is central to the way in which we present the world of research to you throughout this book. The view of research as purposeful is shared by other scientists as well.[1]

Think about what we mean here by "purpose." Purpose drives the decision to engage in research. Assume that you work in a health setting in which you believe the various practices and intervention approaches that you and your colleagues carry out are important and clinically effective in producing a desired outcome. Your administrator is not convinced, however, and costs associated with your practices are beginning to be questioned. You may need to conduct a research project to validate what you are doing and demonstrate the efficacy of the specific treatment approaches that you use. Alternatively, you may need to conduct a research study to help you systematically determine which assistive robotic design is best accepted by elders so that they can age in place in their homes and communities. Similarly, assume that you are concerned about the service needs of a particular group of new immigrants in your community and that you need to obtain a better understanding to develop interventions for this group.

Think also about the following specific examples of how purpose drives the selection of a design:

> Consider a case in which an administrator of a rehabilitation unit in a large teaching and research hospital has just been informed that her inpatient rehabilitation unit may be closed if she cannot demonstrate the value of the department's programs. The administrator decides that she will implement a research project to demonstrate the value of the service to the patients who are being discharged. From the contemporary literature, she selects three criteria for measurement to define valuable intervention: (1) patient satisfaction, (2) rehabilitation staff time spent with each

patient's family in preparation for discharge, and (3) level of daily living skill performance in the occupational therapy clinic before discharge. She selects and measures these three criteria deductively, because she knows that these strengths can be clearly demonstrated by her unit staff. Her purpose in conducting the research is to demonstrate the value of her unit so that it may continue to provide valuable services to all patients. She selects a deductive strategy based on her previous knowledge of the strengths of her programs and the types of positive outcomes she hopes to achieve.

> In another hospital, the rehabilitation administrator has been asked to develop new programming for Asian immigrants who are HIV-positive and for their families. In the absence of a well-developed body of knowledge in this area, the administrator selects an inductive strategy to find out which type of rehabilitation programming will be most valuable and relevant to this ethnic group. She conducts in-depth, unstructured interviews with immigrants who are HIV-positive, their families, and service providers to reveal needs and the methods by which those needs can be addressed within her institution. •

As you can see, purpose is a powerful force that drives the selection of a research strategy. In the first example, the administrator selected a strategy that she, as the researcher, could control and one that was based on the a priori assumptions she was willing to make. In the second example, the administrator selected a strategy that would uncover information that had not been previously determined. Because patient needs, as perceived by patients and families, were shaping institutional programming, an inductive, naturalistic design strategy was selected.

It is not uncommon to have more than one purpose for your study. Consider the example of the health information website. In that example, the presence of disparities in access to Web-based health information was already known. However, the researchers had a hunch that literacy and visual access were major issues not addressed and thus contributing to unequal access to this important health information. So they used experimental-type measurement to verify this hunch and test the comprehension outcomes of their intervention. However, without conducting naturalistic inquiry, they could not have met their purpose of understanding user preference and experience to ensure that the website would be accepted and understood by their target population. To meet these goals, they therefore chose naturalistic methods.

Preference for Knowing

Your preferred way of knowing is a second important consideration when selecting a particular category of research design. Selecting a design strategy is based in large part on your implicit philosophical view; your espousal of the existence and nature of "reality" (ontology); your view of "if we can know" and if so, "how we know what we know" (epistemology); and your comfort level with these or alternative epistemological assumptions. Typically, we do not consciously reflect on our preferred way of knowing. It is usually demonstrated through which research approach makes the most sense to us and feels the most comfortable. Also, investigator personalities often influence the inclination to participate in one of the three traditions.

Level of Knowledge Development

The third consideration in selecting a research design involves the level of knowledge that has been developed in the particular area of interest. When little or nothing is understood about a phenomenon, a more descriptive and/or naturalistic approach to inquiry is indicated. When a well-developed body of knowledge exists and is useful in the opinion of the researcher, designs that can produce predictive findings may be most appropriate and may suit the purposes of the investigator. However, we do not suggest that naturalistic inquiry is chosen only when little knowledge has been developed. It may be possible that even with a well-developed body of knowledge, phenomena are not explained to the researcher's satisfaction. Or perhaps the context is of importance in coming to know about a phenomenon. In either case, one might choose a naturalistic approach to unveil new insights that have not been revealed through well-tested theory. Again, choice is based on a combination of the level of knowledge and the investigator's purpose. We explore the relationship of knowledge to design selection in more detail in subsequent chapters.

Practical Considerations

Finally, practicality cannot be neglected. First, conducting research takes time and money and requires skill. The researcher must consider each of these practical constraints. If you are a clinician, can the inquiry be integrated into your workload? If you are a researcher, how much time can you devote to a study? If you conduct a clinical trial, can you access a sufficient number for your sample? Typically, naturalistic designs such as ethnography and life history are more time consuming than experimental-type designs that can reach many subjects through a survey approach. Moreover, naturalistic analysis often involves several time-consuming steps such as transcriptions of video or audio recordings and iterative analyses.

Second, conducting research is often costly. Financial support may be required to pay researchers, assistants, and participants, as we discuss in Chapter 22. Expensive equipment and software may be needed to collect and analyze data, and costs simply to plan and implement a study often shape research design options.

The degree of researcher knowledge and skill in methodology has a major bearing on choosing a design. As example, if you are versed only in basic statistical analysis, you are limited in the type of experimental-type analysis that you can perform and interpret, unless you can afford a statistician.

A major influence on choosing a strategy is the context in which a study can be conducted. Unless clinical trials are planned, research in health and human services is frequently conducted in the settings in which services are provided. Thus the researcher may have only a sample of convenience available.

Protection of human subjects is the final and perhaps most critical consideration in selection of approach, as we discussed in Chapter 3. Protecting the safety, confidentiality, and autonomy of participants while generating useful and beneficial knowledge must be the researcher's primary concern in design selection.

Table 4-2 summarizes the criteria for selecting designs across the research traditions.

TABLE 4-2 *Criteria for Selecting Designs by Research Tradition*

Criterion	Experimental-Type	Naturalistic	Mixed Method
Practical purpose	Need to control and delimit scope of inquiry	Reveal new understandings	Multiple
Preferred way of knowing	Singular reality, objectively viewed	Multiple, interpreted realities	Multiple
Level of knowledge development	Well-developed theory	Limited knowledge; challenge to current theory	Both

Summary

We have made the following major points in this chapter:

1. Experimental-type research is based in a single epistemological framework of logical positivism and involves primarily a deductive process of human reasoning.
2. Naturalistic inquiry is based in multiple philosophical traditions that can be categorized as pluralistic and holistic in their perspectives and involves inductive and abductive processes of human reasoning.
3. Mixed method research, which is based on several philosophical schools of thought, draws on strategies from both experimental-type and naturalistic inquiry traditions and may involve multiple and varied thinking and action processes.
4. Each tradition has a distinct language and flow of thinking and action procedures.
5. The selection of a strategy is based on your preferred way of knowing, your research purpose, the level and acceptability of knowledge development in the area of interest, and practical constraints.

EXERCISES

1. Select a topic of interest and determine how you might approach it using experimental-type reasoning and the sequence of the 10 essentials.
2. Using the same topic as selected for Exercise 1, suggest how you might approach the topic using naturalistic inquiry.
3. Compare and contrast both approaches, and think of how you will approach your topic using mixed method strategies.

References

1. Tashakkori A, Teddlie C: *Handbook of mixed methods in social & behavioral research*, ed 2, Thousand Oaks, Calif, 2010, Sage.
2. Hoover KR, Donovan T: *The elements of social scientific thinking*, ed 11, Boston, 2011, Cenage.
3. Babbie E: *The practice of social research*, ed 13, Belmont, Calif, 2013, Wadsworth.
4. Padgett D: *Qualitative methods in social work research*, Thousand Oaks, Calif, 2007, Sage.
5. Hume D: *A treatise of human nature: being an attempt to introduce the experimental method of reasoning into moral subjects*, London, 1878, Longmans, Green, & Co.
6. Audi R: *Epistemology*, 2011, Routledge.
7. Russell B: *Introduction to mathematical philosophy*, New York, 1919, Macmillan.
8. DePoy E, Gilson SF: *Human behavior theory and applications: a critical thinking approach*, Thousand Oaks, Calif, 2012, Sage.
9. Cook TD, Campbell DT: *Quasi-experimentation: design and analysis issues for field settings*, Boston, 1979, Houghton Mifflin.
10. Campbell DT, Stanley JC: *Experimental and quasi-experimental designs for research*, Boston, 1963, Houghton Mifflin.
11. Denzin N, Lincoln Y: *Landscape of qualitative research*, Newbury Park, Calif, 2007, Sage.
12. Husserl E: *Ideas: general introduction to pure phenomenology*, New York, 1931, Macmillan (Boyce WR, translator).
13. Denzin N: *Interpretive interactionism*, Thousand Oaks, Calif, 2001, Sage.
14. Denzin N: *Collecting and interpreting qualitative materials*, Thousand Oaks, Calif, 2008, Sage.
15. Byers W: *The blind spot*, Princeton, NJ, 2011, Princeton University Press.
16. Perry J, Bratman M, Fischer JM: *Introduction to philosophy: classical and contemporary readings*, New York, 2012, Oxford University Press.
17. Silverman M: *Facing post-modernity: contemporary French thought on culture and society*, New York, 1999, Routledge.
18. Brewer J, Hunter A: *Foundations of multimethod research: synthesizing styles*, Newbury Park, Calif, 2006, Sage.
19. Hoenig H, Giacobbi P, Levy C: Methodological challenges confronting researchers of wheeled mobility aids and other assistive technologies. *Disabil Rehabil Assistive Technol* 2:159–168, 2007.

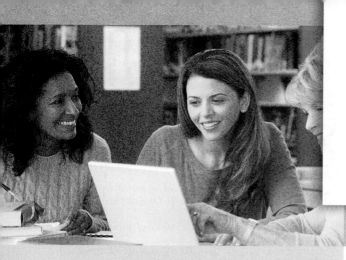

Chapter 5
Framing the Problem

Where do you begin now that you are ready to participate in the research process? An important initial challenge in the conduct of research is selecting a topic and, within that, stating a specific problem that is meaningful, appropriate for scientific inquiry, purposeful, and engaging.

By "meaningful," we suggest that the identified research problem should lead to an inquiry that either yields new knowledge or verifies existing knowledge that is useful to the investigator, his or her profession or social group, and/or the consumer or public.

By "appropriate," we mean that the selection of a problem can be submitted to a systematic research process and that the research will yield knowledge to help solve the identified problem. First, let us look at the word problem. Different from popular vernacular, we use the term "problem" in the philosophical sense and define it as a puzzling situation to be engaged and unraveled by research.[1] Not all problems that are relevant to health and human service providers can be addressed through or require systematic inquiry. For example, research cannot tell us about morals or what our preferences for a work area should be.

By "purposeful," we suggest that health and human service research be designed with a purpose that may serve investigators, consumers, professionals, funders, policy makers, or others concerned with health and human services and the health of the public. As we discuss throughout the book, purpose not only is a driving factor in topic selection, but shapes each essential.

Finally, "engaging" refers to the passion, interest, or compelling need to conduct the research. As we have indicated, if you do not have a good personal, professional, or scholarly reason for engaging in the process, your research may not be completed to your satisfaction. We have seen too many projects that have gone unfinished and not shared, so make sure that when you start your project, you are committed to its rigorous completion.

Most people are able to identify a broad topic of interest to them. However, after doing so, they often

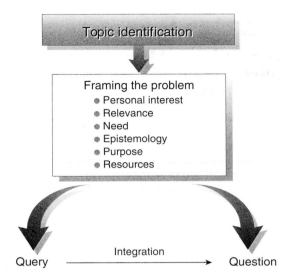

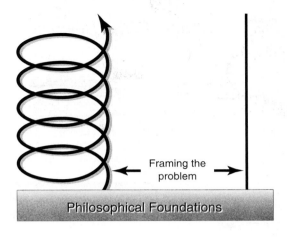

Figure 5-1 Framing the problem: thinking sequence.

find that articulating a specific research problem within that topic of interest is more difficult. The challenge of specifying a particular research problem is due in part to unfamiliarity with the research process and how problem formulation guides that process. This chapter is designed to remediate that barrier and provide the knowledge that you will need to accomplish this essential.

The way in which a research problem is framed influences and shapes all subsequent thinking and action processes of research. More specifically, as depicted in Figure 5-1, this essential leads to a design tradition, and then the development of a specific research question in the experimental-type tradition of research, to a line of query in one of the naturalistic traditions, or to a question and query that integrate both research traditions. Thus, problem identification is not simply a matter of identifying or stating a specific problem; one must also have a clear understanding of the relationships among topic, problem formulation, research question/query, and action processes in order to frame a meaningful, appropriate, purposeful, and engaging problem statement.

Formulating a problem statement is also influenced by the personal characteristics of the researcher such as his or her personal interest, perceived need, and preferred epistemology.

This chapter examines the thinking processes involved in identifying a topic, framing a research problem, and linking design selection to the purpose of the study.

Identifying a Topic

The first consideration in beginning a research project is to identify a topic from which to pursue a specific investigation. A *research topic* is a broad issue or area that is important to investigate, in our case as a health and human service professional. One topic may yield many different problems and strategies for investigation.

Here are just a few examples of the topics for which research is being generated: posthospital experience, health disparities, depression care, health promotion in diverse communities, pain control, community independence, adaptation to functional limitations, drug abuse, hospital management practices, gender differences in caregiving, impact of interprofessional care, hospital safety practices, self-management of chronic illness, symptom presentation, and health experiences. Others include psychosocial aspects of illness, disablement, or wellness; social networks and health; neighborhood characteristics and mobility; creativity as a source of coping and wellness; technology to enhance function and quality of life; spirituality and impact on health; and end-of-life decision making. •

- Professional experience
- Societal trends
- Professional trends
- Published research
- Existing theory
- Other sources

Given the breadth of fascinating areas in health and human service practice, it is usually easy to identify a topic that is of personal interest or one that is relevant to and important for professional practice. But where do topics and specific researchable problem areas come from? There are six basic sources helpful to professionals in selecting a topic and researchable problem (Box 5-1).

Professional Experience

The professional arena is perhaps the most immediate and important source from which research problems evolve. The ideas, unanswered questions, or "professional challenges" (similar to those posed throughout the book) that routinely arise often yield significant areas of inquiry. A practitioner who engaged in regular reflection or what has been referred to as reflexive intervention[2] can pose many queries in the course of service delivery that may warrant the research process. Many of the themes or persistent issues that emerge in collaboration, teamwork, case review, supervision, or faculty, student, and staff conferences may provide investigators with researchable topics and specific questions/queries. Themes that cut across diverse individuals, such as family involvement or consumer perceptions of their experiences in health and human services, provide topics that may ultimately stimulate the development and focus of specific research problems.

A rehabilitation professional in an inpatient rehabilitation hospital posed to us an observation that she and her staff found intriguing. They observed that many adaptive devices issued to patients for self-care were often left behind by patients in their rooms at the time of discharge. Although she believed patients needed these devices to function independently in their homes, she wondered why patients did not think similarly. When the devices were taken home, she also wondered whether they were used and, if so, whether they enhanced the patients' functioning in their environment. Discussions with practitioners in other hospital sites revealed similar observations and concerns. A review of the literature showed several studies on device abandonment that identified limited functionality of devices as the cause for nonuse.[3] However, even when function was improved, explained, and practiced, devices were still left behind. Here, then, is an identified clinical problem worthy of systematic inquiry. Think about the specific researchable questions that can be pursued to examine device use and abandonment systematically.

Societal Trends

Social concerns and trends reflected in the policies, legislation, and funding priorities of federal, state, and local agencies, foundations, and corporations provide another critical area from which potential inquiries for health and human service investigation emerge. For example, the government reports Healthy People 2020, U.S. Public Health Service documents, establish health-related objectives and priorities for the United States. Similarly, the reports on health care and practice generated by the Institute of Medicine (IOM) also identify priority research areas. The IOM's 2014 publication "Including Health in Global Frameworks for Development, Wealth, and Climate Change"[4] outlined the fundamental changes needed throughout the globe in light of climate trends. Similarly, the IOM publication *Retooling for an Aging America*[5] provides important data about current health care and raises the many difficult problem areas that must be addressed through research, education, and change in health policy. Also, the publications of the World Health Organization (WHO) or Rehabilitation International are helpful to review in order to identify international priorities. These types of documents provide an important source for identifying research problems and specific questions and queries with high public health importance.

Another social arena from which research problems emerge is the set of specific requests for research generated by federal, state, and local governments. Government agencies have numerous established funding streams that provide monetary support to researchers who identify meaningful and appropriate research problems within topic areas relevant to the delivery of health and human services.

> In the arena of health promotion and disease prevention, the Centers for Disease Control and Prevention (CDC) issues various calls for research that focuses on fall risk reduction or identifying risk factors related to secondary disability and its prevention. The Department of Health and Human Services (DHHS) announces various requests for research proposals to study the effects of welfare reform on the health of children living in poverty. The Department of Defense also has various calls for research on breast cancer, traumatic brain injury, posttraumatic stress disorders, and dementia. •

To publicize research priorities set by the federal government, the *Federal Register*,[6] a daily publication of the U.S. government (appearing in both hard-copy and online formats), lists funding opportunities and policy developments of each branch of the federal government. Many libraries receive the hard-copy publication, and the online version can be accessed through the Internet. The *Federal Register* is an invaluable resource to help identify problem areas and funding sources. Numerous other sources list research grant opportunities, including the *National Institutes of Health (NIH) Guide for Grants and Contracts,* the *Federal Grants and Contracts Weekly,* and the *Chronicle of Higher Education, Foundation Center*—just to name a few in the United States. If you are interested in learning about the international and global research issues and questions that are important to grant funders, you can consult the Internet and search your area of interest. Many government sources (e.g., Fulbright Commission; Fogarty Center) and nongovernmental organizations (NGOs) have specific focal areas concerning international investigations. These documents are all sources for understanding societal trends from which to identify topics that have societal meaning, are appropriate for scientific inquiry, and lead to the development of purposeful problem statements.

Professional Trends

Other resources for identifying important research topics and problem areas are the online or hard-copy newsletters and publications of each health and human service profession. Investigators frequently read these resources to determine the broad topic areas and problems of current interest to a given profession. Also, professional associations establish specific short-term and long-term research goals and priorities for their professions.

> The American Occupational Therapy Foundation identified "autism spectrum disorders and health issues related to aging as its FY2014 funding priorities."[7] As a result, the foundation awarded grants to five individuals conducting research in those areas. •

More recently, professional associations have been interested in advancing evidence-based practice,[8] so they have sponsored research endeavors to identify the barriers to using this approach and mechanisms for advancing its integration into daily practice. Examining the goals and policy statements of professional associations provides a good source from which to establish a research direction.

Published Research

The research world itself provides a significant venue for identifying research topics and problem areas. Health and human service professionals encounter research ideas by interacting with peers, attending professional meetings in which researchers report research findings, participating in research projects, and reviewing published research reports. Reading scholarship in print and online professional journals provides an overview of the important studies conducted in an area of interest. Most published research studies identify additional research problems and unresolved issues generated by the research findings as part of the discussion section of the paper. Journals in all formats (e.g., online; bound copies) publish current research findings that are useful and relevant to the helping professions; these include the *Journal of Dental Hygiene, Journal of* the American Medical Association, *Research in Social Work Practice, American Journal of Occupational Therapy, Occupational Therapy Journal of Research, Journal of Nursing Research, Medical Care, Physical Therapy, Qualitative Research in Health Care, The Social Service Review, American Journal of Public Health, Psychological Review,* and *Social Work,* to identify just a few of the most important journals to review and identify current research knowledge in areas relevant to health and human service professionals.

Routinely reading journals related to your profession and areas of interest will also provide you with specific ideas as to what concerns and issues your professional peers believe are important to investigate, as well as the studies that need to be replicated or repeated to confirm the findings. There are many other journals published by the helping professions and related disciplines that may assist in identifying a topic. Substantive topic journals that cross disciplines, such as *Archives of Physical and Rehabilitation Medicine, Psychiatric Services, Journal of Gerontology, Childhood and Adolescence, Topics in Geriatric Rehabilitation, American Journal of Public Health, The Gerontologist,* and *Journal of Rehabilitation,* are just a few of the outstanding journals that provide specific ideas for research studies that need to be conducted in topics relevant to health and human service professionals. New journals are always being developed to capture emerging specific research topics.

Finally, reading articles that provide a comprehensive overview, systematic review, or meta-analysis of a focused body of research is extremely helpful in shaping a research direction. Such articles usually summarize the state of knowledge to date and identify future research needs in a particular research area.

Existing Theory

Theories also provide an important source for generating topics and identifying research problems. As we discuss in Chapter 7, a theory posits a number of propositions and relationships between and among concepts. To be considered a theory, each specified relationship within the theory must be submitted to systematic investigation for verification or falsification. Inquiry related to theory development is intended to substantiate the theory and advance or modify its development by refuting some or all of its principles.

Consider Piaget's well-known theory of cognitive development, advanced in the mid-1920s. Piaget developed his theory of the structural development of cognition by observing his two children. Over 60 years, Piaget, his peers, and other scholars interested in human cognition subjected Piaget's theoretical notions to extensive scientific scrutiny. Hundreds of studies have been conducted to corroborate, modify, or refute Piaget's principles. Further study related to Piaget's theory has been initiated to determine the application of the theory to education and health-related intervention, as well as many other arenas.

Consider another well-known theoretical framework, the stress-health process model. This framework posits that external factors create stressors for individuals who must then appraise their ability and resources to manage these pressures. Individuals who perceive a lack of resources (e.g., skill) to manage stressors may experience increased stress and burden, which if it persists may result in negative health and psychosocial consequences, such as depressed mood.[9] This framework has also generated much research to empirically verify the proposed linkages among stressors, a person's appraisal of them, and related health consequences for different populations such as families providing care to persons with serious chronic and mental illnesses, or individuals who are displaced because of natural disasters. •

Other Sources

There are many opportunities beyond professional and research sources from which to develop topics that can lead to problem statements that are meaningful, require systematic inquiry, and are purposeful. For example, reliable blogs, social network sites, tweets, webinars, and listservs contain ideas and exchanges that can spark inquiry and lead to relevant contemporary topics. Also, collaborating with others in practice, research, or other professional activities can stimulate ideas for topical areas to pursue.

Framing a Research Problem

So now you have some idea as to where to look for and how to identify a topic. Foremost, the topic area must be of keen interest to you because you will be spending a lot of time and energy reading and thinking about it. However, you still face the dilemma of identifying a particular problem within a broad topic area. An endless number of problems or specific issues can emerge from any one topic. Thus, the challenge to the researcher is to identify just one particular area of concern or specific research problem. A specific research problem provides some boundary to the area to be studied. That is, a research *problem statement* identifies the specific phenomenon to be explored, the reason it needs to be examined, and the reason it is a problem or issue. The way in which you frame and state the problem is critical to the entire research endeavor and influences all subsequent thinking and action processes in which you will engage; that is, the way a problem is framed determines the way it will be answered, the type of knowledge generated, and the way the knowledge generated can potentially be used. Therefore, this first research essential should be thought through very carefully. As you become familiar with the entire research process, you will be able to more fully understand the relationships between the selection of a topic and problem statement and the subsequent research processes that occur.

The questions we pose in Box 5-2 can help guide your thinking as you move from selecting a broad topic area to framing a concrete research problem. By answering these reflective questions, you will begin to narrow your focus and hone in on a researchable problem that has meaning, requires systematic inquiry, and is purposeful.

Interest, Relevance, and Need

It is important to be certain that the topic you develop is interesting and engaging to you. As we have noted, research, regardless of the framework and type of methodology used, takes time and can consume your thoughts. In addition, you should be convinced of the relevance of and need for the inquiry. If the problem is not challenging, exciting, relevant, and needed, the process can quickly become tedious and lack meaning for you. Researchers must be passionate about their area of work; otherwise, the effort may seem pointless.

Research Purpose

As discussed we have and will emphasize throughout the book, research should be purposeful. We suggest that there are three levels of purpose that each research project should addresses. The first level is professional. Much of the research in health and human service is initiated to inform professional practice, advance care, and optimize health and psychosocial outcomes of individuals. For example, this level may involve understanding pathways and mechanisms such as the physiological and psychological contributors to pain as a way to improve pain relief interventions; or it may lead you to investigate who is at most risk and in need of specific types if interventions. Or perhaps you might become immersed in developing and testing an intervention to evaluate its efficacy in achieving desired outcomes. You may bring innovation to your profession by examining how new collaborations and technologies can enhance health and wellness and promote compliance with health and fitness routines.

The second level of research purpose is personal. Researchers often have personal reasons for conducting research, or they choose topics that resonate personally with their experiences, relationships, and commitments. Practitioners, administrators, and other health and human service professionals may conduct research for such personal reasons as adding

---

> **BOX 5-2** *Six Guiding Questions in Framing a Problem*
>
> 1. What about this topic is of interest to me?
> 2. What about this topic is relevant to my practice?
> 3. What about this topic is unresolved in the literature?
> 4. What is my preferred way of coming to know about phenomena and this topic?
> 5. What societal or professional purpose does knowing about this topic serve?
> 6. What resources do I have to investigate this topic?

new challenges to their jobs, career advancement, commitment to funding new projects, or a desire for academic collaboration and growth or institutional advancement. Furthermore, a topic of interest may reflect a deep personal concern. For example, some researchers who focus on specific diseases choose the disease on the basis of their own family history or encounter with the condition. Another researcher who was unable to participate in outdoor sports because of poor balance and weakness partnered with engineers to develop aesthetically designed, highly functional fitness equipment for cross country skiing and outdoor hiking.

The third level of purpose for conducting research is theoretical and methodological and reflects issues that emerge from or are missing from the literature (see Chapter 6). For example, in the experimental-type tradition, the researcher may be interested in testing nonlinear systems theory related to human behavior or in describing, explaining, or predicting phenomena through that lens. Here are examples of *purpose statements* within this research tradition:

Descriptive. Little is known about how family systems ebb and flow over time in response to unexpected illness of a child. The present study is a descriptive examination of the family as a non-linear system experiencing an unexpected event and undergoing trial and error to cope.

Explanatory. In order to examine the relationship between adolescent individuation and family cohesion after divorce, this study will examine family dynamics through a nonlinear systems approach.

Predictive. Parents of children with traumatic brain injury often have difficulties coping post injury. This study examines changes in family functioning from a nonlinear systems perspective in order to identify how unexpected events change family function.

Meta-analysis. There is a robust corpus of studies that have tested interventions to support families in which a child has become injured. The purpose of this study is to understand the overall effect of supportive programs on family systems when unpredictable events occur.

In naturalistic-type traditions, the purpose is primarily to understand meanings, experiences, and phenomena as they evolve in the natural setting in which they occur. The following are examples of purpose statements for different naturalistic designs:

Ethnography. The purpose of this study on deafness is to gain an understanding of families' beliefs about deafness, when the parents are deaf and communicate through ASL and the child prefers a cochlear implant.

Ethnography. The purpose of this study is to gain an understanding of the meaning of providing distant day-to-day care to a relative with a chronic illness through technology with the hope that greater understanding of the experience of caregiving will assist health professionals in working together with caregivers to find technological approaches through which they can maintain their work life while still providing care.

Phenomenology. The purpose of the study is to develop a structural definition of health as it is experienced in everyday life of individuals in remission from cancer treatment.

Grounded theory. This study explicates the multidimensional relationships that develop between physicians and patients with chronic illness in order to develop a theory of the processes that affect self-care decisions in patients.

Grounded theory. The purpose of the study is to identify processes used by family members to manage the unpredictability elicited by the need for and receipt of a heart transplant, and hence a theory of this transitional period.

Heuristic inquiry. The purpose of this study is to examine and understand the meaning of chronic illness in families, from the perspective of all family members.

Participatory action research. The purpose of this inquiry is to assess service needs of homeless teens, as investigated and defined by service recipients.

Meta-analysis. The purpose of this inquiry is to seek universal themes and comparisons in the meaning of the home environment in supporting individuals with functional challenges in six countries.

Critical theory. This study gives voice to women who are victims of institutional violence as the basis for understanding their needs and promoting socially just policy responses to this set of informants.

Integrated designs can have multiple purposes that reflect both research traditions or only one tradition. Consider the following examples in which the purpose in each combines both traditions:

> *The purpose of this mixed method study is to reveal the ways in which elder rural women define health and wellness and then test the accuracy of these definitions in a large cohort of the population.*
> *The purpose of this mixed method study is to test the level of posttraumatic stress disorder and then study the meanings of trauma and neglect among young adults who have been raised in two-parent households in which both parents work.*

Epistemology (Theory of Knowledge)

We have discussed how problem formulation and study purpose shape thinking and action processes in research. In addition, your theory of knowledge and preferred way of knowing, or epistemology, will also influence the research direction you pursue and whether you will seek to develop a discrete question that objectifies concepts (experimental-type tradition), or develop a query to explore multiple and interacting factors in the context in which they emerge (naturalistic tradition), or develop an approach that integrates both or multiple traditions. The age-old ontological and epistemological dilemmas, respectively, of "what is knowledge?" and "how do we know?" (discussed in Chapter 4) are active and forceful determinants in how a researcher frames a problem. The researcher's preferred way of knowing is either clearly articulated or implied in each problem statement. You might recall the classic research conducted by Carol Gilligan in which she sought to understand why girls and women scored disproportionately lower on scales of moral development than their male counterparts. By choosing an epistemic pathway different from experimental-type design based on Kohlberg's theory of moral

development, Gilligan's work was already expansive and shaped by induction.[10] In opposition to numerically inferior moral development, Gilligan sought to portray girls in a different light. As you can see, the "how do you know" question was approached by Gilligan in an inductive way, with the potential to reveal new insights and knowledge that could not have surfaced if well-tested theory continued to be applied through logico-deductive research. Now, reexamine the purpose statements listed in this chapter to determine the investigator's preferred way of knowing that is implicitly assumed.

Resources

Resources represent the concrete limitations of the research world. The accessibility of place, group, or individuals and the extent to which time, money, and other resources are necessary and available to the researcher to implement the inquiry are examples of some of the practical constraints of conducting research. These real-life constraints actively shape the development of the research problem an investigator pursues, the scope of the study that can be implemented, and all thinking and action processes.

Summary

There are many considerations in framing an inquiry. These include examining the diverse sources and methods through which investigators identify topics for inquiry. Six questions guide the refinement of a topic into a research problem. These questions organize thinking processes along personal, professional, social, ontological, and practical lines. For example, considering your interest in a research topic is a personal thinking process, whereas assessing existing resources available for conducting a project is a practical thinking process. With regard to the purposive aspects of conducting research, investigators organize their research to meet personal, professional, and methodological goals.

Your preferred way of knowing (epistemology) also plays a key role in framing an inquiry. How a researcher frames a problem has significant implications for the selection of design from the experimental-type tradition, the naturalistic tradition, or an integration of the two, as will be seen in subsequent chapters.

Equipped with an understanding of why and how investigators frame research problems, you are ready to begin the thinking process of examining and critically using literature as a basis for helping you frame a problem statement and develop knowledge.

EXERCISES

1. Select a topic (e.g., spinal cord injury, adaptation to a disabling condition, technology needs of elders) and identify one experimental-type and one naturalistic article related to the topic. Then, compare and contrast the way in which the research problems and queries in each are framed.
2. Identify the purpose statement in each article selected in Exercise 1.
3. In each article, identify the source of the topic.

References

1. McCarthy J: *Some problems of philosophy, empirically considered*, Oxford, UK, 2013, Oxford University Press.
2. DePoy E, Gilson SF: *Evaluation practice*, London, 2009, Routledge.
3. Gitlin LN, Schemm RL, Landsberg L, et al: Factors predicting assistive device use in the home by older persons following rehabilitation. *Journal of Aging and Health* 8(4):554–575, 1996.
4. Institute of Medicine: *Including health in global frameworks for development, wealth, and climate change*, 2014, <http://www.iom.edu/Reports/2014/Including-Health-in-Global-Frameworks-for-Development-Wealth-and-Climate-Change.aspx>.
5. Institute of Medicine: *Retooling for an aging America: building the health care workforce*, 2008, <http://www.iom.edu/reports/2008/retooling-for-an-aging-america-building-the-health-care-workforce.aspx>.
6. Federal Register: <https://www.federalregister.gov>.
7. *American Occupational Therapy Foundation: 2014 press release*, <www.aotf.org/Portals/0/documents/News/Press Releases/03%2012%202014%20AOTF%20OT%20IRG%20Grants%20Announced.pdf>.
8. Turner RJ: *Understanding health disparities: the promise of the stress process model. Advances in the conceptualization of the stress process*, New York, 2010, Springer, pp 3–21.
9. Guastello SJ, Koopmans M, Pincus D: *Chaos and complexity in psychology: the theory of nonlinear dynamical systems*, Cambridge, UK, 2011, Cambridge University Press.
10. Gilligan C: *In a different voice*, Cambridge, MA, 1993, Harvard University Press.

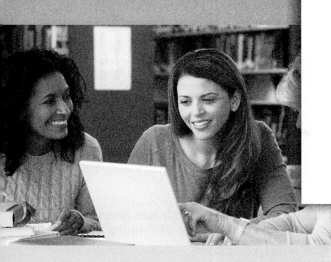

Chapter 6
Developing a Knowledge Base Through Literature and Resources

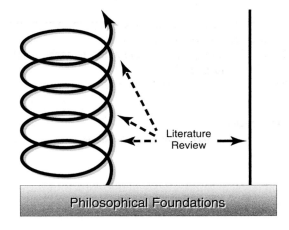

"literature" to refer to the broad spectrum of sources, including print, virtual, image, material, and so forth, that are relevant to an investigation.

Most of us have had the experience of spending long hours at the library or on the Internet poring through literature and materials to discover what others have written about a topic of interest. Although you probably have participated in this type of activity for various classroom assignments, reviewing information for research is more systematic and serves more specific purposes.[1]

One important purpose of reviewing the literature for research is to help sharpen the focus of your initial research interest and the specific strategy you plan to use to conduct a study. Discovering what others know and how they come to know it is an important function of the review when conducted at

With the explosion of the Internet, sources of information and knowledge beyond refereed articles and other scholarship appearing in print have been increasingly accepted as part of the "literature" review. In this chapter, we therefore use the term the initial stage of developing a research idea. The review, when conducted at this stage, involves a process by which the researcher critically assesses text and other relevant material that is directly and indirectly related to both the proposed topic and the potential strategies for conducting the research.

Another purpose of a literature review is to help determine how your research fits within an existing body of knowledge and what your research uniquely contributes to the scientific and knowledge generation enterprise. Reviewing the literature for this purpose occurs as you are formulating your research ideas as well as when you are ready to prepare a report of your findings.

A literature review also serves as a source of data in its own right. For example, in certain forms of qualitative research, literature and other sources are brought in at different points of the research process to emphasize, elaborate, or reveal emergent themes. Likewise, a systematic literature review is used in quantitative, or experimental-type, methodologies to gather data, such as when the review forms the unit of analysis for a meta-analysis (see Chapter 10) or when ranking the level of evidence for a particular issue.

Thus, reviewing the literature is a significant thinking and action process in the world of research. However, it is often misunderstood and undervalued.

In this chapter, we begin our discussion with a presentation of the various reasons to conduct a literature review. We then detail the specific steps involved in conducting a literature review and share strategies that will help you accomplish this task. Because typically there is so much information directly related to any one topic, as well as literature from related bodies of research that also should be examined, the review process may initially seem overwhelming. However, some "tricks of the trade" can facilitate a systematic and comprehensive review process that is feasible, manageable, and even enjoyable.

Why Review the Literature?

There are four major reasons to review literature in research (Box 6-1). Let us examine each reason in depth.

> **BOX 6-1** *Reasons to Review the Literature*
>
> 1. Determine previous research on topic of interest
> 2. Determine level of theory and knowledge development
> 3. Determine relevance of current knowledge base to the problem area
> 4. Provide rationale for selection of research strategy

Determine What Research Has Been Conducted on the Topic of Inquiry

Why should you conduct a study if it has already been done and done well or to your satisfaction? Here, the key words are "done well" and "to your satisfaction." To determine whether the current literature is sufficient to help you solve a professional problem, you must critically evaluate how others have struggled with and resolved the same or a similar question. Many novice researchers think that they lack either the right or the knowledge to be critical of published literature. However, being critical is the very point of conducting the literature review. You examine previous studies to critically determine whether these efforts were done well and whether they answer your question satisfactorily or completely.

An initial review of the literature provides a sense of the previous work done in your area of interest. The review helps identify (1) the current trends and ways of thinking about your topic, (2) the contemporary debates in your field, (3) the gaps in the knowledge base, (4) the ways in which the current knowledge on your topic has been developed, and (5) the conceptual frameworks used to inform and examine your problem.

Sometimes an initial review of the literature will steer you in a research direction different from your original plan.

> Consider the following example. Suppose you want to examine the extent to which mild aerobic exercise promotes cardiovascular fitness in a population of otherwise healthy elders who do regularly participate in a fitness program. You find several studies that already document a positive outcome, but you question the methodologies used by these studies,

including the type of exercise, the research design, and the criteria for inclusion of study participants. Also, you find that many authors suggest further inquiry is necessary to determine the particular exercises that promote cardiovascular fitness, as well as those that maintain joint mobility. Although this area is not what you had originally planned, the literature review refines your thinking and directs you to specific problem areas that need greater research attention than the one originally intended. You need to decide whether replication of the reported studies is important to verify study findings, whether replication with a different sample (e.g., racially and ethnically diverse elder persons not included in previous studies) would be important, and whether your focus should be modified according to the other recommendations specified in the literature (e.g., need to examine different forms of exercise for a wider range of health outcomes). •

Now consider the following example.

An investigator was interested in examining the psychological outcomes of therapeutic riding. She had planned to do a case study inquiry, following one adolescent over a period of 2 years. However, after conducting a literature review, the investigator found 10 case studies of psychological outcomes, each suggesting larger experimental-type studies that could predict outcome in large groups. Given the presence of sound and relevant research, the investigator changed her methodology to meet the recommendations of the previous studies. •

Look at another example of how the literature can initially influence the investigator's research direction. Peters[2] was interested in examining the relationship between "victim blaming" and myths about the causes of domestic violence. He performed an extensive literature review to ascertain what studies had been conducted and what instrumentation would be available for his study. Because he was unable to locate instrumentation on myths about domestic violence, he shifted his initial study to developing and validating an instrument to measure the construct of domestic violence myth acceptance. It was necessary for Peters to shift the research focus to instrument construction as a first research step in addressing his initial question. •

> **BOX 6-2**   *Three Factors to Review Critically*
>
> - Level of knowledge
> - How knowledge is generated
> - Boundaries of a study

Determine Level of Theory and Knowledge Development Relevant to Your Project

As you review the literature, not only do you need to describe and synthesize what exists, but more important, you need to critically analyze the knowledge level, knowledge generation, and study boundaries in each work (Box 6-2).

Level of Knowledge

When you read a study, first evaluate the level of knowledge that emerges from the study. As discussed in Chapter 7, studies produce varying levels of knowledge, from descriptive to theoretical. The level of theory development and knowledge in your topic area and how it has been investigated will strongly influence the type of research strategy you select. As you read related studies in the literature, consider the level of theoretical development. Is the body of knowledge descriptive, explanatory, or at the level of prediction? Typically in general inquiry, and necessarily in experimental-type inquiry, the development of knowledge proceeds incrementally such that the first wave of studies in a particular area will be descriptive and designed to describe the characteristics of a phenomenon. After description is complete, researchers search for associations or relationships among factors that may help explain the phenomenon. On the basis of the findings from explanatory research, attempts may be made to study the phenomenon from a predictive perspective by either testing an intervention or developing causal models to explain the phenomenon further.

Identifying the level of knowledge in the area of interest helps you identify the next research steps.

Since the 1990s, a rich body of literature on family caregiving has been generated at each of the three knowledge levels and in many disciplines, including family studies, social work, occupational therapy, nursing, and gerontology. Initially, descriptive research was necessary to identify the phenomenon of caregiving and describe the physical and psychological concomitants of this activity. Explanatory research then showed the role of gender, relationship, culture, and other factors in caregiver appraisals of their experiences. More recently, predictive studies have focused on evaluating complex causal models to predict long-term outcomes of caregiving, as well as testing interventions that attempt to reduce the negative consequences of providing extended care, such as those providing technological assistance.[3] •

How Knowledge Is Generated

After you have determined the level of knowledge of your particular area of interest, you need to evaluate how that knowledge has been generated. In other words, you need to review the literature carefully to identify the research strategy or design used in each study. Many people tend to read the introduction to a study and then jump to the discussion section or set of conclusions to see what it can tell them. However, it is important to read each aspect of a research report, especially the section on methodology. As you read about the design of a particular study, you critically examine whether it is appropriate for the level of knowledge that the authors indicate exists in the literature and whether the conclusions of the study are consistent with the design strategy. This important critical analysis of the existing literature is a major part of literature review that you need to feel fully empowered to perform so that you not only provide a sound rationale for your study but also do not limit the viability of your own work. You may be quite surprised to find that, unfortunately, scholarship is full of research that demonstrates an inappropriate match among research question, strategy, and conclusions.

As an example, a recent study presented by a doctoral student in a research forum sought to examine the extent to which enhancing accessibility to mental health counselors through email predicted the strength of an alliance between the two. However, in his research plan he chose to measure frequency of email contact and alliance. He therefore found that he could only make claims about a relationship but not about prediction. •

BOX 6-3	*Questions to Ask as You Read a Study*

1. Are the research methods congruent with the level of knowledge reviewed by the investigators in their report?
2. How well do the research procedures adequately address the proposed research question?
3. Is there compatibility or fit among literature, procedures, findings, and conclusions?

As you read a study, ask yourself the three interrelated questions in Box 6-3. The answers to these questions will help you understand and critically determine the appropriateness of the level of knowledge generated in your topic area. This understanding in turn will help to shape the direction of your own research.

Boundaries of a Study

It is important to determine the boundaries of the studies you are reviewing and their relevance to your study problem. By "boundaries" we mean the "who, what, when, and where" of a study.

If you do not find any literature in your topic area, you may choose to identify an analogous body of literature to provide direction in how to develop your strategy. For example, if you are studying narrative as a clinical tool for helping clients with newly acquired vision impairments and cannot find research specifically in this area, you might find studies of this phenomenon in literature on acquired mobility or neurological conditions.

Now suppose you are interested in testing the efficacy of a hypertension reduction program in a rural setting, and published studies report positive outcomes for a range of interventions. On closer examination, however, you discover that these studies have been conducted in urban areas in which outdoor walking can occur on sidewalks. Moreover, the studies include primarily male participants with backgrounds different from the population you plan to include in your study. Therefore, it will be important to examine studies that test health promotion interventions relevant to rural settings and to include participants with characteristics similar to the intended targets of your study. By extending the literature review in this way, you will obtain a better understanding of the issues and design considerations that are important for the specific boundaries of your study. Also, you may discover that the level of theory and knowledge development in hypertensive risk reduction programs is advanced for one particular population (e.g., urban men) but undeveloped in respect to another population (e.g., rural women). •

geographies, and the fit between family needs and available community transportation services, are important in determining outcome. This comprehensive review supports the need to conduct a predictive study to examine the interaction of variables. •

Determining the boundaries of the literature helps you to evaluate the level of knowledge that exists for the particular population and setting you are interested in studying. The National Institutes of Health (NIH) has been vigilant about boundaries, recognizing that many studies are applied to populations that have not participated in the study. In efforts to redress this problem, NIH has instituted policies to include populations such as women, children, and minorities who have not been included in research.

Determine Relevance of the Current Knowledge Base to Your Problem Area

Once you have evaluated the level of knowledge advanced in the literature, you need to determine its relevance to your topical area and focus.

Let us assume you are considering conducting an experimental-type study. In order to do so, your literature review must contain research that points to a theoretical framework relevant to your topic and research that identifies specific variables and measures for inclusion in your study. Your literature review must also yield a body of sufficiently developed knowledge so that hypotheses can be derived for your study. In other words, in the experimental-type tradition, the literature provides the rationale and structure for everything that you investigate and for all action processes.

For each variable you choose to include in your study, even demographics, you must support or justify your inclusion of the variable on the basis of sound literature. Just think of all the extraneous information that could be introduced into a research study. For theoretical, ethical, and methodological soundness, experimental-type approaches require supportive literature for all variables.

Consider research involving the testing of interventions designed to support family caregivers of persons with dementia. You find literature that identifies, tests, and verifies what interventions are needed to enhance safety in the home. Given the weight of evidence that families experience great distress and express the need to learn new strategies to manage dementia care, particularly as the disease progresses, the intervention approach and use of a randomized trial was well substantiated. •

If your literature review reveals a clear gap in existing knowledge or a poor fit between a phenomenon and current theory, you probably should consider a strategy in the naturalistic tradition. Or if your literature review reveals useful theory but you feel it is too narrow to fully investigate your work, you might choose mixed methods, both to validate current theory and build on it with inductive strategies.

Suppose you are planning to conduct a study to identify the factors that predict residential placement by family members of older adults with mobility impairment who live in rural communities. You review the literature and find that single predictors, such as the aging member's satisfaction with current living arrangements, the available technology to assist in household care and communicate with family in other

To develop an assistive robotic awareness and education program for rural elders as a means to facilitate aging in place, you consult the literature. However, although there are many theory-based and well-tested interventions for other conditions and ages, you are not able to find any studies of need or intervention success with elders who reside in rural towns. In light of this large gap in the literature, you conduct a naturalistic inquiry to ascertain the awareness of these devices and willingness to use them among rural older adults. However, as you collect data, you find the uncanny valley literature, which proposes that a human-like (anthropomorphic) appearance of robotic devices may interfere with acceptance.[4] You consult the literature to obtain theoretical detail and measures so you can then test that theory, mixing inductive and deductive strategies.

The concepts and constructs contained in this initial formulation would include elders, rural community, aging in place, and acceptance of assistive robotic technology. These terms would be your first keywords, to be used in a computer database or library catalog search. •

| **BOX 6-4** | *Six Steps to Conducting a Literature Review* |

Step 1: Determine when to conduct a search
Step 2: Delimit what is searched
Step 3: Access databases for periodicals, books, documents, and other resources
Step 4: Organize the information
Step 5: Critically evaluate the literature
Step 6: Write the literature review

Once the addition of foundational work to literature and theory is found, researchers will have the rationale for selecting more diverse and complex design approaches to subsequent and related studies.

Provide a Rationale for Selection of the Research Strategy

After you have determined the content and structure of existing theory and knowledge related to your problem area, the next task is to determine a rationale for the selection of your research design. A literature review for a research grant proposal or a research report is written to directly support both your research and your choice of design. You must synthesize your critical review of existing studies in such a way that the reader sees your study as a logical extension of current knowledge in the literature. Look at Box 6-2 once again. The rationale for conducting an experimental-type design is well supported by the existence of case studies as well as the recommendations that are made by the investigators in their conclusions.

We now turn to the mechanics of how to conduct a literature search; then we offer guidelines for developing a written rationale.

How to Conduct a Literature Search

Conducting a literature search and writing a literature review are exciting and creative processes. However, there may be so much literature and other resources in the area of interest that the review process can initially seem overwhelming. Six steps can guide you in the thinking and action processes of searching the literature, organizing sources, and taking notes on the references that you plan to use in a written rationale (Box 6-4).

Step 1: Determine When to Conduct a Search

The first step in a literature review is the determination of when a review should be done. In studies in the experimental-type tradition, a literature review always precedes both the final formulation of a research question and the implementation of the study. In the experimental-type tradition, definitions of all variables studied and the level of theoretical complexity underpinning an inquiry must be presented for a study to be scientifically sound and rigorous. (We discuss "rigor" in greater detail in subsequent chapters.)

In the tradition of naturalistic inquiry, the literature may be reviewed at different points throughout the project. Although defining variables and instrumentation is not relevant and thus is not the function of literature review in this tradition, examining information serves multiple purposes in naturalistic methods.[5] For example, the literature may be used as an additional source of data and included as part of the information-gathering process that is subsequently analyzed and interpreted. Another purpose of the literature review in naturalistic inquiry is to inform the direction of data collection once the investigator has initiated a study. As discoveries occur in data collection, the investigator may turn to the literature for guidance about how to interpret emergent themes and identify other questions that should be asked in the field.

For example, consider the following scenario.

Two investigators were interested in examining barriers to outdoor fitness participation (specifically, distance walking and jogging) in individuals with temporary and permanent mobility impairments (such as knee and hip pain or replacement, or impairment due to cerebrovascular accident). They consulted the literature, initially planning to conduct an experimental-type design, and found research on limited functionality of durable medical equipment (DME)[6] as the reason for abandonment. However, when the guidance from the research was followed promoting more functional features being added to DME, such as ergonomic grips and larger tires on walkers, no discernable difference in acceptance and use of mobility equipment was realized. Because the research was not productive in guiding intervention for their demographic group, they turned to naturalistic inquiry to answer their query. By conducting open-ended individual and group interviews, they found that the stigmatizing appearance of supportive and adaptive mobility aids was the primary barrier to full participation in outdoor sports. On the basis of this finding, they developed a large-scale survey to confirm these findings in a broader segment of their population and to test the extent to which contemporary design synthesized with comfort and functionality would promote adoption of device use for safe, fully participatory outdoor fitness.[7] •

To the extreme are forms of naturalistic research in which no literature is reviewed before or during fieldwork. In a classic study of prison violence using an endogenous research design (discussed in more detail in Chapter 11), Maruyama[8] and the research team of prison inmates did not believe that a review was necessary or relevant to the purpose of their study.

Usually, however, researchers working in the naturalistic-type tradition review the literature before conducting research to confirm the need for a naturalistic approach. For example, in the study by DePoy and Gilson[7] discussed earlier, the literature provided the rationale for their approach.

Although an extensive review of the literature conducted before undertaking any further thinking

or action processes refines the research approach and design, investigators are continually updating their literature review throughout their studies.

Step 2: Delimit What Is Searched

Once you have decided when to conduct a literature review, your next step involves setting parameters as to what is relevant to search; after all, it is not feasible or reasonable to review every topic that is "somewhat related" to your problem. Delimiting the search, or setting boundaries to it, is an important but difficult step. The boundaries you set must ensure a review that is comprehensive but still practical and not overwhelming.[1]

One useful strategy across all traditions is to base a search on the core concepts and constructs contained in the initial inquiry.

Similarly, these lexical concepts (concepts that are expressed as words) will help you begin a search using these variable names as keywords (words or phrases that are used in online searches to identify and categorize work that contains these specific concepts) to seek literature and determine how your topic has already been studied. As Internet searches become the rule rather than the exception, the precise selection of keywords is a critical skill to develop in order to hone and refine your search, as well as for efficiency.[9]

Step 3: Access Databases for Periodicals, Books, and Documents

For us, the excitement of searching and finding nuggets of literature and other sources is a great gift. But we are often faced with the dilemma of how to proceed to access diverse sources when time is limited. Fortunately, the ubiquity of the Internet creates a venue even from one's home not only for accessing formal print materials but for any type of resource that can be imaged and beyond. The disadvantage of Web-based sources is their enormity and their variability in systematic rigor. Given that so many libraries and search engines provide opportunities for human interaction and guidance, the overwhelming and uncertain nature of information can be tamed. Of course, we are not suggesting that entering and working within the physical space of a library is not valuable. To the contrary, the library and other collections often contain the only sources to inform your research. So get ready to go to the computer at the library or access your library through a computer or mobile device from your home to search *databases*. Library searches have become technologically sophisticated and are a big advantage over previous searching mechanisms such as card catalogues, which are now housed in antique stores. However, the most valuable resource for finding references in the library is still the reference librarian, who may be on site or online. Working with an experienced librarian is the best way to learn how to navigate physical and virtual libraries, find the best search words for your area of interest, and access the numerous databases that open the world of literature to you.

You have many choices for beginning your search. You can access literature through an online database or through other indexes and abstracts. You can still browse hard copies of journals, although libraries are turning increasingly to e-journals. You can peruse museum exhibits on site or on-line, lurk on listservs, or actively participate in dialogue to direct your search. In health and human service research, you will more likely begin your search within four categories of materials: books, online and paper journal articles, online resources such as collections of papers and scholarly blogs, and government documents. You may also find gray literature such as newspapers, news Web sites, and newsletters useful, especially those from professional associations.[10] In addition, you can construct a literature search based on the references listed in the research studies and resources you obtain. However, do not depend exclusively on what other authors identify as important. References from other articles may not represent the broad range of studies you may need to review, or the most current literature. A year or more may pass between submission of a manuscript and its publication; therefore, the citations that precede each article may be outdated unless you are seeking historical references.

Searching Periodicals, Journals, and Scholarly Books

Most researchers begin their search by examining online and paper periodicals, journals, and scholarly books. To begin your search, it is helpful and time-efficient to work with the online databases. Searching databases can be rewarding, but you must know how to use the system. You can search databases by examining subjects, authors, or titles of articles.

To illustrate the range of options, Figure 6-1 presents a screen capture of the website home page of Fogler Library at the University of Maine. Note the multiple methods of obtaining information listed on this single Web page. The user can conduct a single search (One Search) that accesses all data bases simultaneously, can select from diverse search sources listed alphabetically, and can even chat with a reference librarian online.

One of our favorite databases is Project Muse.[11] As reflected in the narrative excerpted from its description, Project Muse is particularly productive for finding legitimate full text and image books, articles, collections and other resources relevant to all phases of Examined Practice. Note the criteria of peer review and high quality scholarship in the excerpt.

Project MUSE is a leading provider of digital humanities and social science content for the scholarly community. Since 1995 the MUSE journal collections have supported a wide array of research needs at academic, public, special, and school libraries worldwide. MUSE is the trusted source of complete, full-text versions of scholarly journals from many of the world's leading university presses and scholarly societies, with over 120 publishers currently participating. UPCC Book Collections on Project MUSE, launched in January 2012, offer top quality book-length scholarship, fully integrated with MUSE's scholarly journal content. Project MUSE's mission is to excel in the broad dissemination of high-quality scholarly content. Through innovation and collaborative development, Project MUSE anticipates the needs of and delivers essential resources to all members of the scholarly community.

- High quality, peer-reviewed, stable content
- Content written by the most prestigious authors and scholars in their fields
- Books and journals from non-profit scholarly publishers, including university presses and societies
- Once content goes online in MUSE, it stays online, permanently[11]

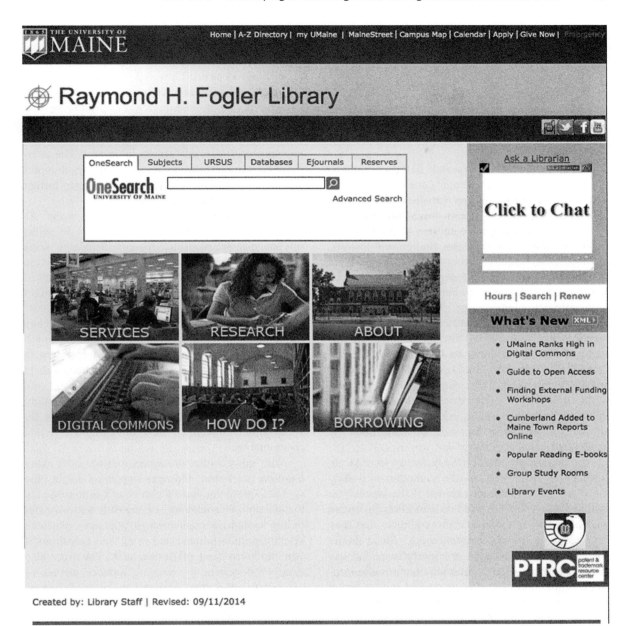

Created by: Library Staff | Revised: 09/11/2014

Figure 6-1 Screen Capture of Home Page of Fogler Library, University of Maine.

BOX 6-5 *Experience of Disabled Women Who Experience Domestic Violence*

....

Keywords:
disability
women
domestic violence

Let us first consider a search based on subject. Begin by identifying the major constructs and concepts of your initial inquiry (as discussed earlier). Then, translate these into keywords, terms which are used to identify works that contain the named concepts. In addition to the title, author, and abstract, most journals require authors to specify and list keywords that reflect the content of their study. Each database groups these studies according to these keywords.

For example, Box 6-5 presents part of the title of a study on disability and domestic violence and key words depicting the focus of the research. Without these keywords, this study containing disability would not be likely to be identified in a search on domestic violence. This example illustrates how valuable keywords are in adding dimension to a study, ensuring that its future dissemination and use in research can be maximized.

You can obtain help from a reference librarian in formulating keywords, or the computer will help direct you to synonymous terms, if the words you initially select are not used as classifiers. You can always consult a thesaurus for synonyms that may lead to more productive searching. Most online systems are user-friendly, are interactive, and use smart searching—that is, the computer provides step-by-step directions on what to do and will examine terms that are contained in or analogous to the terms you interest in your initial search. If you search any of the keywords listed in Box 6-5, you will find significant studies in that topic area. Omit "disability" as a keyword and see how your search changes.

Let us return to the example of the mobility fitness device study to show the importance of keywords. We will begin our search with the keywords/terms "fitness," "mobility device," and "elder." The combination of terms is critical in delimiting and focusing your search. For example, when we searched Google Scholar, an online database of journal and newspaper articles available to the public, we first entered the keyword "fitness." The computer indicated 249,000 sources in the past 5 years relevant to the subject of fitness. A review of all these sources obviously would be too cumbersome. We then entered our second keyword, "mobility device," at a prompt that requested further delimiting. The computer then searched for works containing both topics and indicated 20,600 articles. The final term further decreased the number of sources.

This search raises another important issue. As database options expand, it is important to select options that are feasible. We conducted the same search on the Nursing and Allied Health Collection database that we accessed through the University of Maine. The keyword "fitness" yielded 2396 articles over the past 5 years. Adding the term "elder" decreased the number of articles to 56. The final key term, "mobility device," reduced the number to 12. Because this small number of articles appeared in only one database, we then expanded our search to check other databases including engineering and entered the word "adaptive." This word brought us to a new literature, one that was productive for identifying research on new devices, safety, and functionality.

After your chosen databases indicate how many citations are found, the next step is to display the sources. Often you have a choice of examining only the citation, the abstract, or the full text. If your online system is connected to a printer, you can select a print command and print your selections if you prefer to read off-screen text. You may also search the system by entering authors' names or words you believe may appear in the titles of sources. This entry expands your search to relevant articles that may not have included the combination of keywords initially used. Your computer, tablet, or smartphone will search the references and compile a list of sources from which to choose.

In some cases, it is more efficient to ask the librarian to assist you. Large databases, such as the Education Resources Information Center and Medline, although accessible without assistance, can be easily accessed in this manner. Librarians are also adept at selecting keywords that are productive and targeted to your topic. Remember, with contemporary technology, you do not have to be on site at the library to get real-time assistance. As we noted earlier, many university library websites have live chat functions that allow you to interact with a librarian as long as you have Internet access.

You also may want to do a search in important indexes and abstracts, some of which are not available online, such as some library holdings of special collections, to ensure that you have fully covered the literature relevant to your study. In health research, indexes and abstracts are numerous and continue to increase as a result of the omnipotence of the Internet. We have listed just a few that we have found valuable in Box 6-6.

The many abstracting and indexing services include *Ulrich's International Periodicals Directory*, which was recently developed as a global source for libraries and researchers in all areas of the world. Ulrich.net is especially useful because it lists all periodicals and databases in which these periodicals are indexed.

One major directory of abstracts that is not frequently used but is extremely helpful in locating sources is *Dissertation Abstracts Online* (Dialog, LLC n.d.).[12] We mention this source because a literature review in a dissertation is usually exhaustive, and thus obtaining a dissertation in your topic area may provide a comprehensive literature review and bibliography that is immediately available to you.

Another strategy is to identify whether an article has been published that comprehensively reviews the literature in your area of interest. A literature review or a meta-analysis of studies on a particular area provides an excellent way to search the literature. Also, these reviews usually identify gaps in the literature and make recommendations as to next research steps.

Several other search engines are worth considering. BASE is a browser devoted to open source scholarship (Bielefeld University Library, 2004-2013).[13] To access the Deep Web of hidden sources, or those not always indexed and accessible on more commonly used search engines, Deep Web browsers are extremely valuable. Deep Web search engines such as TOR allow anonymous searching as well.

BOX 6-6 *Useful Indexes and Abstracts*

Biomedical Reference Collection: Basic
CINAHL with Full Text
Health Source: Consumer Edition WEB
Health Source: Nursing/Academic Edition
MEDLINE
Nursing & Allied Health Collection: Basic
Physical Education Index
PubMed
SPORTDiscus
STATIRef
Other useful databases:
AccessScience
AHFS Consumer Medication Information
CAB Direct
Cochrane Collection Plus
Directory of Open Access Journals
FSTA: Food Science & Technology Abstracts
Global Health (CABDirect)
Google Scholar
Health and Safety Science Abstracts
IngentaConnect
JSTOR
Nature
Nurtition Abstracts and Reviews. Series A: Human and Experimental (CABDirect)
PILOTS (Published International Literature on Traumatic Stress)
POPLINE
PsycARTICLES
PsycINFO
PubMed Central
Review of Aromatic and Medicinal Plants (CABDirect)
Risk Abstracts
Science Citation Index (Web of Science)
ScienceDirect
Taylor & Francis online journals
TOXNET
Web of Knowledge
Web of Science

Another important feature of the Internet is that one can now access knowledge presented in languages in which the reader's literacy is low. Google Translate, BabelFish, and other automated translation tools, although not perfected for full accuracy, open a global universe of sources to the knowledge seeker.

Images can also be searched on sites such as Google Image. You can browse your computer or mobile device for an image, upload it to the search engine and find identical or similar images. This type of search is particularly valuable in finding certain types of research in which images and material culture are the topical focus.

A final set of Internet browsing sources worth noting is the academic and scholarly open sources repositories such as Digital Commons, ResearchGate, and Academia.edu. These sites provide open access to work posted by the author. The advantages of such tools include immediate and open access to full-text documents and even works in progress. Remember, however, that careful scrutiny and evaluation are warranted, given that peer review is not a requisite criterion for this material.

Some Unconventional Gems

In addition to the known and identified search engines and browsers discussed earlier, you can use some unconventional methods through which knowledge can be sought. One of our favorite ways to sample book material is Amazon's "Look Inside" feature. Using this tool, you can often access introductory chapters and search for keywords in order to decide if a purchase is warranted. Publishers' websites allow a range of browsing from sampling excerpts to examining the table of contents of their book collections.

Blogging, vlogging, and social media should be considered cautiously but not eliminated from your search. These sources can provide well-developed knowledge as well as data guiding you to new research topics. As example, three Facebook pages, The Women of Advanced Style: Age and Beauty, Disabookability, and Disability Arts, were used as data sources by researchers in informing redesign research for mobility equipment for elders.

Finally, we discuss Wikipedia, the online encyclopedia that can be edited by anyone. Similar to any repository, Wikipedia entries need to be evaluated by the reader for rigor. However, to some extent, Wikipedia has a built-in evaluation of its own sources. In a search for knowledge to inform the problem of elder abandonment of mobility devices, this message appeared:

*This article **needs additional citations for verification**. Please help improve this article by adding citations to reliable sources. Unsourced material may be challenged and removed. (Disability Studies, 2013)*

Wikipedia is an encyclopedia and thus if you use it purposively and critically, it provides an efficient source for brief summaries of topical areas.

Most beginning investigators are concerned with the number of sources to review. Although there is no magic number, most researchers search the literature for articles written within the previous 5 years. A search is extended beyond 5 years to evaluate the historical development of an issue or to review a breakthrough or classic article. The depth of a review depends on the purpose and scope of your study. Most investigators try to become familiar with the most important authors, studies, and papers in their topic area. You will have a sense that your review is comprehensive when you begin to see citations of authors you have already read, or if you are not finding material that leads to new learning. Also, do not hesitate to contact a researcher who has published in your topic area; ask about the researcher's recent work (which may not be published yet) and recommendations on specific current articles for you to review. You can also access the curriculum vitae of a researcher or, if the individual is noteworthy, an article on his or her work may be found on Wikipedia.

Step 4: Organize Information

With your list of sources identified by your searches, you are ready to retrieve and organize them. We usually begin by reading abstracts of journal articles or samples or reviews of book contents to determine their value to the study. On the basis of the abstract or table of contents, we determine the level of relevance of scholarship as highly relevant to not relevant. Determining relevance helps you narrow the reading task so that it is manageable and productive.

Although it is not necessary to complete searching before accessing sources, we suggest that an efficient way of seeing a broad landscape of knowledge is through creating a list or a taxonomy before more in-depth exploration of single sources. This task can be accomplished manually or digitally. We find that "tagging" a source is useful and quick in identifying it as part of a body of content. Tagging is a digital step through which a file is located in a larger category by name and/or color. Digital databases located on local or cloud repositories provide simple to sophisticated organizing tools as well.

Because it is not possible to remember all the important information presented in reading, it is critical to document the type of information (research or theory paper, for example), the content, the conceptual framework, methodology, and the relevance of each source to your study. As with organizing citations and sources, there are many schemes for documenting. You may find that manually taking notes on index cards is effective because the cards can be shuffled and reordered to fit into an outline. However, we prefer to take notes electronically. For example, apps such as Index Card[14] are invaluable if you prefer note cards that can be automated and used to prepare a report. But if paper and pen note writing is preferred, scanning tools with optical character recognition can import notes into a computer or tablet so that they can be aggregated and shared. Writing notes directly on a tablet screen is also an option in apps such as Note Taker.[15] Systems that both annotate and allow note taking are increasing in number and popularity. For example, RefWorks[16] is offered in many university libraries. This powerful tool not only automates referencing, but provides the option for notations as well as sharing. References can be imported into formal reports and maintained in a cumulative searchable, manipulable database. Using this tool requires an active Internet connection. However, there are other apps and software that can be used offline. Whatever method you use,

always be sure to cite the full reference. We have all had the miserable experience of losing the volume, page number, or URL of a critical source and then spending hours trying to find it later.

Although investigators organize and write notations in their own way, we offer two strategies—using a chart and using a concept/construct matrix—to help you organize your reading. These two organizational aids will also assist in the writing stage of your review.

Charting the Literature

For a *literature review chart,* you select pertinent information from each work you review and record it using a chart format. To use a chart approach, you need to determine the categories of information you will extract from each resource to record or place on the chart. The categories you choose should reflect the nature of your research project and how you plan to develop a rationale for your study. For example, if you are planning an experimental fitness study for elders with diabetes, your review may need to highlight the limited number of adequately designed exercise studies with this particular population. Therefore, the categories of your chart might include the designs of previous studies and the health status of the samples. Table 6-1 shows an excerpt from such a chart. This chart would be used to structure a review of research on exercise intervention studies for healthy older adults and to evaluate research designs and specific outcomes of previous studies.

Charting research in this way allows you to reflect systematically on the literature as a whole and critically evaluate and identify research gaps.

Charting tools can be as simple as Excel, which allows you to create fields for each reference, or table

TABLE 6-1   *Excerpt from Literature Review Chart*

Author (Date)	Sample Boundaries	Design	Dependent Constructs	Claims
Blumenthal et al (1982)	24 elder adults from retirement homes (mean age 69 years)	No group control	Mood (profile of mood)	No change
			Temperament (Thurstone scale)	No change
			Self-report of improvement	40% improved
			Personality type	No change

| TABLE 6-2 | *Excerpt from Gilson's Concept/Construct Matrix* |

Concept 1	Concept 2	Concept 3	Concept 4	Concept 5
Disability	Campus architecture	Accessibility	Spatial policy	Wheeled mobility

functions contained in word processing apps such as Word, Pages, or Open Office.

Concept/Construct Matrix

The *concept/construct matrix* organizes information that you have reviewed and evaluated by key concept/construct (the x axis) and source (the y axis). Table 6-2 shows an excerpt from a concept matrix.

In this naturalistic study of access architectures on college campuses, Gilson[15] began his literature review by searching three major constructs: disability, campus architecture, and accessibility. Two other constructs, spatial policy and wheeled mobility, were also identified in the literature on campus architectures. Gilson integrated these constructs into his theoretical discussion of existing knowledge, and they were added to the concept matrix. •

As you begin to write the literature review, the concept/construct matrix facilitates quick identification of the scholarship that addresses the specific concepts/constructs you need to discuss. This approach also provides a mechanism to ensure that you review each core construct of your area of inquiry in the literature and systematically link to the others.

Step 5: Critically Evaluate the Literature

This step is the most important for you when conducting your literature review. By "critical," we do not simply mean determining what is deficient about sources as the complete analysis of the strengths and limitations of a study.[18] Simply repeating what is in the literature and decimating it does not constitute a critical review.[16] Several guiding questions can help you critically evaluate the literature you read. Use the questions in Table 6-3 to guide your reading of the research literature and the questions in Box 6-7

| BOX 6-7 | *Guiding Questions for Evaluating Nonresearch Sources* |

1. What way of knowing and level of knowledge are presented?
2. Was the work presented clearly, unambiguously, and consistently?
3. What is the purpose of the work? Is the purpose implicit? Is it stated? How does the purpose influence the knowledge discussed in the work?
4. What is the scope and application of the work?
5. What support exists for the claims being made in the source?
6. What debates, new ideas, and trends are presented in the work?
7. What are the strengths and weaknesses of the work?
8. What research queries, or questions, emerge from the work?

to assist your evaluation of "nonresearch" literature. Your responses to these evaluative questions will inform your research direction.

An evaluation of nonresearch sources involves examining the level of and support for the knowledge presented. Nonresearch sources include position papers, theoretical works, editorials, debates, curated exhibits, and gray literature.[19] As mentioned earlier, another important resource is work that presents a critical review of research in a particular area. These published literature reviews provide syntheses of research as ways of summarizing the state of knowledge in particular fields and identifying new directions for research.

Step 6: Write the Literature Review

Now that you have searched, obtained, read, and organized your literature, it is time to prepare the actual review. You may need to summarize your review for a proposal to seek approval from your institution's office for protection of human subjects, for a proposal to seek funding to support your research, or to justify the conduct of your study for a manuscript that describes the completed research project. A good literature review presents an overview of the relevant work on your topic and a critical evaluation of the works. There is no recipe for

TABLE 6-3   *Evaluating Research Articles Experimental Type: Naturalistic Inquiry*

_____ Was the study clear, unambiguous, and internally consistent?
_____ What is (are) the research question(s)? Are they clearly and adequately stated?
_____ What is the purpose of the study?
_____ How does the purpose influence the design and the conclusions?
_____ Describe the theory that guides the study and the conceptual framework for the project. Are they clearly presented and relevant to the study?
_____ What are the key constructs identified in the literature review?
_____ What level of theory is suggested in the literature review? Is it consistent with the selected research strategy?
_____ What is the rationale for the design found in the literature review? Is it sound?
_____ Does the design of the project fit the level of theory? Is relevant knowledge presented in the literature review?
_____ Diagram the design.
_____ Does the design answer the research question(s)? Why or why not?
_____ What are the boundaries of the study? How are the boundaries selected?
_____ What efforts did the investigator make to ensure validity and reliability?
_____ What data collection techniques were used? Is the rationale for these techniques specified in the literature review and/or in the methods section?
_____ How does data collection fit with the study purpose and study question?
_____ How are the data analyzed? Does the analysis plan make sense for the study? How does the analysis plan fit with the study purpose and study question?
_____ Are the conclusions supported by the study?
_____ What are the strengths of the study?
_____ What level of knowledge is generated?
_____ What use does this knowledge have for health and human service practice?
_____ Are there ethical dilemmas presented in this article? What are they? Did the author(s) resolve the dilemmas in a reasonable and ethical manner?
_____ Was the study clear, unambiguous, and credible?
_____ What is (are) the research query(ies)? Are they clearly and adequately stated?
_____ What is the purpose of the study?
_____ How does the purpose influence the design and the conclusions?
_____ Describe the theory that guides or emerges from the study.
_____ What are the key constructs identified in the literature review or emerging from the study?
_____ What level of theory is suggested in the literature review? Is it consistent with the selected research strategy?
_____ What is the rationale for the design found in the literature review? Is it sound?
_____ Does the design of the project fit the level or acceptability of theory? Is relevant knowledge presented in the literature review?
_____ Does the design answer the research query(ies)? Why or why not?
_____ What are the boundaries of the study? How are the boundaries selected?
_____ What efforts did the investigator make to ensure trustworthiness?
_____ What information collection techniques were used? Where is the rationale for these techniques specified, and is it sound?
_____ How does information collection fit with the study purpose and study query?
_____ How are the data analyzed? Does the analysis plan make sense for the study? How does the analysis plan fit with the study purpose and study query?
_____ Are the conclusions supported by the study?
_____ What are the strengths of the study?
_____ What level of knowledge is generated?
_____ What use does this knowledge have for health and human service practice?
_____ Are there ethical dilemmas presented in this article? What are they? Did the author(s) resolve the dilemmas in a reasonable and ethical manner?

- Introduction
- Discussion of each related concept, construct, principle, theory, and model in current literature
- Brief review of related study designs and their results
- Critical appraisal of current related research and knowledge
- Integration of various works reviewed
- Fit of investigator's study with the collective knowledge related to the topic under investigation
- Overview and justification for study and design

BOX 6-9   *Suggested Outline for Writing Narrative*

I.   Introduction (overview of what the review covers)
II.   Review of specific concepts
III.   Description of how each concept has been studied
IV.   Overview of studies
V.   Design
VI.   Results
VII.   Critical evaluation
VIII.   Critical summary of current knowledge and gaps in literature
IX.   Integration of concepts; relationships proposed in studies
X.   Identification of research needs
XI.   Rationale for study and design
XII.   Overview and niche for proposed study

writing a narrative literature review. Most investigators, whether working in an experimental-type or naturalistic tradition, include in their narratives the categories of information shown in Box 6-8. One suggested outline for writing the narrative of a literature review is presented in Box 6-9.

Summary

The literature review is a critical evaluation of existing literature and sources relevant to your study. Because it is a critical evaluation, reviewing the literature is a thinking process that involves piecing together and integrating diverse resources. The review provides an understanding of the level of theory and knowledge development that exists about your topic. This understanding is essential so that you can determine how your study fits into the construction of knowledge in the topic area.

The literature review is also an action process through which concepts are organized and sources are logically presented in a written review. The literature review chart and concept/construct matrix are two organizational tools that will help you conceptualize the literature and prepare an effective review, one that convinces the reader that your study is necessary, and it represents the next step in knowledge building. Remember, the primary purposes of writing a literature review and including it in the written report of your research are to establish the conceptual foundation for your research, establish the specific content of your study, and, most important, provide a rationale for your research design.

Also, keep in mind that a systematic review of the literature can also function as a research methodology. Chapter 11 describes two methodologies that use published literature as the unit of analysis.[6]

EXERCISES

1. You are interested in studying the outcome of a joint mobilization program which is designed to increase the range of motion of the lower extremities of children with spinal cord injuries. Identify the keywords you will use to conduct a search for relevant literature.
2. Select a research article and develop a concept/construct matrix from the literature presented. What level of knowledge and theory development is presented for each concept/construct? For each study, was the selected design appropriate for the level of knowledge in the literature?
3. Identify a specific area of research that interests you and the specific related constructs. Conduct a keyword search for each construct using a relevant database. How many articles do you identify for each construct searched? How would you refine your keyword search?

References

1. Kiteley R, Stogdan C: *Literature reviews in social work*, Thousand Oaks, Calif, 2014, Sage.
2. Peters J: Measuring myths about domestic violence: development and initial validation of the Domestic Violence Myth Acceptance Scale. *J Aggress Maltreat Trauma* 16:1–21, 2008.
3. Wegerer J: *7 ways technology helps family caregivers*, July 22, 2013. http://www.aplaceformom.com/blog/2013-7 -21-technology-family-caregivers.
4. Burleigh TJ, Schoenherr JR, Lacroix GL: Does the uncanny valley exist? An empirical test of the relationship between eeriness and the human likeness of digitally created faces. *Comp Hum Behav* 29:759–771, 2013.
5. Creswell JC: *Qualitative inquiry and research design: choosing among five approaches*, ed 3, Los Angeles, 2013, Sage.
6. Bateni H, Maki B: Assistive devices for balance and mobility: benefits, demands, and adverse consequences. *Arch Phys Med Rehabil* 86:134–145, 2005.
7. DePoy E, Gilson S: *Disability as designed and branded*, London, 2014, Routledge.
8. Maruyama M: Endogenous research: the prison project. In Reason P, Rowan J, editors: *Human inquiry: a sourcebook of new paradigm research*, New York, 1981, Wiley.
9. Mertens DM: *Research and evaluation in education and psychology*, Thousand Oaks, Calif, 2014, Sage.
10. Bengtson J: *Grey literature 101*, 2013. http://libguides.health .unm.edu/content.php?pid=200149.
11. Project Muse: *Project Muse*, 2013. http://muse.jhu.edu.
12. Dissertation Abstracts: *Proquest*. 2014. http://dissexpress .umi.com/dxweb/search.html.
13. BASE: *Bielefeld Academic Search Engine*. 2004–2014. http:// www.base-search.net/about/en/.
14. DenVog, LLC: *Index Card*. 2013. https://itunes.apple.com/us/ app/index-card/id389358786.
15. Software Garden: *Note Taker*, 2014. https://itunes.apple.com/ us/app/note-taker-hd/id366572045?mt=8.
16. RefWorks: *RefWorks*, 2009. http://www.refworks.com.
17. Gilson SF, DePoy E: The student body. *Res Social Sci Disabil* 6:27–44, 2011.
18. Bressler C: *Literary criticism: an introduction to theory and practice*, ed 5, New York, 2011, Longman.
19. Huffine R: *Value of grey literature to scholarly research in the digital age*, June 15, 2010, Elsevier. http://cdn.elsevier.com/ assets/pdf_file/0014/110543/2010RichardHuffine.pdf.

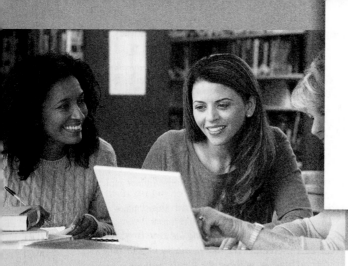

Chapter 7
Theory in Research

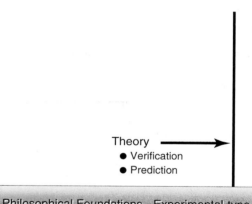

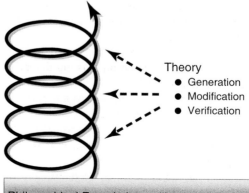

Think of a particular field of inquiry or a particular research question or query of interest to you, and ask yourself the following two questions:

• What knowledge exists about this phenomenon?

• What theories have been developed to explain or have been used to understand the phenomenon?

You will want to keep asking these basic questions as you engage in the research process and explore different problems of interest. For each research question or query that you pose, the way in

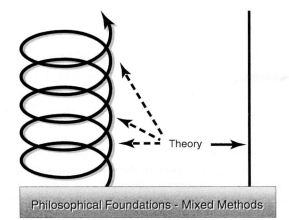

Philosophical Foundations - Mixed Methods

which you answer these basic questions will largely determine the types of research actions (e.g., design strategy, analysis, and reporting) that you will implement. As discussed in previous chapters, the level of knowledge and *theory* development in a particular field shapes how a research question or query is framed and a design strategy is implemented. Theory therefore has a critical role in both experimental-type and naturalistic research as well as in mixed method methodologies.

Why Is Theory Important?

When people hear the word "theory," they often feel overwhelmed and assume that the term is not relevant to their daily lives or is too abstract and complicated to understand. However, think about how difficult life would be without theory. Theory informs us each day in many aspects of our lives, from knowing how to prepare for the weather to guiding our professional practice. For example, predicting the weather is based on existing theory. The meteorologist looks at present weather conditions and past weather patterns and makes a prediction in the form of a forecast. But is theory a truth? From this example, the message is a resounding "no," because what is theorized to happen in the atmosphere is built on conceptual models.

In health and human service delivery, you make a decision about which intervention to use with a patient or client on the basis of theory. You use a theory to guide your decisions, even though you may not be fully cognizant that you are actually doing so.

As discussed in Chapter 1, a primary purpose of research is directly linked to theory. In experimental-type designs, one primary purpose of research is to test theory using deductive processes. Let's say you want to understand why a particular group of women refuse noninvasive cancer screenings (e.g., breast examinations). You may draw on various theories such as the Health Belief Model to examine the relationship between health beliefs and health practices in this group of women. Without use of a theoretical framework, you would not know which variables to measure and examine.

In naturalistic inquiry, a purpose of the design is theory generation or contribution to the elaboration of an existing theory using induction or abduction. For example, let's say you want to understand the experiences and coping strategies of families caring for children with severe chronic illnesses. You review the extant literature and believe that existing stress process and coping theories do not adequately capture the experiences of this population. You may start with those theories to frame your initial questions, and then your analyses may purposely expand on or modify the theories. Alternatively, you may conduct a study with the explicit purpose of developing new theory from the ground up, so to speak, in an area for which theory development is lacking, an existing theory does not adequately apply to the population being studied, or the theory inadequately accounts for factors known to affect the behavior or experiences of interest.

This chapter introduces another important point as it concerns the relationship between research and theory: that is, you must have a theoretical framework to conduct adequate research. This is the main theme of this chapter and a basic premise of this text. You will find that there are still too many published works in the literature that are atheoretical. We believe such studies are enumerative and thus have limited utility. By enumerative, we mean that they merely count. For example, the census relies on the conduct of counting categories of residents in the United States but does not theorize anything about the population. It may provide a slice in time look at who lives in the United States, but the "so what" question is not directed by theory. The purpose of research in testing, verifying, and advancing theory is thus not met by such activities, although it may look as if research is being conducted. As Kurt Lewin, the father of modern social psychology once said: "There is nothing so practical as a good theory."[2]

As discussed throughout this text, research involves what we refer to as thinking (e.g., theory identification/criticism, problem statement formulation) and action processes (e.g., setting boundaries, data collection, analyzing information). Critical to the thinking processes of research is understanding human experience and phenomena. At the heart of this thinking process is identifying theories or parts of theories that can help organize ideas and the phenomena of interest to study. Even though we may not realize it, theory frames how we ask, look at, and answer a research question or query. Theory provides conceptual clarity and the capacity to connect the new knowledge obtained through the action process of data collection to the vast body of knowledge to which it is relevant. Without theory, we do not have conceptual and hence practical direction.

Data that are derived without being conceptually embedded in theoretical contexts do not advance our understanding of human experience and ultimately are not useful other than for counting. Remember, "usefulness" is an important component of our definition of research. An important point is that theory helps a researcher see the big picture or the forest instead of just a tree. That is, it helps the researcher make sense of details and place them within a larger conceptual context. If we only focus on a single tree or detail, we lose sense of the whole and how that one detail or observation functions or relates to a larger body of knowledge. Also, without putting the single tree or datum within context, we lose an understanding of the conceptual, textured picture (forest).

Let us examine more closely why theory must inform or shape research actions by considering the meaning and use of common terms such as "race" and "ethnicity" in the United States.

Not every country considers categories such as race and ethnicity. However, as mentioned earlier, every 10 years the U.S. government conducts a national census in which characteristics of individuals, families, and neighborhoods are counted by collecting information. Since the 1970s, there has been a significant debate about the need and rationale for recording race and ethnicity.[3] However, there is no consensus about a clear, theoretically based definition and thus a measure of race and ethnicity in the census. That is, no one really knows what the terms "race" and "ethnicity" mean; there is great conceptual confusion. As Ahmad and Sheldon stated in their classic work, "[T]he 'ethnic' question in the census is both rigid and externally imposed. It uses a culturalist, geographic, and 'nationalist' notion of race dressed up as ethnicity."[3] Therefore, some have argued that the gathering of race and ethnicity data is atheoretical and thus can be dangerous; it may lead to inaccurate analysis and development of policies or social actions that are consequently inappropriate.[4]

Nevertheless, given our present social structure and how health and social policy are formulated, knowledge about racial and ethnic categories can be important for program planning. Thus, collecting information about race and ethnic categories must be based first on a careful consideration of the definition and use of these terms as theoretical constructs, their supported relevance in the literature, and then on appropriate ways to *operationalize* or measure the theoretically based definition. Only a theoretically based approach can avoid potential harm to significant numbers of people by ungrounded and vague use of these important terms. •

What Is Theory?

By now you might be asking, "So what is theory?" Definitions range from traditional views of theory as systems to organize, describe, and predict a single reality; to abstract systems of language symbols that provide multiple interpretations and ideas of phenomena; to ideological foundations for social action.[5]

We draw on Kerlinger's classic definition of theory because we believe it is the most comprehensive and useful for investigators and students of research. Kerlinger defines theory as "a set of interrelated constructs, definitions, and propositions that present a systematic view of phenomena by specifying relations among variables, with the purpose of explaining or predicting phenomena."[6] In this definition, a theory is a set of related ideas that has the potential to explain or predict human experience in an orderly fashion, and it is based on data. The theorist develops a structural map of what is observed and experienced in an effort to promote understanding and facilitate the ability to predict outcomes under specific conditions. Through deductive research approaches or empirical investigations, theories are either supported and verified or refuted and falsified. Through inductive approaches, theories are incrementally developed to explain and give order to observations of human experience. Abduction seeks the best explanation from an array of possibilities.[7]

As implied in Kerlinger's definition, four interrelated structural components are subsumed under theory and range in degree, or level, of abstraction. Although numerous taxonomies for the parts of a theory have been proposed,[5] we suggest that the four basic structures of theory are *concepts, constructs, relationships,* and *propositions* or principles. Let us first examine the meaning of "abstraction" and then discuss each level.

Levels of Abstraction

Abstraction often conjures up a vision of the ethereal, the "not real." However, "abstraction" as it relates to theory development depicts a symbolic representation of shared experience. For example, if we all see a form that has fur, a tail, four legs, and barks, we name that observation a "dog." We have shared in the visual experience and have created a symbol (the word "dog") to name our sensory experience.

All words are merely symbols to describe and communicate experience. Words are only one form of abstraction; different words represent different *levels of abstraction,* and a single word can represent multiple levels of abstraction.

Figure 7-1 displays the four levels of abstraction within theory and their interrelationships. Shared experience is the foundation on which abstraction is built. It is important to recognize that we do not use the term "reality" as the foundation. Reality implies that there is only one viewpoint from which to build the basic elements of a theory. In contrast, this text is based on the premise that humans experience multiple realities and multiple perspectives about the nature of reality. Therefore, levels of abstraction must be built on shared experience, defined as the consensus of what we obtain through our senses. For experimental-type researchers who work deductively, shared experience is usually thought of as sense data, or that which can be reduced to observation and measurement. For researchers working inductively and abductively in the naturalistic tradition, shared experience may include meanings and interpretations of human experience. In mixed methods, both perspectives are integrated in some fashion.

Let us use the example of the "furry being with four legs and a tail that barks" to illustrate the multiple meanings that can be attributed to shared experience. Shared experience tells each of us that this is a dog, but the word "dog" may also carry with it diverse meanings, such as fear or happiness.

Each type of experience is equally important to acknowledge, as are the different meanings attributed to a single word.

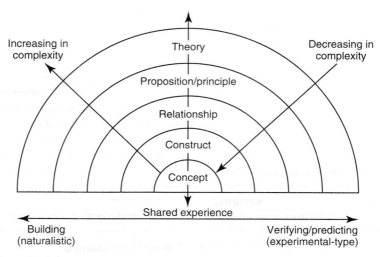

Figure 7-1 Levels of abstraction.

Concepts

As depicted in Figure 7-1, a concept is the first level of abstraction and is defined as a single, first-order symbolic representation of an observable or experienced referent.[5] By first order, we mean that there is no abstract level between shared experience and concept. Concept is directly inferred from observations and other sense data. Concepts are the basic building blocks of communication because they provide us with the means to tell our experiences and ideas to one another. Without concepts, we would not have language.[5] In the case of the "furry being," the word "dog" can function as a concept. At this basic level of abstraction, the term "dog" describes an observation shared by many. The words "furry," "tail," "four legs," and "bark" are also concepts because they are directly sensed.

In experimental-type research, concepts are selected before a study is started and are defined to permit direct measurement or observation. In naturalistic research, concepts are derived primarily through direct observations and continual engagement with the phenomenon of interest in the context in which it occurs. Mixed methods inquiry makes use of both approaches.

Constructs

A construct, the next level of abstraction, does not have an observable or a directly experienced referent

in shared experience. Meanings become important to consider at this level of abstraction, because two individuals who articulate the same construct may attribute disparate meanings to it. If we look again at the term "dog" as a construct rather than a concept, the word may mean "fear" to some and "happiness" to others. Although we stated earlier that "dog" is a concept, in this case, "dog" functions as a construct because what is observable is not the communicated meaning. Rather, the meaning of the term takes on the feelings evoked by "dog," such as fear or happiness.

Fear and happiness are also examples of constructs. What may be observed are the behaviors associated with fear or happiness—that is, someone who sweats, shakes, and turns pale at the site of a dog or someone who smiles, approaches, and pets the dog, respectively. These observations of both feelings are synthesized into the constructs of fear and happiness. Thus, fear and happiness are not directly "observed" but are surmised by observations of human behavior and are based on a constellation of behavioral concepts. "Health," "illness," and "professional" are also examples of constructs in that they are not directly observable or able to be sensed, but must be inferred from other indicators.

Categories provide additional examples of constructs. The category of "mammal" or "canine" is an example of a construct. Although each category or construct is not directly observable, it is composed of a set of concepts that can be observed.

Other examples of constructs relevant to health and human service inquiry include quality of life, wellness, life roles, rehabilitation, poverty, disability, health disparity, depression, functional status, and psychological well-being. Although not directly observable or able to be sensed directly, each is made up of parts or components that can be observed or submitted to measurement. Think about the construct of "quality of life": Which concepts make up this construct? Some may include health status, self-efficacy, activity engagement, economic security, or positive mood. If you consider that even this relatively low level of abstraction is multifaceted, you can begin to understand why health and human service research is so complex.

Relationships

So far, we have been discussing single-word symbols or units of abstraction. At the next level of abstraction, single units are connected to form a relationship. A relationship is defined as an association of two or more constructs or concepts.[8] For example, we may suggest that the size of a dog is related to the level of fear that a person experiences. This relationship has two constructs, "size" and "fear," and one concept, "dog." Think again about the construct of "quality of life" and consider the concepts that form it and their relationship. Now consider the relevance of this relationship for a specific population with whom you work or in which you have an interest (e.g., elderly, children with mobility impairments, individuals with spinal cord injury, prisoners). For example, research suggests that quality of life in older adults is related to the extent to which functional limitations curtail activity participation.[9] Thus, the relationship between two concepts, impairment and activity restriction, is critical to the construct of quality of life as it pertains to older adults living at home.

Propositions (Principles)

A proposition is the next level of abstraction. A proposition, or principle, is a statement that governs a set of relationships and gives them a structure.[8] For example, a proposition suggests that fear of large dogs is caused by negative childhood experiences with large dogs. This proposition describes the structure of two sets of relationships: (1) the relationship between the size of a dog and fear and (2) the relationship between childhood experiences and the size of dogs. It also suggests the direction of the relationship and the influence of each construct on the other. Let's revisit the construct of quality of life. Can you develop a proposition based on the relationship between functional difficulty and activity limitation? One proposition may be that quality of life is affected by the extent to which having a functional difficulty limits participation in valued activities. That is, having a functional difficulty leads to limited quality of life to the extent that activities in which one wants to participate are affected or curtailed.

> A theory related to the "furry being" may be that "fear of large dogs derives from childhood experiences." Therefore, the fear can be cured by psychoanalysis that aims to mediate the negative effects of childhood experiences. This theory explains the phenomenon "fear of dogs"; it is verifiable and can lead to prediction. If, through research, we can support a positive relationship between childhood experiences, fear of dogs, and the effectiveness of psychoanalysis in reducing that fear, we can predict this relationship in the future and control its outcome. •

Design Selection and the Four Levels

Now let's consider how these levels of abstraction relate to the selection of a particular research design or approach to studying a phenomenon of interest.

Remember—abstraction is the symbolic naming, representation, and frequent communication of shared experience. The further a symbol is removed from shared experience, the higher the level of abstraction. Each level of abstraction moves farther away from shared experience (see Fig. 7-1). Thus, the higher the level of abstraction, the more complex your design becomes. This principle is based on common sense. If the scope of your study is to examine a basic experience or concept (how many people get the flu in a particular season), then a descriptive study scrutinizing prevalence rates would be necessary. In contrast, if the scope of your study is to examine a construct, a more complex investigation may be necessary to evaluate indicators of the elements of the construct. For example, suppose you are interested in determining the level of cognitive recovery in a group of people with head injuries. This type of investigation is an inquiry into the construct of "cognitive recovery" and requires that one construct be defined and measured in your population. Complexity is encountered in the research process with the lexical definition of the construct, which describes its meaning in words. Once you select a definition, the rest of the research process is relatively straightforward.

Let's say instead that you want to move into the realm of propositions and determine the extent to which the person's age at the time of injury affects recovery rate. In this type of investigation, you would define the construct lexically (in words), define "recovery," and state the nature of the relationship between recovery and the concept of "age." As you add more constructs, such as "level of severity of injury" and "status before injury," your design increases in complexity.

Assume you are interested in understanding the behaviors that place rural teenagers at risk for contracting human immunodeficiency virus (HIV). Because most knowledge on HIV risk in the adolescent population focuses on urban teenagers, you have limited theory, or sets of constructs, to investigate. Consequently, you may simply collect data by asking questions and observing behaviors of the referent group. As your observations proceed, however, you find many factors emerging that have an impact on rural teenage behavior and risk. The complexity of your research approach increases as you focus on discovering and interpreting the meaning of specific patterns or relationships among constructs that you observe.

Although concepts, constructs, relationships, and propositions or principles provide the basic language and building blocks of any research project, each research tradition handles the levels of abstraction differently.

Role of Theory in Design Selection

How does theory shape the selection of research design strategies? When theory is well developed and conceptually fits the phenomenon under investigation, deductive studies will likely be implemented, as in the tradition of experimental-type research. When theory is poorly developed or does not fit the phenomenon under study, inductive and abductive studies that generate theory may be more appropriate, as in the tradition of naturalistic inquiry. Mixed methods are used for both purposes. The degree of knowledge development and relevance of a theory for the particular phenomenon under investigation determines in part the nature and type of research that is appropriate.

The relationship of theory and design can be illustrated by considering the Gilligan-Kohlberg example that we discussed in Chapter 5. Recall that the classic theory of moral development advanced by Lawrence Kohlberg suggested three basic levels of moral reasoning that develop and unfold throughout the life span: preconventional, conventional, and postconventional.[10] Many investigators have accepted this theory as truth and have attempted to characterize and predict the moral reasoning of different populations using measures anchored on this developmental theory. Based on these studies, populations and individuals have been categorized according to the level of moral reasoning they exhibit. This information served a valuable conceptual framework in promoting our understanding of morality in humans. The characterization of moral reasoning based on Kohlberg's theory is an example of a deductive relationship between theory and research; that is, the theory has been accepted as accurate, and subsequent studies intend to verify and advance the application of the theory in varied populations.

However, as we noted, in many studies of moral reasoning in adults based on Kohlberg's theoretical framework, women were reported to reason at a lower level than men. Researchers therefore concluded that women were not as morally advanced as men. Although this conclusion makes no sense, this type of deductive "illogic" is common practice, particularly when a theory is developed for one group and automatically applied to another without consideration of its "fit."

Recognizing this illogic with regard to women, researchers using different theoretical frameworks have begun to tackle the issue. For example, researchers using a feminist framework have not accepted Kohlberg's theory as true for women because it is intuitively contrary to what is experienced and believed. These researchers, including Gilligan,[11] have argued that although knowledge has been well developed in this area, Kohlberg's theory does not seem to fit or to be relevant to the experiences of women. Therefore, investigations of moral reasoning in women as well as for other groups (e.g., individuals from diverse racial and ethnic groups) have been developed by applying inductive research strategies. Collectively these studies have shown that women and other groups are not less moral than men but rather base their moral decision making on criteria that were substantially different from those initially identified by Kohlberg's theory and those operationalized in the scales developed to reflect his theory. Thus, research shows that Kohlberg's notions do not explain moral reasoning for a particular group—women. By using inductive strategies, researchers have been able to identify and illustrate the processes by which women and other groups reason and function, and thus new theory has been developed that reflects diverse thought processes. Given that Kohlberg developed his theory of moral reasoning by studying white men, the deductive strategy was most valuable in expanding knowledge of the moral reasoning in this group, but not necessarily in women or others from different backgrounds. Use of an inductive research strategy illustrates the relationship between theory and naturalistic inquiry; in other words, naturalistic inquiry is extremely valuable as a *theory-generating* tool and also can be used to verify or refute a theory.

Another example more relevant to health and human service practice involves the *International Classification of Functioning, Disability, and Health* (ICF).[12] In response to difficulties encountered by experimental-type researchers in applying ICF concepts and classifications to culturally diverse populations and countries, the World Health Organization and National Institutes of Health jointly implemented the Cultural Applicability Research (CAR) study initiative. The purpose of CAR was to develop guidelines for implementing classification schemas and instrumentation across cultural groups. CAR identifies the contextual, multilevel consequences of applying diagnostic conditions and provides empirical knowledge to inform use and interpretation of ICF taxonomy.[8] Since its inception, CAR has been applied widely to other domains of health, well-being, and flourishing.

These examples show the limitations of applying theory and knowledge developed on one group to other diverse groups and how this generates both inductive and deductive systematic inquiry in health and human service research.

Now you have a sense of the meaning of theory and how it relates to research knowledge development and the selection of design strategies. Let us now consider the role and relationship of theory and research for each of the specific research traditions.

Theory in Experimental-Type Research

Experimental-type researchers begin with a theory and seek to simplify and reduce abstraction by making the abstract observable, measurable, and predictable (see Fig. 7-1). This process of *theory testing* typically involves specifying a theory and then developing testable hunches or hypotheses. A *hypothesis* is linked to a theory and is a statement about the expected relationships between two or more concepts that can be tested. A hypothesis indicates what is expected to be observed and represents the researcher's "best hunch" as to what may exist or may be found on the basis of the principles of the theory.

Consider Achey's[13] work, in which she is using attribution error theory to examine why women with physical impairments have been excluded from human trafficking research and intervention. Achey found literature that illustrates how attitudes and institutional barriers create socially disabling conditions that exclude women with physical impairments from basic rights, safety, and resources available to their nondisabled counterparts. Of particular relevance to her study are the myths, attributions, and inaccurate beliefs—attribution error—that prevail and thus create these barriers.[14,15]

Given the role of attribution error as an ongoing barrier to the extinction of sexual abuse of all women, Achey[13] hypothesized attribution error as predictive of the omission of women with physical impairments from human trafficking research and services. Specifically she proposes that the role of myth about embodied disablement is institutionally and socially operative in preventing adequate and humane responses to halt human trafficking for her population of interest.

Based on this theory, hypotheses can be written in two forms, nondirectional or directional (see Chapter 8). Here is an example of a nondirectional hypothesis that can be derived from defensive attribution theory:

> There is a relationship between attribution error, in which women with physical impairments are seen as asexual and thus could not be victims of trafficking with the frequency of inclusion of this population in research.

A hypothesis can also indicate the direction or nature of a relationship between two concepts or constructs, as in the following example of a directional hypothesis:

> As the strength of perceived myth of the asexuality of women with physical impairments increases, provider willingness to serve these women in victim services decreases.

Consider yet another example using stress process theories. Although there are different versions, stress process theories seek to explain individual reactions to and consequences of chronic stressors. These theories basically posit the following; individuals may confront various objective stressors such as poor health, financial difficulties, or caregiving challenges that persist over time. Individuals must evaluate whether the external demands posed by these stressors are a potential threat and if so, whether the individuals have sufficient coping mechanisms to manage them. If individuals perceive external demands as threatening and their coping resources as inadequate, they may experience burden, upset, or distress. The appraisal of stress is assumed to subsequently contribute to negative emotional and behavioral responses (e.g., depression) that in turn place individuals at risk for poor health and psychiatric symptoms. Numerous research studies with specific hypotheses reflecting each point along the stress process pathway can flow from this framework.[16] One major hypothesis stemming from this theory is that use of positive coping strategies or other resources and/or the minimization of external stressors can reduce negative consequences on physical and psychosocial health. That is, the more an individual uses positive coping strategies such as problem solving versus emotive coping (wishing the problem would go away), the more likely it is that the individual will experience reduced stress and positive health outcomes. This hypothesis is based on one of the tenets of this framework, that if individuals cognitively reframe their situation and employ strategies that lower their perceived stress, they will cope more effectively. Stress process theories have been applied to a wide range of populations such as individuals with chronic conditions, family caregiving, or individuals exposed to chronic stressors such as those exposed to displacement due to natural disasters.

Here is yet another example. The Life Span Theory of Control is based on the premise that control over one's immediate life space or personal environment and daily activities is an important human invariant that transcends cultural groups.[17] This theory suggests that humans, by their nature, must exert some level of control over behavior-event contingencies in everyday life. Applied to the field of rehabilitation, the theory suggests that persons with physical difficulties resulting in limitations in performing daily activities may be threatened by or experience loss of control. This threat of or actual loss of control may in turn result in feelings of anxiety, which may lead to depression unless strategies, either cognitive or behavioral actions, are implemented to help the person achieve control between behavior and outcomes or a sense of efficacy. By using strategies that enhance control, people experience a sense of enhanced well-being, and positive outcomes are attained.

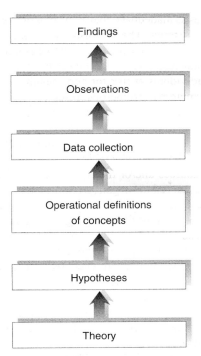

Figures arranged bottom to top with upward arrows:

Theory → Hypotheses → Operational definitions of concepts → Data collection → Observations → Findings

Figure 7-2 Using theory in experimental-type research.

On the basis of this theory, what do you think are some of the hypotheses that may be generated and tested? One directional hypothesis might be that use of adaptive technology enhances self-efficacy in people who have activity limitations resulting from physical impairments. Now, can you think of other meaningful hypotheses based on this theory?

Consider the hypotheses you thought of and those we suggested. What can you conclude about a hypothesis? As shown in Figure 7-2, a hypothesis is the initial reduction of theory to a more concrete and observable form. On the basis of the hypothesis, the researcher develops an operational definition of a concept so that it can be measured by a scale or other instrumentation. The operational definition of the concept further reduces the abstract to a concrete, observable form. Thus, in contrast to a lexical definition that defines a concept by words (which are other concepts), an operational definition of a concept defines it by specifying the exact procedures for measuring or observing the phenomenon. In the example of attribution error theory, the investigator

needs to operationalize the concept of myth. The process of operationalizing a concept is not easy or straightforward. Likewise, in the example of personal control theory, the investigator needs to operationalize self-efficacy and behavioral outcomes. Each researcher may develop his or her own way of operationalizing these key concepts. These definitions, however, must come from existing theory. For example, we could theorize depression as cognitive-behavioral and operationally define it by the number of self-deprecating statements made about oneself over a specified period of time. However, if we were using a psychoanalytic theoretical framework in which depression is lexically defined as internalized anger, we would operationally define it as observed hostile behavior towards oneself. The process of operationalization is discussed in greater detail in Chapter 17, in which we examine issues related to measurement and instrument construction and selection.

Using an operational definition, the researcher makes observations that result in data points, which are then analyzed. Analysis determines whether the findings verify, falsify, or modify the theory. Operationalization is the fundamental premise of the scientific process. Reducing abstraction to measurable components is used primarily to test relationships among concepts of a theory, and it is ultimately used to determine the adequacy of a theory to make predictions and thus control the phenomenon under study.

Box 7-1 lists the basic characteristics of the use of theory by experimental-type researchers. The process, referred to as logical deduction, begins with an abstraction and then focuses on discrete parts of phenomena or observations. Constructs are defined and simplified and then operationalized into concepts that can be observed to allow measurement. This process moves from a more abstract to a less abstract level, more concrete and observable level.

Common Theories Used in Health and Human Service Research

Box 7-2 lists five common categories of theories used in health and human service research. These are, of course, not the only theoretical categories that can be or are used in research, but merely provide

> **BOX 7-1** *Six Characteristics of Use of Theory in Experimental-Type Research*
>
> 1. Logical deductive process
> 2. Primarily uses theory testing
> 3. Movement from theory to lesser levels of abstraction
> 4. Assumes unitary reality that can be measured
> 5. Assumes knowledge through existing conceptions
> 6. Focus on measurable parts of phenomena

> **BOX 7-2** *Five Categories of Theories Used in Health and Human Service Research*
>
> Longitudinal developmental—theories that propose that humans develop and unfold in a typical fashion over the life span
>
> Environmental theories—theories that attribute human experience to interior and exterior environmental factors
>
> Categorical theories—theories that locate humans as members of diverse categories (e.g., race, ethnicity, gender, disability)
>
> Systems theories—theories that see humans in context in which movement or change in one element affects the whole
>
> New and emerging theories—postmodern and post-postmodern theories that propose human experience as interpretive and integrate previously distant disciplines (e.g., art and physics, strengths theory and engineering, disability theories and design)

common exemplars that illustrate basic constructs and the types of knowledge that can be generated. For a helpful compendium of relevant theories, see DePoy and Gilson.[18]

The theories presented in Table 7-1 also highlight the evolution and refinement that theories may undergo. As new data emerge and propositions are tested, falsified, and modified, theories often undergo incremental modifications. For example, Heckhausen and colleagues originally proposed the Life-Span Theory of Control in 1995,[19] but in 2010, they presented an expanded version of the theory, the

Motivational Theory of Life-Span Development.[17] Within disability theory, medical views of disability, which characterized disability as embodied deficits, were challenged with social theories that portrayed disability as a set of attitudinal, institutional, and physical barriers to functioning rather than embodied deficit.

Theory in Naturalistic Inquiry

Whereas theory testing is the primary goal of researchers in the experimental-type tradition, researchers working in the naturalistic tradition are usually developing or expanding on theory from observations. Thus, in naturalistic inquiry, the researcher begins with understanding, examining a shared experience, and then represents that experience at increasing levels of abstraction by constructing or identifying from the ground up concepts, constructs, and principles to understand the phenomena under study. In this approach, definitions of concepts and constructs are not necessarily set before a study is initiated; rather, definitions emerge from the data collection and analytical processes. In many of the orientations of naturalistic research, the aim is to "ground" or link concepts and constructs to each observation or datum. This theory-method link,[16] or grounded-theory approach, is described in a classic work by Glaser and Strauss in this way:

> *Generating a theory from data means that most hypotheses and concepts not only come from the data, but are systematically worked out in relation to the data during the course of the research. Generating a theory involves a process of research.*[20]

As discussed later in this text, each strategy classified as naturalistic inquiry is based on a different set of assumptions about how we come to know human experience. However, all researchers in the naturalistic tradition tend to use qualitative methodologies to ground theory in observations. That is, definitions of concepts and then constructs emerge from the investigative process and analysis of the documentation (the data) of shared experience. On the basis of emergent concepts and their relationships, the investigator develops theory to understand,

TABLE 7-1 Exemplar Theories used in Health and Human Service Research

Theory	Brief Explanation of Model	Potential Hypotheses Testing the Theory
1. Health Belief Model[21]	People will be motivated to avoid a health threat if they believe they are at risk (*perceived susceptibility*) for the disease/condition and if they deem it serious (*perceived severity*). These two necessary conditions—perceived susceptibility and perceived severity—converge to describe *perceived threat*, the central construct of HBM. Perceived threat is also influenced by *cues to action*, which are environmental stimuli such as advertising campaigns and relatives who have the disease; cues to action extend this individual-level theory into an ecological perspective. An individual's decision to engage in health behaviors is further influenced by the counterbalance between *perceived barriers* and *perceived benefits*. All of these factors, moderated by demographic characteristics, comprise the HBM. In 1988, Rosenstock and colleagues[28] added to the model an additional construct—*self-efficacy*—to capture individual perceptions of confidence to perform a behavior.	In 12 months, the incident cases of sexually transmitted diseases (STDs) among teenagers in New York City will decrease by 10% if an advertising campaign is launched that includes messages of empowerment and also emphasizes that teenagers are at elevated risk for STDs and that STDs carry pernicious health consequences. Further, health departments must increase access to free condoms and describe the potential health benefits derived from contraceptives.
2. Protection Motivation Theory[22]	According to PMT, three central and necessary components of a fear appeal include: (1) *magnitude of noxiousness*; (2) *probability of occurrence*; and (3) *efficacy of recommended response*. Cognitive processes are crucial in that they mediate the relationship between fear appeal and attitude change.	Among patients enrolled in a randomized controlled trial testing the efficacy of prescription XYZ in managing high blood pressure, treatment adherence will be poor (i.e., below 70%) if participants do not believe that high blood pressure will lead to any deleterious health outcomes (e.g., congestive heart failure).
3. Health Action Process Approach[23]	Theorizes that *intention to change* is the most potent predictor of whether an individual will actually change his or her undesirable behavior to a more desirable one. Within this framework, HAPA proposes two stages of motivation: (1) *preintentional motivation*; and (2) *postintentional volition*. Preintentional processes (e.g., outcome expectancies, risk perception, action self-efficacy) result in the emergence of intention, whereas postintentional processes (e.g., maintenance self-efficacy, planning) result in the actual behavior being enacted.	Men and women will be more likely to quit drinking if they are not only aware of the potential negative health risks such as liver cirrhosis and believe in their ability to quit, but also have a detailed plan on when and how they will quit and if they feel they can self-regulate if they get a craving or see others drink.
4. Theory of Reasoned Action[24]	An individual will engage in a health behavior if he or she has the *intention* to do so. Intention is composed of two main elements, *attitudes* and *subjective norms*. Attitudes are operationalized as the belief that one's behavior will result in positive health outcomes (*behavioral beliefs*) and is also dependent on the degree to which one values these positive health outcomes (*evaluation*). Subjective norms are operationalized as the appraisal of whether others will approve or disapprove of one's behavior (*normative beliefs*) and whether or not the individual is affected by these normative beliefs (*motivation to comply*).	Motivational Interviewing will be efficacious in promoting daily exercise among men with osteoporosis if participants want a reduction in pain and if they believe exercise will lead to a reduction in pain; further, effect sizes will be largest if participants' family members and friends whose opinions are valued are solicited to help implement and maintain health-promoting behaviors (i.e., exercise).
5. Theory of Planned Behavior[25]	TPB is incremental to TRA with the addition of the construct *perceived behavioral control*. Perceived behavioral control is conceptualized as the degree to which an individual perceives a specific behavior as either easy or difficult to enact.	Building off of the example above, patients with osteoporosis may have functional limitations, so an efficacious Motivational Interviewing intervention must also increase one's self-efficacy, demonstrating that even simple exercises within the participant's capabilities may have the power to increase well-being.

TABLE 7-1 *Exemplar Theories used in Health and Human Service Research–Cont'd*

Theory	Brief Explanation of Model	Potential Hypotheses Testing the Theory
6. Life-Span Theory of Control[26] 7. Motivational Theory of Life-Span Development[27]	This theory suggests that threats to or actual losses in the ability to control important outcomes such as performing self-care may activate individuals to use strategies to buffer threats and losses. Strategies are categorized as primary behaviorally oriented control or secondary cognitive-oriented control strategies. To the extent that control-oriented behavioral and cognitive strategies are used that are directed toward attaining health or functional goals, threats to or actual losses of control may be minimized and positive affect and health enhanced or achieved.	Greater use of compensatory control strategies (e.g., seeking help from others) mediates the relationship between greater functional limitations and decreased caregiver burden.

explain, and give meaning to social and behavioral patterns.

Although each design structure describes this process somewhat differently, Figure 7-1 illustrates the basic idea of the inductive process.

In some naturalistic inquiries, theory is used much as in experimental-type research. Once immersed in observations, the investigator frequently draws on well-established theories to explain these observations and make sense of what is being observed. Consider how the previous discussion of attribution error might provide the ethnographer with an understanding of cultural views of sexual trafficking of women with physical impairments. In the process of observing how groups perceive, describe, and respond to victims of trafficking, the ethnographer may be reminded of attribution error theory that seems to fit with the data set. Thus, the theory is applied to the data set as an explanatory mechanism. However, the use of theory in this example occurs after the data have been collected and analyzed. When an investigator is proceeding inductively, theory does not guide data collection and is not imposed on the data; rather, the data may suggest which theory, if any, might be relevant to understanding and explaining observations.

This is not to say that naturalistic inquiry is atheoretical. Theory use, however, has a different function than in experimental-type research. All research begins from a particular theoretical framework based on assumptions of human experiences and realities and how we can come to know them. This theoretical framework is not substantive or content specific, but is structural and process oriented and frames the research approach assumed by the investigator.

Theory can be used in naturalistic inquiry in many ways. One way is that the researcher may begin a study by using a substantive theoretical framework to explore its particular meaning for a specific group of people or in specified situations. For example, an investigator might examine how individuals with mobility impairments adapt to their physical changes to achieve control in their environment and the meaning of control for this group. In this case, as in most naturalistic traditions, the function of the substantive theory is to place boundaries on the inquiry rather than fit the data into the theoretical framework by reducing concepts to predefined measures.

Alternatively, one or more theories may be used to explain emerging themes or to understand observations. Finally, the purpose of a naturalistic study may be to generate a theory of a particular human behavior or health problem. Theory generation serves primarily to reveal the multiple meanings and subjective understandings of the phenomena under study. In this process of theory construction, knowledge emerges from informants or study participants with concepts and constructs grounded in observations. Revisit Gilligan's work for an illustration. She conducted open-ended interviews with women and girls to inductively develop a theory of "female" moral reasoning.[11] In the global context, naturalistic research is increasingly used to generate theory about geographies and cultures that have not

BOX 7-3 *Five Characteristics of Theory in Naturalistic Inquiry*

1. Inductive and abductive processes
2. Primarily generates theory
3. Movement from shared experience to higher levels of abstraction
4. Assumes discovery of meaning through multiple subjective understandings
5. Focus on depicting complexity

TABLE 7-2 *Use of Theory Among the Three Research Traditions: Experimental-Type, Naturalistic, Mixed Methods*

Deductive	Inductive and Abductive	Mixed Methods
Theory testing	Theory validating	Both
Decrease level of abstraction	Increase level of abstraction	Both

been studied. Naturalistic theory building ensures that the theory emerges from what is observed rather than being imposed where it may not be accurate.

Box 7-3 summarizes the basic characteristics of the use of theory in naturalistic inquiry. As we illustrate, the treatment of theory occurs primarily within inductive and abductive processes that move from shared experience to higher levels of abstraction.

Theory Use in Mixed Methods

As you may have surmised by now, theory use in mixed methods can occur in many ways. It may be that the researcher starts with a hypothesis that when tested is unsupported. In this case the researcher may turn to inductive theory building to develop an accurate understanding of what was not revealed in logico-deductive research. Or, even in the presence of existing theory, a researcher may think that it is not sufficiently expansive to explain a diverse set of groups. If a researcher begins by developing a theory through naturalistic inquiry, testing it using experimental designs would be indicated.

> Consider this example. Achey[13] is planning to test the hypotheses presented earlier in her study of attribution error creating barriers for women with physical impairments to be included in research and services. However, she also plans to expand on the nature of the beliefs and myths by conducting a mixed method study. If she understands both the magnitude of attribution error and then the content of it, she is well positioned to develop an educational intervention for preservice health professional students. •

Table 7-2 presents an overview of the use of theory in experimental-type, naturalistic, and mixed method research traditions.

Summary

In this chapter, we have discussed the following five major points:

1. Theory is fundamental to the research process. Although one can count, one cannot do any type of research without having a theoretical framework.
2. Theory consists of four basic components that reflect different levels of abstraction. These levels are concepts, constructs, relationships, and propositions (principles).
3. The level at which a theory is developed and its appropriateness to the phenomenon under study determine in part the nature and structure of research design.
4. Experimental-type research moves from greater to lesser levels of abstraction by reducing theory to specific hypotheses and operationalizing concepts to observe and measure as a way of testing the theory.
5. Naturalistic inquiry moves from less abstraction to more abstraction by grounding or linking theory to each datum that is observed or recorded in the process of conducting research.

EXERCISES

1. Select an experimental-type article and determine the level of abstraction presented in the literature

review. Identify all parts of the theory that are presented in the article.

2. In the same article, search for the important constructs (those that have been subjected to measurement), find their lexical definitions, and determine how the authors have operationalized them.

3. Select a naturalistic article and examine the use of theory in the study. What level of abstraction is developed in the article?

4. Select a mixed method study and examine the use of theory. What levels of abstraction are present in the article and how did mixed methods treat these abstracts?

5. Compare how theory is used in each article. How are they similar? How do they differ?

References

1. Corveleyn J, Luyten P, Blatt S, et al: *The theory and treatment of depression*, New York, 2005, Routledge.

2. Smith M: *Kurt Lewin: groups, experiential learning and action research*, 2001. <http://infed.org/mobi/kurt-lewin-groups-experiential-learning-and-action-research>.

3. Ahmad W, Sheldon T: Race and statistics. In Hammersley M, editor: *Social research: philosophy, politics and practice*, Newbury Park, Calif, 1992, Sage, p 30.

4. Ashcroft B, Griffiths G, Tiffin H: *Post-colonial studies: the key concepts*, New York, 2013, Routledge.

5. Corvellas H: *What is theory? Answers from the social and cultural sciences*, Copenhagen, 2013, Copenhagen Business School Press.

6. Kerlinger FN: *Foundations of behavioral research*, ed 2, New York, 1973, Holt, Rinehart & Winston.

7. Tavory I, Timmermans S: *Abductive analysis: theorizing qualitative research*, Chicago, 2014, University of Chicago Press.

8. Wilson J: *Thinking with concepts*, Cambridge, Mass, 1966, Cambridge University Press.

9. Pernambuco CS, Rodrigues BM, Bezerra JC, et al: Quality of life, elderly and physical activity. *Health* 4:2013. Available at: <http://dx.doi.org/10.4236/health.2012.42014>.

10. Kohlberg L: *The psychology of moral development*, New York, 1984, Harper & Row, p 6.

11. Gilligan C: *In a different voice*, Cambridge, Mass, 1993, Harvard University Pres.

12. *International classification of functioning, disability, and health*, Geneva, 2014, World Health Organization. Available at: <http://www.who.int/classifications/icf/en>.

13. Achey N: *Fundamental attribution error as a disability abuse framework*, Dissertation proposal, 2014.

14. Kim E: Asexuality in disability narratives. *Sexualities* 14:479–493, 2011.

15. Plummer SB, Findley PA: Women with disabilities' experience with physical and sexual abuse: review of the literature and implications for the field. *Trauma Violence Abuse* 13:15–29, 2012.

16. Binstock R, George L: *Handbook of aging and the social sciences*, London, 2011, Elsevier.

17. Heckhausen J, Wrosch C, Schulz R: A motivational theory of life-span development. *Psychol Res* 117:32–60, 2010.

18. DePoy EG, Gilson SF: *Human behavior theory and applications: a critical thinking approach*, Thousand Oaks, Calif, 2012, Sage.

19. Heckhausen J, Schulz R: A life-span theory of control. *Psychol Rev* 102:284–304, 1995.

20. Glaser B, Strauss A: *The discovery of grounded theory: strategies for qualitative research*, New York, 1967, Aldine.

21. Rosenstock IM: The health belief model and preventive health behavior. *Health Edu Behav* 2:354–386, 1974.

22. Rogers RW: A protection motivation theory of fear appeals and attitude change. *J Psychol* 9:93–114, 1975.

23. Schwarzer R: Modeling health behavior change: How to predict and modify the adoption and maintenance of health behaviors. *Applied Psychol* 57:1–29, 2008.

24. Ajzen I, Fishbein M: *Understanding attitudes and predicting social behavior*, Englewood Cliffs, NJ, 1980, Prentice-Hall.

25. Ajzen I, Madden TJ: Prediction of goal-directed behavior: attitudes, intentions, and perceived behavioral control. *J Experiment Soc Psychol* 22:453–474, 1986.

26. Heckhausen J, Schulz R: A life-span theory of control. *Psycholog Rev* 102:284–304, 1995.

27. Heckhausen J, Wrosch C, Schulz R: A motivational theory of life-span development. *Psychol Rev* 117:32–60, 2010.

28. Rosenstock IM, Strecher VJ, Becker MH: Social learning theory and the health belief model. *Health Edu Behav* 15:175–183, 1988.

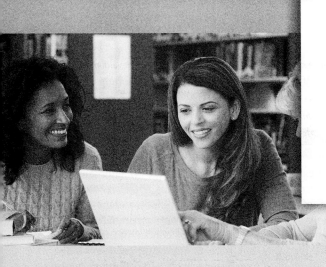

Chapter 8
Formulating Research Questions and Queries

Up until now you have learned about specific thinking and some action processes, such as the role of theory in research (Chapter 7), ways to identify and frame research problems (Chapter 5), and the purpose of and methods for conducting the literature review (Chapter 6). All of these processes are part of the important work of refining the structure and content of any type of inquiry. Now you are ready to move beyond these initial starting blocks as we examine how to develop specific questions within the experimental-type tradition and queries within the naturalistic tradition. Developing a *question* or *query* represents the first formal point of entry into a study.

We have just used two distinct terms, "question" and "query," to describe these initial formal points of entry into a study. These terms reflect the different approaches to research used in each tradition and in mixed methods. Your research question or query will guide all other subsequent steps and decisions, such as how you collect information and what other types of procedures you will follow.

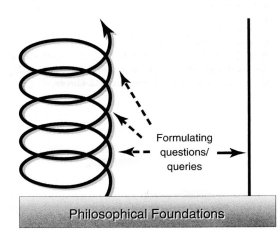

Formulating questions/ queries

Philosophical Foundations

Questions in Experimental-Type Design

In experimental-type research, entry into an investigation requires the formulation of a very specific question with a prescribed structure. That is, from a broad topic of interest, you narrow your scope to articulate a specific question that will guide the conduct of the investigation. This question must be concise and focused. It establishes the boundaries or limits framing the concepts, individuals, or phenomena to be examined in the study. The question also must be posed a priori, or before engaging in the research process, because it becomes the foundation or basis from which all subsequent research action processes are developed and implemented and by which the rigor of the design is determined. As discussed in other chapters, rigor in experimental-type design basically determines the worth of a study based on the degree to which the design answers the research questions in a stable manner. So, without an articulated research question, design rigor is the guess of the reader, because the exact question being answered has to be assumed or extrapolated from narrative about research aims and so forth. We therefore encourage you to identify and carefully articulate your research questions so that your reader does not have to be a soothsayer.

The purpose of the research question in the experimental-type tradition is to articulate not only the concepts that will be studied, but also their structure and scope, and to define the set of boundaries. The research question leads the investigator to highly specified design and data collection action processes that involve a form of observation or measurement to answer the question as it is specified. Research questions are developed deductively from the theoretical principles that exist and are presented in the literature.

Each type of question reflects a different level of knowledge and theory development concerning the topic of interest. Questions that seek to describe a phenomenon, referred to as Level 1 questions, are asked when little to nothing is empirically known about the topic. Level 2 questions explore relationships among phenomena and are asked when descriptive knowledge is known and formally articulated, but relationships are not yet understood. Level 3 questions test existing theory or models and are asked when a substantial body of knowledge is known and well-defined theory is developed.

Level 1: Questions That Seek to Describe Phenomena

Questions that aim to describe phenomena are referred to as Level 1 questions. Level 1 questions are *descriptive questions* designed to elicit descriptions of a single topic or a single population about which there is theoretical or conceptual material in the literature but little or no empirical knowledge. This level of questioning leads to exploratory action processes with the intent to precisely describe an identified and defined phenomenon.

Return to the mobility device example discussed in Chapter 4. Suppose you are a therapist working in a rehabilitation center. One of your responsibilities is to introduce clients to a range of adaptive mobility equipment that clients may need or may find useful at home. You notice, however, that some of your older clients appear hesitant to use this equipment, and you are not convinced that they will continue to use the issued assistive devices once they are home. Because this has important practice, policy, and cost implications, you and your department consider this concern important enough to investigate.

Your first step is to conduct a comprehensive literature review. You might start with a keyword search, such as "adaptive equipment," "assistive mobility devices," and "rehabilitation." Although some literature has been developed over the past several years,[1,2] it is not yet adequate in its development to explain patterns of use and nonuse, particularly among elders discharged from rehabilitation services. Because of the minimal literature development on abandonment, you decide that the first step is to design a Level 1 study to describe patterns of equipment use in the home after rehabilitation and to identify reasons for use and nonuse among clinical populations, such as older people with recent strokes or hip fractures, who would benefit from the use of equipment over time. Your initial Level 1 research questions are:

1. What is the frequency of use of adaptive mobility devices by older individuals who have been diagnosed

with strokes and discharged to their home following rehabilitation?

2. What are the reasons for use and nonuse of assistive mobility devices by this population at 3, 6, and 9 months after discharge?

Now suppose you were interested in advancing higher educational opportunities for students with diverse sensory impairments in graduate health career education. Although a body of knowledge exists regarding the attitudes of occupational therapy faculty toward including students with disabling conditions in occupational therapy education, little is known about the attitudes of other public health faculty toward including this student population in graduate education. Therefore, research based on a Level 1 question will be meaningful and appropriate to describe the attitudes of public health faculty toward accepting and teaching students with diverse impairments in their graduate classes. Level 1 questions focus on a description of one concept or variable in a population. To describe a variable, which can be defined as a characteristic or phenomenon that has more than one value, you first derive a lexical definition of the concept from the literature and operationalize or define it in such a way as to permit its measurement. Thus, Level 1 questions focus on measuring the nature and/or magnitude of a particular phenomenon in the population of interest.

In response to the changing context of practice, a study conducted by Hoppes and Hellman[3] examined the attitudes of occupational therapy students toward community practice. Although there was a growing body of literature on the need to educate students for community practice, Hoppes and Hellman were concerned that "students' voices have seldom been heard in the discussion about assimilating community engagement into occupational therapy education." To inform progressive occupational therapy education that would be meaningful to students, these investigators initiated a descriptive study to answer the following research questions:

1. Do students believe there are specific actions they can take to address community needs?
2. Do students feel a moral obligation to help in their communities?

BOX 8-1 *Level 1: Descriptive Research Questions*

1. What are the most commonly applied for assistive devices in an elder population of Swedish residents who apply for grants for these devices?
'2. For elders with depressive symptoms, to what extent do impairment, functional status, and severity of depressive symptoms change over 3 years?
3. What is the incidence of a history of family problems in the area of substance use, psychopathology, compulsive disorders, and violence? To what extent are there significant differences in student histories of family problems by age, gender, or race/ethnicity?

---

3. How do students perceive the costs and benefits of helping in their communities?
4. To what extent are students aware that needs exist in their communities?

To answer these questions, the investigators identified specific items on the Community Service Attitudes Survey that measured each of the variables named in the four Level 1 questions (actions to address community needs; moral obligation to help communities; perceived costs and benefits of community helping; and awareness of needs in communities). Occupational therapy students were named as their population of interest. Box 8-1 presents additional examples of Level 1 questions. Note that they answered the questions "what?" and "how much?" (As we discuss later, the wording of the first two questions posed by Hoppes and Hellman, although seen frequently in this type of lexicon, is not correct for experimental-type questions.)

As you can see, the focus of a Level 1 question is on "what," "how," and "how much." Level 1 questions focus on the description of one concept or variable in a defined population. A variable is defined as a characteristic or phenomenon that has more than one value. To describe a variable, you first derive a lexical definition of the concept (description of the term in words) from the literature and then operationalize it (define a concept by how it will be measured). For example, suppose you were interested in understanding the degree of skill in computer use in a population of well adults over the age of 85. The variable would be skill in computer use. You would therefore consult the literature to find a fitting lexical definition of skill in computer use and then operationalize it so that numbers could be used as descriptive of skill.

We indicated earlier that the questions posed by Hoppes and Hellman[3] were not phrased correctly. That is because research questions in experimental design cannot have yes or no answers but must allow for a range of options, even if the findings result in absence or presence. Level 1 questions therefore focus on measuring the nature of a particular phenomenon in the population of interest. The following stems are frequently used in these questions: "What is the extent of" or "How is," followed by the variable and the one population of interest. As shown in the examples, only one population is identified. Notice that these stems all provide for a larger range than yes or no responses. Also, single concepts are examined in each study, such as assistive devices, functional status, computer skill, and family disorders. Each of these concepts can be defined so as to permit their measurement—that is, they can be examined empirically.

Level 1 questions describe the parts of the whole. Remember, the underlying thinking process for experimental-type research is to learn about a topic by examining its parts and their relationships. Level 1 questioning is the foundation for clarifying the presence of parts, their magnitude, and/or their specific nature. In the scheme of levels of abstraction, Level 1 questions target the lowest levels of abstraction: concepts and constructs (see Chapter 7).

As discussed in later chapters, Level 1 questions lead to the development of descriptive designs, such as surveys, exploratory or descriptive studies, trend designs, feasibility studies, need assessments, and case studies.

Level 2: Questions That Explore Relationships Among Phenomena

The Level 2 *relational questions* build on and refine the results of Level 1 studies. Once a "part" of a phenomenon is described and there is existing knowledge about it in the context of a particular

population, the experimental-type researcher may pose questions that are relational. Level 2 reflects relational questions and builds on and refines the results of Level 1 studies. The key purpose of Level 2 questioning is to explore relationships among phenomena that have already been identified and described. Here the stem question asks, "What is the relationship?" or a variation of this (e.g., "association"), and the topic contains two or more concepts or variables. "What is the relationship between exercise capacity and cardiovascular health in middle-aged men?" In this case, the two identified variables to be measured are exercise capacity and cardiovascular health. The specific population is middle-aged men. As you can surmise, Level 1 research must have been accomplished for the two variables to be defined and operationalized.

> Suppose you are involved in establishing exercise programs for adults as part of their cardiac care. Although you know there is much evidence to support the cardiovascular benefits of aerobic exercise in general, you do not know much about the exercise capacity of middle-aged men, and this group has become your primary clinical population. Thus, you may be interested in asking a Level 2 question such as, "What is the relationship between exercise capacity and cardiovascular health in middle-aged men?" In this case, the two identified variables that are measured are exercise capacity and cardiovascular health. The specific population is middle-aged men. As you can surmise, Level 1 research must have been accomplished for the two variables to be identified, defined, and operationalized. •

Returning to the example of attitudes of public health faculty, suppose we now want to know the relationship between attitudes and numbers of students admitted into public health majors. We would pose a Level 2 question such as, "What is the relationship between faculty attitudes and number of public health majors with mobility impairments?" This Level 2 question would lead us to measure and look at the association between two variables, attitudes and number of majors admitted to public health programs. Suppose we found that negative attitudes were related to low numbers of public health majors

---

BOX 8-2 *Level 2: Relational-Type Questions*

1. What is the relationship among use of assistive devices, living arrangements, and level of difficulty performing activities of daily living in a sample of applicants to a home modification program?
2. What is the relationship among depressive symptoms, impairment status, functional status, and use of assistive devices?
3. To what extent are there differences in student histories of family problems by age, gender, or race/ethnicity?

---

with mobility impairments. We would be able to claim an association but not a causal relationship between the two variables.

Let us revisit the Level 1 examples and see how they can be modified to become Level 2 questions. Suppose we have conducted studies to address the Level 1 questions in Box 8-1. If we continue our research agenda in each of these areas of inquiry, we would be ready for the relational questions in Box 8-2.

Level 2 questions address relationships between variables. Studies with this level of questioning represent the next level of complexity above Level 1 questions. These questions continue to build on knowledge in the experimental-type framework by examining their parts, their relationships, and the nature and direction of these relationships. Level 2 questions primarily lead to research that uses passive observation design, as discussed later in the text. Refer to the levels of abstraction in Chapter 7 and see where Level 2 questions fit in the schema of building theory and knowledge in the experimental tradition.

Level 3: Questions That Test Knowledge

Level 3 questioning builds on the knowledge generated from research conducted in Level 1 and Level 2 investigations. A Level 3 question asks about a cause-and-effect relationship among two or more variables, with the specific purpose of testing knowledge or the theory underpinning the knowledge. We

refer to this level inquiry as a *predictive question.* Given the findings of the Level 2 question, it would be important to know whether attitudes are causal of barriers to public health education for students with mobility impairments. A Level 3 question would therefore be indicated. Building on the knowledge already generated, we now would be able to ask the following question: "To what extent do faculty attitudes have an influence on the number of students with mobility impairments who are accepted into public health majors?" The resultant study will test the theoretical foundation proposing that negative attitudes create educational barriers and exclusion of otherwise qualified students, and the study will be able to predict the opportunity for these students to be accepted into public health majors on the basis of faculty attitudes. At this level of questioning, the purpose is to predict what will happen and provide a theory to explain the reason(s). On the basis of a Level 3 question, specific *predictive hypotheses*, statements predicting the outcome of one variable on the basis of knowing another, are formulated. Action based on this knowledge can be taken to promote educational opportunity if you know where, why, and how to intervene.

At Level 2, we asked the question, "What is the relationship among the attitudes of occupational therapy faculty and the number of students with disabilities admitted into occupational therapy education programs?" Assume that in conducting this relational-type study, we find an association between faculty attitudes and number of students with disabilities. That is, our study shows that programs in which the occupational therapy educators have positive attitudes tend to have a higher enrollment of students with disabilities than programs with faculty having negative attitudes. Building on this knowledge, you can now ask a Level 3 question such as the following: "To what extent do faculty attitudes influence the number of students with disabilities who are accepted into occupational therapy programs?" Such a study would test the theory underpinning the reasons that positive attitudes promote opportunity for students with disabilities. Also, the study would be able to predict the opportunity for disabled students to be accepted into occupational therapy programs on the basis of faculty attitudes. •

In a Level 3 question, it is already established that two concepts are related, based on previous research findings (from Level 2 research). The point of study at Level 3 is to test these concepts in action by manipulating one to affect the other. Level 3 is the most complex of experimental-type questioning. Once the foundation questions formulated at Levels 1 and 2 are answered, Level 3 questions can be posed and answered to develop knowledge—not only of parts and their relationships, but of how and why these parts interact to cause a particular outcome. Level 3 questions examine higher levels of abstraction, including principles, theories, and models.

Consider these examples of possible questions:

1. In a population of adults with mobility impairments, what age, geographic, and device appearance characteristics predict acceptance and use of adaptive mobility devices for safe engagement in regular fitness activity?
2. To what extent do age and previous experience with using a computer predict willingness to use a mobile tablet for communicating with friends and family in a population of rural adults who cannot drive?

Knowledge generated from these types of Level 3 studies would provide guidance for safe participation in fitness activity for individuals with mobility impairments and for promoting virtual communication for rural individuals who do not drive.

Now consider another type of Level 3 question.

> 🔍 For the past 15 years of research on family caregiving, many Level 1 studies have described the experience of caregiving by families of children and older adults with a wide range of physical and cognitive impairments. Also, on the basis of Level 1 findings, there is a rich body of knowledge at Level 2. For example, numerous studies show that women and spouses tend to show more distress and burden with caregiving than other family members. Given the knowledge of stress associated with caregiving and different relational patterns that have emerged, more recent research has tested the Level 3 type of questions. These studies, using basic stress theories, have sought to predict caregiving outcomes over time and to test specific theory-based interventions to alleviate the burden associated with the role of caregiver. Such Level 3 questions include the following:
>
> To what extent does a home-based skills-training intervention improve communication patterns between children with physical impairments and their mothers?
> To what extent does participation in a virtual support group reduce emotional burdens among women caring for family members with dementia?

To answer a Level 3 question, research action processes capable of revealing causal relationships among variables must be implemented. A true experimental design or a variation would need to be conducted.

Now consider the following example:

> 🔍 Suppose you are working in a middle school and are asked to develop a program to reduce and prevent obesity. Because of the popularity of smartphones in this age group, your program involves providing a free mobile app and wireless sensing device for wirelessly tracking and recording level of physical activity for youth who enroll in a regular, supervised sports and fitness program. You begin by selecting the children at highest risk for obesity: those who are already overweight. You implement an experimental program for children between the ages of 11 and 15 who meet the weight criterion for being overweight but not obese. To ascertain the success and viability of expanding the program to all children, you now want to know whether the experimental program met the aims of reducing weight and increasing fitness. You pose the following question:
>
> To what extent does participation in the experimental intervention predict fitness improvement and weight loss in overweight youth between the ages of 11 and 15?
>
> To answer your question, you would randomly select and assign your sample (we discuss sampling in Chapter 14) and introduce the experimental condition—the intervention—to one group and not the other. You then compare each group on a measure of exercise participation. •

TABLE 8-1		Questions at Three Levels in Experimental-Type Research	
Level	Stem	Level of Abstraction	Design Possibilities
1	What is ...?	Concepts and constructs	Survey
	What are ...?		Exploratory Descriptive Case study Needs assessment
2	What is the relationship ...?	Relationships	Survey
			Correlational, passive
			Observation
			Ex post facto
3	Why ...?	Principles Theories	Experimental designs Quasi-experimental designs
		Models	

BOX 8-3 Helpful Rules in Developing a Research Question

1. At Level 1, examine a variable in one population.
2. At Level 2, examine the relationship between a minimum of two variables.
3. If there is a cause or effect to be investigated, pose the question at Level 3.
4. If the words "cause," "effect," or any of their synonyms appear in the question, eliminate these words, or specify what they are and how they vary.
5. All variables must be written so that they vary.
6. At Level 3, there must be two variables that specify a cause and effect.
7. If a Level 3 question is written, make sure it is both ethical and possible to manipulate the causal variable. If not, rewrite the question at Level 2.

Data from Brink PJ, Wood MJ: *Basic steps in planning nursing research: from question to proposal*, ed 7, Boston, 2011, Jones & Bartlett.

Developing Experimental-Type Research Questions

As you see, question formulation for experimental-type research is relatively straightforward. You can refer to Table 8-1 as a basic guide in helping you develop research questions at the three levels. Also, Box 8-3 provides helpful rules for developing questions at the appropriate level.

Keep in mind that one challenge in developing an experimental-type research question, particularly for new researchers, is proposing a question that is (1) very specific, (2) not too broad, and (3) feasible to study. One tendency is to develop a question that is too "big." If your question can be broken down into subquestions, you know you have not yet developed an appropriate research question.

Hypotheses

As discussed in previous chapters, experimental-type researchers frequently engage in studies that involve *hypotheses*. A classic definition of hypothesis is "a proposition to be tested or a tentative statement of a relationship between two variables."[4]

As the definition implies, hypotheses are primarily necessary and developed for Level 2 and Level 3

questions. For a Level 1 question, the experimental-type researcher usually has a "hunch" about the expected distribution of a single variable; however, a statement about a single variable is not a hypothesis. By definition, a Level 1 question does not have the essential elements of at least two variables and a statement of expected relationship.

Although a hypothesis is a researcher's best hunch about a phenomenon, this "guess" does not emerge from thin air. Rather, it must be based on existing literature and theory and must stem from the research question guiding the study.

Hypotheses serve important purposes in experimental-type research. First, they form an important link between the research question and the design of the study. In essence, hypotheses rephrase the research question and turn it into a testable or measurable statement. Second, hypotheses may identify the anticipated direction of the proposed relationship between stated variables. Information regarding directionality of a relationship between variables is usually not contained in the actual research question.

There are two types of hypotheses, nondirectional and directional. *Nondirectional hypotheses* post a relationship or prediction but do not give you more information. *Directional hypotheses*, as indicated by the name, not only propose a relationship or prediction, but posit the way in which variables are related. As an example, in formulating a hypothesis on the causal relationship between faculty attitudes and educational opportunity in public health majors, we might state a nondirectional hypotheses such as:

Faculty attitudes are related to low admission rates.

A directional hypotheses might look like:

Negative faculty attitudes are associated with lower admission rates for students with mobility impairments in public health curricula.

Consider this research question: "What is the relationship between the attitudes of occupational therapy faculty and the number of students with disabilities admitted into occupational therapy education programs?" In this study, the investigator may hypothesize that there will be an association between faculty attitudes toward inclusion and the number of students with disabilities admitted into programs. However, the direction of this expectation is not stated. If the investigator formulates a directional hypothesis, it may appear as follows: "It is hypothesized that positive faculty attitudes will be associated with a greater number of admissions of students with disabilities." •

Notice that this statement does not suggest or state an expected cause but rather states a direction in a proposed relationship.

Now consider the hypothesis for the following Level 3 question: "To what extent do faculty attitudes influence the number of students with disabilities who are accepted into occupational therapy programs?" The researcher is interested in predicting admission rates as a result of faculty attitudes. The researcher may structure a project in which programs and faculty with positive attitudes are compared with programs and faculty with unfavorable attitudes. If other variables are controlled and a design is developed in which causal relationships are ascertained, the following hypothesis may be stated:

There will be a significant difference in admission rates between programs with and programs without positive faculty attitudes toward inclusion of students with disabilities.

Based on a literature review and prior empirical findings, the researcher may choose to state the directional hypothesis as follows:

There will be significantly fewer students admitted to programs with unfavorable faculty attitudes than to programs with favorable faculty attitudes toward inclusion. •

A third and critical purpose of hypotheses is that these purposefully constructed statements "set the stage" for the type of statistical analyses that will be used. We discuss these logical thinking processes and actions later in the book.

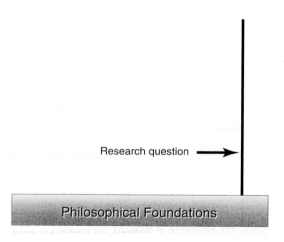

Table 8-2 provides examples of hypotheses for each type of experimental-type research question.

Research Queries in Naturalistic Inquiry

Now we turn to a completely different approach to formulating research. In naturalistic inquiry, formal entry into a study requires the initial development of a broad query. Although various philosophical perspectives inform inquiry within naturalistic research, as previously discussed, and although the task of framing the problem and query are somewhat differ-

TABLE 8-2   *Examples of Hypotheses by Level of Question*

Level	Question	Nondirectional/Hypothesis	Directional Hypothesis
1	What is the pattern of use and reasons for nonuse of mobility aids among elders with mobility impairments?	No hypothesis is possible.	Expected distribution: older adults with mobility impairments will use mobility aids with high frequency.
2	What is the relationship between the attitudes of faculty toward disability and the actual number of admissions of students with disabilities?	There will be an association between attitudes and the number of student admissions.	Positive faculty attitude will be associated with a greater number of admissions of students with disabilities.
2	What is the relationship between gender and depression in spousal caregivers of elders with physical disabilities?	The level of depression in female spouses will be different from the level of depression in male spouses.	Female spouse caregivers will be more depressed than male spouse caregivers.
3	To what extent do faculty attitudes influence the number of students with disabilities who are accepted in occupational therapy programs?	There will be a significant difference in admission rates between programs with and programs without positive faculty attitudes toward inclusion.	Significantly fewer students are admitted to programs with faculty who have unfavorable attitudes than to programs with faculty who have favorable attitudes toward inclusion.

ent among varied approaches, there is some underlying similarity to query development.

Researchers in the naturalistic tradition generally begin by identifying a topic and a broad problem area or specifying a particular phenomenon from which a query is pursued. We thus use "query" to refer to a broad statement that identifies the phenomenon or natural field of interest and to distinguish naturalistic and experimental-type traditions in this action step.

The natural field (which can be physical, conceptual, or even virtual) where the phenomenon occurs

> The phenomenon of interest may refer to symbolic patterns of interaction in a cultural group, the experience of disability, the meaning of pain, or diverse interpretations of material objects such as adaptive equipment. •

forms the basis for discovery, from which more specific and limited questions evolve in the course of conducting the research. Thus, the initial entry into the study is based on a query statement that identifies the phenomenon of interest and the location and population or community that will be the focus. Then, once the study has been initiated and as new insights and meanings are obtained, the first problem statement and query are reformulated. On the basis of new insights and issues that emerge in the field, the investigator formulates smaller, more concise

subquestions that are subsequently pursued. These smaller questions are contextual; that is, they are derived inductively from the context itself and are rooted in the investigator's ongoing efforts to understand the broad problem area. In turn, each smaller question that is posed may lead the investigator to use a different methodological approach. This interactive questioning–data gathering–analyzing–reformulating of the questions and initial query represents a critical and core action process of naturalistic inquiry.

Let us examine the process by which a research query is developed and then reformulated in three qualitative methodological approaches within the naturalistic tradition. As you read on, think about what is common among formulation and reformulation of queries and how these processes differ from experimental-type questioning.

Classic Ethnography

As the primary research approach in anthropology,[5] ethnography is concerned with describing and interpreting cultural patterns of groups and understanding the cultural meanings people use to organize and interpret their experiences and more recently consumption and response to images within visual culture.[6] In this approach, the researcher assumes a "learning role" to interpret and experience different cultural settings and materials.[7] The information gathered bridges the world and culture of the researcher to that of the researched. After the ethnographer has identified a phenomenon and cultural setting, a query is pursued.[8] There is always a strong descriptive element in ethnography, so the ethnographic query implicates what the ethnographer is to describe. You haven't posed an ethnographic question until it is clear what the ethnographer is to look at and to look for at least with sufficient clarity to initiate an inquiry.

In discussing his own experiences, Wolcott[9] stated that the aims of ethnography are contained within the researcher's queries. The researcher is obligated to uphold the highest ethical standards, and to respect and view ethnographic questions as emergent from the context and thus are necessarily often unplanned.

As you can see, experimental-type questions and hypotheses stand in stark contrast to the interpretative-opened, purposive query posed initially by the ethnographer.

As the processes of data gathering and analysis proceed in tandem, specific questions emerge and are pursued. These questions emerge in the field as a consequence of what Agar[10] classically labeled as *breakdowns,* or disjunctions, a concept that we still find useful and central to ethnographic inquiry. "A breakdown is a lack of fit between one's encounter with a tradition and the schema-guided expectation by which one organizes experience."[10] A breakdown represents the difference between what the investigator observes and what he or she expects to observe. These differences stimulate a series of questioning and further investigation. Each subquestion is related to the broader line of query and is investigated to resolve the breakdown and develop a more comprehensive understanding of the phenomenon in its entirety. An ethnographic query therefore establishes the phenomenon, the setting of interest, or both. The query also sets up the thinking and action processes necessary to understand the boundaries of the study and the phenomenon under investigation.

To summarize, once a query has been posed, questioning occurs simultaneously with collecting information and making sense of it. One process drives the other. The interactive questioning, data gathering, and analytical waltz results in the reformulation and refinement of the problem and the structuring of small subquestions. These subquestions are then pursued in the field (defined broadly)

to uncover underlying meanings and cultural patterns.

Health and human service professionals have used ethnographic methods, such as interviewing and participant observation (discussed more fully in subsequent chapters), to examine cultural variations in response to impairment, accessibility, adaptation, health services utilization, health care practices, and other related areas.

> The health or human service professional conducting an ethnography may start with a general query such as, "How is pain expressed differently by men and women?" or "How are individuals with severe impairments able to live independently, and what are their patterns of adaptation to varying degrees of community accessibility?" •

Phenomenology

The purpose of the phenomenological line of inquiry is to uncover the meaning of a human experience or phenomenon typically of more than one individual, through the description of those experiences as they are lived by individuals.[11]

Phemonenology "emphasizes studying empirical phenomena directly, as they are perceived by the senses"[11] and thus does not call for independent interpretation by the investigator. The entry into the context to be studied from this perspective is the identification of the phenomenon of interest.

> For example, pain, resilience, aging in place, wellness, homelessness, and sadness may be phenomena that are relevant to the helping professions. From the articulation of the phenomenon, a research query is generated, such as the following:
>
> 1. What is the meaning of being homeless for middle-aged women?
> 2. What is the meaning of fear for persons with traumatic injury?
> 3. What is the meaning of aging in place to community residents?
> 4. What are the common elements in experiencing a feeling of well-being among poor, rural, elder persons?

This approach is different from ethnography in that phenomenological queries focus on particular experiences (e.g., grief, birth of a child, aging, wellness, divorce, illness, and impairment) from the perspective of the individuals and do not seek to understand group or cultural patterns. However, similar to ethnography, the research begins with a broad query. On the basis of what the investigator learns through the action of conducting the research, subquestions and specific inquiries are developed that further inform the overarching query related to the meaning of experience for the individuals participating in the study.

As example, Vickers used a phenomenological approach to explore the experience of people with multiple sclerosis who have left work.[12] Different from assumptions that loss of health and function from the disease was the primary cause of unemployment, Vickers found that this phenomenon was experienced in diverse ways with diverse meanings beyond the disease process.

Grounded Theory

Grounded theory is a method in naturalistic research that is used primarily to generate theory.[13] The researcher begins with a broad query in a particular topic area and then collects relevant information about the topic. As the action processes of data collection continue, each piece of information is reviewed, compared, and contrasted with other information. From this constant comparison process, commonalities and dissimilarities among categories of information become clear, and ultimately a theory that explains observations is inductively developed. Thus, queries that will be answered through grounded theory do not relate to specific domains but rather to the structure of how the researcher wants to organize the findings (Box 8-4).

As you can see, each query indicates that the research aim is to reveal theoretical principles about the phenomenon under study. Grounded theory can also be used to modify existing theory or to expand on or uncover differences from what is already known. In the two queries in Box 8-5, grounded theory is structured to address current theory from a new and inductive perspective.

BOX 8-4 *Examples of Grounded-Theory Queries That Generate Theory*

- What theoretical principles characterize the experience of women who become homeless?
- What similarities and differences can be revealed among ways in which traumatically injured individuals experience their acute care hospitalization?
- How do Native Americans residing in a rural New England community define and maintain their health?

BOX 8-5 *Examples of Grounded-Theory Queries That Modify Theory*

- How can the current theory of moral development be expanded or modified to explain the moral development of Native American children and adolescents?
- What is the relevance of current theory on career development in white middle-class male children and black middle-class female children?

Narrative

Although there is no single definition of narrative,[12] all have two common elements, storytelling and meaning making. In general, narrative methods are interpretive strategies used in diverse disciplines and fields but are particularly popular in postmodern and post-postmodern studies such as interdisciplinary health care robotics and biological art.[14] Synthesizing the diverse definitions of narrative, we define it as a naturalistic method in which stories are told and inductively analyzed for meaning. Stories can be generated by an individual or group in response to a query or can exist in the form of text or even image. However, regardless of the form, the data must tell a story that can be interpreted. According to Squire,[15] narrative queries are particularly useful when knowledge is not known or is insufficient to describe a phenomenon. Squire also suggests that narrative queries may serve to illuminate difficult phenomena or those not easily discussed. However, regardless of the form or function, the data must tell a story that can be interpreted. Mensinga[16] demonstrated five different approaches to narrative, all of which investigated career choice. Although the studies themselves did not identify specific queries, the initial entry point into each was a broad statement about the evolution of career choice and its meaning to the informants who generated the stories. Life history is a type of narrative in that it tells a story about the chronology of a life and the meaning of events within that life. Queries specific to life history address part or a whole longitudinal life and the events (turnings) within it that shaped decisions and pathways.

Developing Naturalistic Research Queries

Ethnography, phenomenology, and grounded theory reflect distinct approaches in naturalistic inquiry. Queries developed within each methodology and design reflect a different purpose and a preferred way of knowing and are shaped by the particular resources available to the investigator. Nevertheless, underlying each of these approaches is an essential iterative process of query–subquestion–reformulation that is central to the structuring of the research enterprise in naturalistic inquiry.

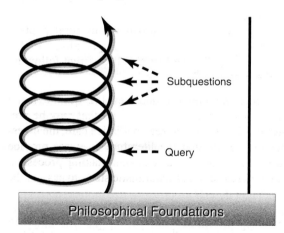

Integrating Research Approaches

Asking questions and posing queries often co-occur in mixed methods. Table 8-3 includes this category in summarizing experimental and naturalistic question/query formulation. As noted, mixed method or integrated designs combine different research

TABLE 8-3	Form and Function of Question/Query Formulation Across Research Traditions		
	Experimental-Type	Naturalistic Inquiry	Mixed Method Design
Form	Focused question	Broad query	Both, or either
Function	Define variables, population, and level of inquiry	Identify phenomena of interest and context	Both, or either

traditions and approaches and, by their nature, may be complex. As such, these designs may rely on the formulation of a query, a question, or both and may order the formulation of these in diverse ways to accomplish the overall research purpose.[17,18]

Consider the following examples to highlight the differences in approach among the experimental-type and naturalistic research traditions and mixed method design.

In determining the extent to which and how the design of a mobility device resolved the problem of abandonment, you conduct a mixed method outcome assessment guided by the following questions and queries:

1. To what extent do elders abandon an aesthetically designed mobility device compared to a typical "medicalized walker" with equivalent functionality?
2. What meanings are perceived by elders regarding the aesthetic design of mobility devices?

Question 1 reflects the structure of an experimental-type level 2 question. Note that it asks for association between abandonment frequency and design by crafting a comparison group approach to inquiry. Question 2 seeks meaning of object, or what we have introduced as object reading.[7]

As shown, integrated designs can be complex. Therefore it is important for you to clearly articulate the specific questions and queries that are posed jointly and to delineate how each contributes to the other.

In your elder study, which the questions above guide, the advantage of a mixed method inquiry is its capacity not only to ascertain use but to delve into the visual world and meanings that prevent elders from following safety practices.

We have already introduced single subject and case study design. Briefly, these inquiries focus on a single unit of analysis that may be studied as holistic or embedded with multiple parts.[19] Single subject and case study research is particularly useful throughout in that it is designed to generate findings as well as theory through collecting and analyzing data through more than one approach. Moreover, because single subject design refers to one phenomenon and does not aim to examine groups and subpopulations within groups (unless a group is framed as a single entity), these mixed method designs are feasible and robust within the daily context of health and human service practice. Single subject design is particularly useful in clinical practice. If you wanted to know how a client was progressing in clinical practice, you might ask the following mixed method question:

What progress does the client feel she is making (query) and how is it exhibited in her mood assessment (Level 1 type question)?

These two forms (question and query) illustrate structured and unstructured questioning characteristic of single subject thinking and action.

Now suppose you want to study socialization of older frail adults who are aging in place. Your purpose is to understand how virtual communication device acceptance affects the psychological well-being of the adults who for the most part remain at home. You pose a specific question, such as, "What is the relationship between computer acceptance, use, and social interaction in a population of frail older adults living in their own homes?" Can you guess which type of question this is? If you guessed Level 2 in the experimental-type tradition, you are correct. This question narrows the area of concern of relationships between use of virtual communication and psychological well-being of frail adults living in their homes. •

Following the implementation of the Affordable Care Act (ACA),[20] a health care research team is interested in studying disparities in access to end-of-life health care among individuals whose income is just above the poverty line. On the basis of the large body of literature on access to health care prior to enactment of the ACA, the researchers conduct a secondary analysis of case data to answer the following Level 1 experimental-type question:

What is the income level of patients in palliative care?

In this study, the investigators find that there is a disproportionate underrepresentation of low-income individuals in palliative care, and they thus set out to investigate why.

Once again, relying on theory and research that has been generated in similar studies conducted before the ACA,[20] the investigators develop a study in which they identify the variables of provider recommendation and geographic diversity that promote or inhibit palliative care and pose the following Level 2 questions:

1. How is provider recommendation related to a family's decision to seek palliative care for a dying family member in a low-income population?
2. What differences in urban versus rural populations exist in decisions to seek palliative care?
3. How are palliative care trends different following the passage of the ACA?

While the Level 1 and Level 2 questions are productive in identifying variables that may be predictive of a decision to seek palliative care, the investigators decide that the literature does not provide sufficient theory about decision-making processes. They therefore plan a naturalistic study to answer the following queries:

1. How do low-income families who now have health insurance through an ACA plan decide to seek palliative care for their loved ones?
2. What experiences and life circumstances are important in decisions to seek or not to seek palliative care?

The investigators in this example initially isolated constructs and variables relevant to their areas of study that favor experimental-type design. The constructs posed in the research question were identified from reading the research literature, from practice experience, or from federal funding initiatives that define the ACA, poverty level, and related health benefits and that suggest geographic differences. Thus, Level 1 and Level 2 questions were appropriate. However, once decision-making processes and experiences became central to the research agenda, the investigators moved to an epistemological framework based in naturalistic tradition. They proceeded inductively, on the basis of a pluralistic framework that proposes multiple decision pathways, experiences, new legislation and benefits, and realities that need to be discovered and understood to derive a comprehensive view of the decision to seek palliative care in the current health care context. Based on an understanding of different realities of and choices to pursue end-of-life options that will emerge in the course of the study, comprehensive guidelines can then be developed and further evaluated.

Summary

There are many ways to frame a research problem. Each approach to problem formulation and query or question development differs according to its research tradition. In experimental-type design, the question drives each subsequent research step. Refinement of a research question occurs before any further action processes can be implemented. Conciseness and clarity are critical to the conduct of the study and are the hallmarks of what makes the research question meaningful and appropriate. Experimental-type questions are definitive, structured, and derived deductively before the researcher engages in specified actions. They all must contain three elements: the variable or variables, the level of questioning, and the population to be studied.

In naturalistic inquiry, the query establishes the initial entrance and boundaries for the study but is reformulated in the actual process of collecting and analyzing data. The researcher fully expects and prepares for new queries and subquestions to emerge in the course of conducting the study. That is, refinement of query and question emerges from the action of conducting the research. The development of specific questions occurs inductively and emerges from

the interaction of the investigator within the field or with the phenomenon of the study. Thus, an initial research question and query have different levels of meaning and implications for the conduct of studies in experimental-type design and naturalistic research. Research queries and subquestions are dynamic, ever changing, and derived inductively.

Integrated studies use the strengths of both experimental-type and naturalistic traditions to pose questions and queries that can reveal, describe, relate, or predict.

EXERCISES

1. To test your understanding of the differences between levels of questioning in experimental-type designs, select a problem area in which you are interested. Frame the problem in terms of Level 1, Level 2, and Level 3 questions.
2. Using the problem area you selected, formulate a broad query to pursue within a naturalistic design.
3. Review your different problem statements and specific queries or questions. Identify the different assumptions that each makes about level of knowledge, preferred way of knowing, and required resources to conduct the study. Use the table below to assist you.
4. Select three research articles in the literature and identify each research question or query. After you have identified them, characterize the nature of each using the table below.

Question/ Query	Assumed Level of Knowledge	Preferred Way of Knowing	Required Resources
1.			
2.			
3.			

References

1. Bateni H, Maki B: Assistive devices for balance and mobility: benefits, demands, and adverse consequences. *Arch Phys Med Rehabil* 86:134–145, 2005.
2. Lauer A, Longenecker Rust K, Smith RO: ATOMS Project Technical Report. Factors in assistive technology device

abandonment: replacing "abandonment" with "discontinuance," *ATOMS*. 2001–2012. http://www.r2d2.uwm.edu/atoms/.

3. Hoppes S, Hellman CM: Understanding occupational therapy students' attitudes, intentions, and behaviors regarding community service. *Am J Occup Ther* 61:527–534, 2007.

4. Neuman WL: *Social research methods: qualitative and quantitative approaches*, ed 7, New York, 2012, Pearson.

5. Agar M *An ethnography by any other name*, 2006. http://www.qualitative-research.net/index.php/fqs/article/view/177/395.

6. Harper D: *Visual sociology*, New York, 2012, Routledge.

7. Candlin F, Guins R: *The object reader*, London, 2009, Routledge.

8. Creswell J: *Qualitative inquiry and research design: choosing among five approaches*, ed 3, Los Angeles, 2013, Sage.

9. Wolcott H: *Ethnography lessons: a primer*, Walnut Creek, Calif, 2010, Left Coast Press.

10. Agar M: *Speaking of ethnography*, Newbury Park, Calif, 1986, Sage, p 21.

11. Bakker H: Phenomenology. In Mills AJ, Durepos G, Wiebe E, editors: *Handbook of case study research*, Thousand Oaks, Calif, 2010, Sage, pp 674–678.

12. Vickers MH: Why people with MS are really leaving work: from a Clayton's choice to an ugly passage. *Rev Disabil Studies Int J* 4:43–57, 2008.

13. Wertz FJ, Charmaz K, McMullen LM, et al: *Five ways of doing qualitative analysis: phenomenological psychology, grounded theory, discourse analysis, narrative research, and intuitive inquiry*, New York, 2011, Guilford Press.

14. Caraballo L, Farman A: *Out of hand: materializing the post-digital*, Museum of Art and Design, New York, October 31, 2013.

15. Squire C: *Narrative research: an interview with Corrine Squire*, Thousand Oaks, Calif, 2013.

16. Mensinga J: Storying career choice: employing narrative approaches to better understand students' experience of choosing social work as a preferred. *Qual Soc Work* 8:193–209, 2009.

17. Creswell J, Plano Clark V: *Designing and conducting mixed methods research*, Los Angeles, 2011, Sage.

18. Tashakorri A, Teddlie C: *Handbook of mixed methods in social and behavioral research*, ed 2, Thousand Oaks, Calif, 2010, Sage.

19. Yin R: *Care study research*, Los Angeles, 2014, Sage.

20. U.S. Department of Health & Human Services: *Affordable Care Act*, April 6, 2014. http://www.hhs.gov/healthcare/rights.

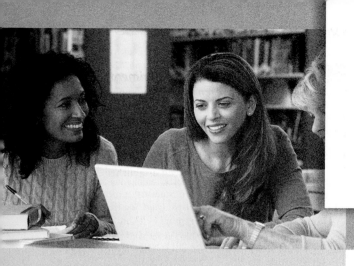

Chapter 9
Language and Thinking Processes

We now are ready to explore the language and thinking of researchers who use the range of designs relevant to health and human service inquiry. As discussed in previous chapters, significant philosophical differences exist between experimental-type and naturalistic research traditions. Experimental-type designs are characterized by thinking and action processes based in deductive logic and a positivist paradigm in which the researcher seeks to identify a single reality through systematized observation. This reality is understood by reducing it to its parts, observing and measuring the parts, and then examining the relationship among these parts. Ultimately, the purpose of research in the experimental-type tradition is to predict what will occur in one part of the universe by knowing and observing another part.

Unlike experimental-type design, the naturalistic tradition is characterized by multiple ontological and epistemological foundations. However, naturalistic designs share common elements that are reflected in researchers' language and thinking processes. Researchers in the naturalistic tradition base their thinking in inductive and abductive logic and seek to understand phenomena within the context in which they are embedded. Thus, the notion of multiple realities and the attempt to characterize holistically the complexity of human experience are two elements that pervade naturalistic approaches.

There are many different types of mixed method designs. However, they similarly draw on and integrate the language and thinking of both experimental- and naturalistic-type traditions. In this chapter, we examine the philosophical foundations, language, and criteria for scientific *rigor* for experimental-type, naturalistic traditions and mixed methods. "Rigor" is a term used in research that refers to the procedures that are used to enhance the research process and judge the integrity of the research design. As you read this chapter, compare and contrast the two traditions and their integration in terms of how they address rigor.

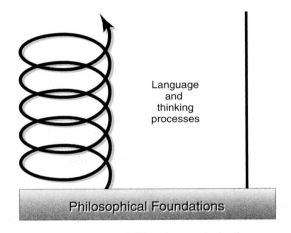

Experimental-Type Language and Thinking Processes

Within the experimental-type research tradition, there is consensus about the adequacy and scientific rigor of research processes. Thus, all designs in the experimental-type tradition share a common language and a unified perspective as to what constitutes an adequate *design*. Although there are many definitions of research design across the range of approaches, all types of experimental-type research share the same fundamental elements and a single, agreed-on meaning (Box 9-1).

In experimental-type research, design is the plan or blueprint that specifies and structures the action processes of collecting, analyzing, and reporting data to answer a research question before any action occurs. As Kerlinger stated in his classic definition, design is "the plan, structure, and strategy of investigation conceived so as to obtain answers to research

> **BOX 9-1** *Characteristics of Experimental-Type Research*
>
> • Based in one epistemology
> • Historically accepted as the "scientific method" for discovering "fact"
> • Evaluated and described by a unified and an agreed-on vocabulary that is well established

questions and to control variance."[1] "Plan" refers to the blueprint for action or the specific procedures used to obtain empirical evidence. "Structure" represents a more complex concept and refers to a model of the relationships among the variables of a study. That is, the design is structured in such a way as to enable an examination of a hypothesized relationship among variables. This relationship is articulated in the research question. The main purpose of the design is to structure the study so that the researcher can answer the research question or questions.

In the experimental-type tradition, the purpose of the design is to control or restrict extraneous influences on the study. By exerting such control, the researcher can state with a degree of statistical assuredness that study outcomes are either the consequence of the manipulation of the independent variable (e.g., true experimental design) or the consequence of that which was observed and analyzed (e.g., nonexperimental design). In other words, the design provides a degree of certainty that an investigator's observations are not haphazard or random but reflect what is considered to be a true and objective reality. The researcher is thus concerned with developing the most optimal design that eliminates or controls unwanted influences, what researchers refer to as disturbances, variances, extraneous factors, or situational contaminants. The design controls these disturbances or situational contaminants through the implementation of systematic procedures and data collection efforts, as discussed in subsequent chapters. The purpose of imposing control and restrictions on observations of natural phenomena is to ensure that the relationships specified in the research question(s) can be identified, understood, and ultimately predicted.

The element of design is one major element that separates research from the everyday types of observations and thinking and action processes in which each of us engages. Design in the experimental tradition instructs the investigator to "do this" or "don't do that." It provides a mechanism of control to ensure that data are collected objectively, in a uniform and consistent manner, with minimal investigator involvement or bias. The important points to remember are that the investigator remains separate from and uninvolved with the phenomena under study (e.g., to control one important potential source of disturbance or situational contaminant) and that procedures and systematic data collection provide mechanisms to control and eliminate bias.

Sequence of Experimental-Type Research

Design is pivotal in the sequence of thoughts and actions of experimental-type researchers (Fig. 9-1). All actions stem from the thinking processes of formulating a problem statement, a theory-specific research question that emerges from scholarly literature, hypotheses (if indicated), and expected outcomes. More specifically, design dictates the nature of the action processes of data collection, the conditions under which observations will be made, and, most important, the type of data analyses and reporting that will be possible.

Do you recall our previous discussion on the essentials of research? In that discussion, we illustrated how a problem statement indicates the purpose of the research and the broad topic the investigator wants to address. In experimental-type inquiry, the literature review guides the selection of theoretical principles and concepts of the study and provides the rationale for a research project. This rationale is based on the nature of research previously conducted and the level of theory development for the phenomena under investigation. The experimental-type researcher develops a literature review in which the specific theory, scope of the study, research questions, concepts to be measured, nature of the relationship among concepts, and measures that will be used in the study are discussed and supported. Thus, the researcher creates a design that builds on both the ideas that have been formulated previously and the actions that have been conducted in ways

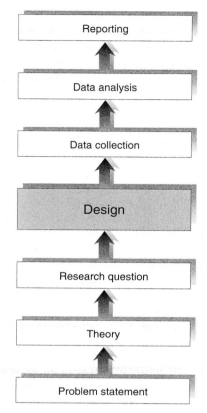

Figure 9-1 Sequence of experimental-type research.

that conform to the rules of scientific rigor in this tradition.

The choice of design not only is shaped by the literature and level of theory development but also is dependent on the specific question asked and resources or the practical constraints, such as access to target populations and monetary and staff considerations. There is nothing inherently good or bad about a design. Every research study design has its particular strengths and weaknesses. The adequacy of a design is based on how well the design answers the research question that is posed. This is the most important criterion for evaluating a design. If the design does not answer the research question, then regardless of how rigorous it may appear, the design is not adequate. For example, the randomized controlled trial is often upheld as the most rigorous design. However, that is only the case for a specific research question that seeks to test the efficacy of a particular intervention, service, or program. Trying to apply this type of design to another type of research question or when it would be unethical to randomly assign persons to one group or another would not be an appropriate design choice.

It is also important to identify and understand the relative strength and weakness of each design element. Methodological decisions are purposeful and should be made with full recognition of what is gained and what is not by implementing each design element. The researcher evaluates whether the strengths of a particular design element outweigh the weaknesses it may pose. Then, at the reporting stage of a study, the researcher clearly articulates the limitations of the study. Every study has a specific limitation or weakness. Identifying that weakness up front and early on in the research process is important so that one can more fully understand the knowledge gained, place findings within an appropriate context, and apply the knowledge ethically and purposively.

Structure of Experimental-Type Research

Experimental-type research has a well-developed language that sets clear rules and expectations for the adequacy of design and research procedures. As shown in Table 9-1, nine key terms structure experimental-type research designs. Let us examine the meaning of each.

Concepts

A concept is defined as the words or ideas that symbolically represent observations and experiences. Concepts are not directly observable; rather, what they describe is observed or experienced. Concepts are "(1) tentative, (2) based on agreement, and (3) useful only to the degree that they capture or isolate something significant and definable."[2] For example, the terms "grooming" and "work" are both concepts that describe specific observable or experienced activities in which people engage on a regular basis. Other concepts, such as "personal hygiene" or "sadness," have various definitions, each of which can lead to the development of different assessment instruments to measure the same underlying concept.

TABLE 9-1   *Key Terms in Structuring Experimental-Type Research*

Term	Definition
Concept	Symbolically represents observation and experience
Construct	Represents a model of relationships among two or more concepts
Conceptual definition	Concept expressed in words
Operational definition	How the concept will be measured
Variable	Operational definition of a concept assigned numerical values
Independent variable	Presumed cause of the dependent variable
Intervening variable	Phenomenon that has an effect on study variables
Dependent variable	Phenomenon that is affected by the independent variable or is the presumed effect or outcome
Hypothesis	Testable statement that indicates what the researcher expects to find

Constructs

As discussed in Chapter 7, constructs are theoretical creations based on observations but cannot be observed directly or indirectly.[3] A construct can only be inferred and may represent a larger category with two or more concepts or constructs.

The construct of "function" may be inferred from observing concepts such as grooming, personal hygiene, dressing, bathing, and work or asking individuals to appraise their function in discrete areas. Similarly, "quality of life" is a construct composed of different concepts such as emotional well-being, physical well-being, and purposeful or meaningful engagement in activities. However, the construct of function or quality of life is not observable unless it is broken down into its component parts or concepts. Because concepts and constructs are abstract, measures of these single-order abstractions are definition dependent. So if we define depression as anger turned inward, we would operationalize it with items that sought to quantify how much anger one expressed toward oneself. But if we defined depression as self-degrading thoughts about oneself, we would seek to measure those. As you can see, neither is right or wrong, but each leads to a different measure and thus different knowledge.

Definitions

The two basic types of definitions relevant to research design are conceptual (lexical) definitions and operational definitions. A *conceptual definition*, or lexical definition, stipulates the meaning of a concept or construct in words (other concepts or constructs) and the relationship to other concepts or constructs and a theoretical framework. An *operational definition* stipulates meaning of a lexical definition by specifying how the concept is observed or experienced. Operational definitions "define things by what they do." Thus, in the experimental-type tradition, the operational definition specifies how the construct will be measured.

> The construct of "self-care" may be conceptually defined as the activities that are necessary to care for one's bodily functions, whereas it is operationally defined as observations of an individual engaged in bathing, dressing, and grooming or the individual's own appraisal of his or her level of difficulty and independence or dependence in performing self-care activities. If the lexical definition chosen by the researcher were different, then the operational definition would also differ. Can you now see the importance of the literature review and theory selection in experimental-type design? The theory shapes not only the topical area but how the design and particularly measurement is structured. •

Variables

A *variable* is a concept or construct to which numerical values are assigned. By definition, a variable must have more than one value even if the investigator is interested in only one condition.

> If an investigator is interested in evaluating the adequacy of self-care routines of persons with motor impairments who are employed, both self-care routine and employment are variables. Self-care routine may have multiple values of relevance to the investigator, such as the level of dependence, safety and efficiency of performance, and perceived difficulty. The investigator needs to determine which of the potential

values that may be attributed to self-care would be of most interest in the inquiry. As indicated earlier, measurement is definition dependent, and now we add the choice of delimiting a variable. Thus, there are different ways to measure self-care routines, and each approach can lead to a different understanding. Likewise, employment status can have multiple values (e.g., employed vs. not employed, number of hours working outside the home), and the investigator needs to determine how to operationalize this variable to best match the theory guiding the research, the study's purposes, and the specific query that is posed. Thus, there is not a single approach to operationally defining a variable, and the decision to use one format versus another must be carefully determined. •

There are five basic types of variables that are used in experimental-type forms of inquiry: independent, intervening, mediating, dependent, and moderating. A variable can have any one of these roles depending on the research question, theory, and hypothesis (if indicated).

An *independent variable* "is the presumed cause of or influence on the dependent variable, the presumed effect."[3] Thus, a *dependent variable* (also referred to as "outcome" and "criterion") refers to the phenomenon that the investigator seeks to understand, explain, or predict. The independent variable almost always precedes any change in the dependent variable. The independent variable is also referred to as the "predictor variable." An *intervening variable* (also called a "confounding" or an "extraneous" variable) is a phenomenon that has an effect on the study variables but that may or may not be the object of the study.

> Let's say you are conducting a study of the adequacy of self-care routines of employed individuals with motor impairments. In this case, employment status represents the independent variable, whereas level of difficulty performing self-care routine represents the dependent variable. Intervening variables in this study may include any other variable that potentially influences either the independent or the dependent variable, such as family support, type and degree of disability, or motivational status. •

Investigators treat intervening variables differently depending on the research question. For example, an investigator may only be interested in examining the relationship between the independent and dependent variables and may thus statistically control or account for an intervening variable. The investigator would then examine the relationship after statistically "removing" the effect of one or more potential intervening variables. However, the investigator may want to examine the effect of an intervening variable such as degree of impairment on the relationship between the independent (employment status) and dependent variables (difficulty performing self-care routines). For this question, the researcher would employ statistical techniques to determine the interrelationships.

In the latter scenario, the intervening variable is considered a "mediator." A mediator is a variable through which an independent variable works to have its effect on a dependent variable. Mediators are theoretically grounded and routed in a multivariate analytic framework for testing hypotheses that concern causal relationships. In a mediation model, it is hypothesized that an independent causal variable leads to changes in an observed mediating variable, which in turn causes changes to an outcome or dependent variable.[4] The independent variable may have a direct effect on the dependent variable, or its effect may be indirect and occur only through its effect on changes to the mediator, or it can have both a direct and indirect effect. These potential relationships are shown in Figure 9-2.

A mediator framework suggests a temporal (time-based) ordering of occurrences such that the independent variable takes place at one point in time, followed by the mediator variable, which then subsequently has a causal effect on a dependent variable that occurs at another point in time. This sequence suggests that longitudinal data sets or data sets with multiple data collection opportunities are best suited for mediation versus a cross-sectional data set in which there is only one point in time for data collection.

Let's say you are testing a depression treatment for a group of older adults with chronic illness. You hypothesize that the treatment (the independent variable) will have a direct effect on the outcome (reducing depressive symptoms) and this impact will also be mediated by the extent to which participants are "behaviorally activated" (e.g., they are actively engaged in positive problem solving and action-oriented solutions to daily challenges). You believe that the intervention that involves depression education and helping participants achieve behavioral goals is effective to the extent it enhances the behavioral activation level of participants.[5] Here the mediation variable would be a level of behavioral activation.

Yet another type of variable is called a "moderator." A moderator is an independent or predictor variable that may interact with another independent variable. Let's say the number of chronic conditions that individuals have (independent variable) is directly related to perceived quality of life (dependent variable). This relationship, however, may differ for men and women, with women experiencing lower perceived quality of life than men. In this case, gender moderates the effect of chronic conditions on perceived quality of life.

A moderator can also be a mediator depending on one's theory and hypothesis. For example, let's say that the relationship between the number of chronic conditions and perceived quality of life is affected by activity level. Individuals with chronic illness who have high levels of activity perceive a higher quality of life than those with low activity levels. In this case activity level would be a moderator. However, chronic conditions may have a negative impact on perceived quality of life if they decrease the ability to engage in previously valued activities. In this case, activity participation mediates the effects of chronic conditions and quality of life.

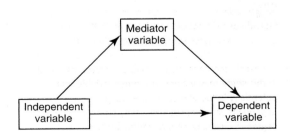

Figure 9-2 A Classic Mediation Model.

Hypotheses

A hypothesis is defined as a testable statement that indicates what the researcher expects to find, given the theory and level of knowledge in the literature. A hypothesis is stated in such a way that it will either be accepted or fail to be accepted by the research process. The researcher can develop either a directional or a nondirectional hypothesis (see Chapter 8). In a directional hypothesis, the researcher indicates whether she or he expects to find a positive relationship or an inverse relationship between two or more variables. A positive relationship is one in which both variables increase and decrease together to a greater or lesser degree.

> In a positive relationship, the researcher may hypothesize that the employed individual with a strong disability identity has greater self-esteem than the unemployed individual with a strong disability identity. Yet another positive relationship might be that individuals with chronic illness who are actively engaged in meaningful activities have greater perceived quality of life than individuals with chronic illness who are not involved in meaningful activities. In these examples, the hypothesis tests the movement of both variables in the same direction. •

In an inverse relationship, the variables are associated in opposite directions (i.e., as one increases, the other decreases). An inverse relationship may involve a hypothesis similar to the following:

> An individual with multiple chronic conditions who has high level of engagement in meaningful activities will demonstrate fewer depressive symptoms than an individual who is not actively engaged in activities. •

In this statement, the expectation is that as the variable "engagement level" increases, depressive symptoms will decrease.

Now that we have defined the key terms that are essential to experimental-type designs, let us review the way they are actually used in this form of inquiry.

Experimental-type research questions narrow the scope of the inquiry to specific concepts, constructs, or both. These single-order abstractions are then lexically or conceptually defined through the literature and operationalized as variables that will be investigated descriptively, relationally, or predictively. The hypothesis (when indicated for Level 2 and 3 questioning) establishes an equation or structure by which independent and dependent variables are examined and tested.

Plan of Design

The plan of an experimental-type design requires a set of thinking processes in which the researcher considers five core issues: bias, manipulation, control, validity, and reliability.

Bias

Bias in this tradition is defined as the potential unintended or unavoidable effect on study outcomes. When bias is present and unaccounted for, the investigator may not be able to fully ascertain whether the study findings are accurate or instead reflect unanticipated and unintended influences that confound a study and the conclusions that can be drawn from it. Many factors can cause bias in a study (Box 9-2). We already discussed one source, the "intervening variable."

Another cause may be *instrumentation*. Instrumentation refers to the ways in which data are obtained in experimental-type approaches. The two major sources of bias inherent in instrumentation are inappropriate data collection procedures and inadequate questions.

Assume you are a health and human service professional working in a community health center.

BOX 9-2 *Possible Sources of Bias in an Experimental-Type Study*

- Selection of inappropriate instrumentation
- Sample selection process that favors a particular unintended group
- Improper training of interviewers
- Deviation from the plan and from structure of the design

Your supervisor, the agency administrator, is conducting a survey of worker satisfaction. To obtain information from employees, the supervisor decides to interview people. Knowing that this person is your superior, how likely are you to provide responses to job satisfaction questions, particularly knowing that your performance evaluation is next month?

> Here is another example. Let's say you are testing an innovative program to improve medication compliance among young adults who test positive for human immunodeficiency virus (HIV). Suppose the person who provides the program also is the person who asks participants whether they are taking their medications before, during, and after the program. If you were a participant in the program, you might not feel comfortable disclosing your noncompliance. You might not want to disappoint the person after developing a relationship with him or her. •

In the situations just portrayed, the procedures for data collection are problematic and introduce bias into the study.

> Now consider how the way in which questions are asked to obtain the data can influence or bias responses. Suppose this question is asked: "Don't you agree that this is a great place to work?" Alternatively, suppose the question is asked: "As you know, not taking medications can be dangerous. To what extent have you been adhering to your medication regimen?" Certainly these questions are poorly phrased; both imply socially and politically correct responses and in essence urge the responders to agree or report positive responses. Now consider this question: "Don't you think that the physical environment and the climate are excellent here?" In this case, the question is confusing and ambiguous. What does "the climate" refer to? Does it signify the weather? The emotional climate? The social climate? In this case, the responder is prompted or guided to produce a socially desirable response. It is also not clear what is being asked.
> Or suppose the instrument is a survey in which you are asked about work satisfaction and are provided with instructions to select the answer of the following which best reflects your opinion:
> 1. I am very satisfied
> 2. I am somewhat satisfied

> Certainly, if you are not satisfied, you have no option to indicate that sentiment within the structure of responses provided by the researcher. •

Interview or survey questions that elicit a socially correct response, or that do not provide a range of responses sufficient to answer the research questions, and questions that are vague, unclear, or ambiguous introduce bias into the study design.

Sampling is another major source of bias.

> Suppose that only the supervisor's social friends were selected as the targeted sample to participate in the satisfaction studies and are viewed as representative of the agency population. Such a sample would not represent the overall level of job satisfaction for all employees. In this example, the characteristics of the sample serve as potential bias and thus influence the outcomes of the study.
> Or let's say the HIV medication support program only enrolled persons who were already "compliant" with following their regimen. The results could not be generalized to all young adults with the diagnosis of HIV. •

> Improper or uneven training of data collectors and interviewer "drift," in which an interviewer strays from the interview protocol from fatigue or overfamiliarity, can bias study outcomes as well. •

> In the same study of employee satisfaction, if multiple persons collect information about job satisfaction but each asks the survey questions differently or in a nonuniform manner, interviewer procedures may introduce bias. •

Experimental-type designs are characterized by detailed and precise plans and procedures that are established before conducting the study. Thus, any deviation from the original plan for data collection and analysis may be a potential source of bias. The violation of standard procedures is an important point in the study at which bias may be introduced.

Suppose that the agency director decided to collect data regarding the level of job satisfaction of agency employees on Monday. Monday was selected because all employees were normally available. However, the data collection was accomplished on Tuesday because Monday was a holiday. On Tuesday, all home-based service providers were in the field and therefore were not surveyed for their degree of job satisfaction. This deviation in the plan could have significantly affected the study outcome, because a large segment of the agency employee population would have been omitted from the study. •

An essential part of planning a design is to introduce systematic procedures to minimize or eliminate as many sources of bias as possible. As you read subsequent chapters, think about the potential sources of bias. Also, as you conduct your own studies or read and analyze published studies, consider findings and conclusions in light of potential bias.

Let's say you have participated in a program designed to help you more effectively manage your diabetes. The facilitator of the program is conducting an evaluation of the program's effectiveness in accomplishing this aim. The facilitator asks each program participant to respond to a brief questionnaire before beginning the program and then on its completion. Although you liked the facilitator, you do not think the program was informative, nor did it change your ability to manage your disease. How likely are you to express your true feelings about the program if the facilitator is asking you the postevaluation questions? How can you design the pre- and postprogram data collection differently to avoid imposing bias? •

Manipulation

Manipulation is defined as the action process of maneuvering the independent variable so that the effect of its presence, absence, or degree on the dependent variable can be observed. To the extent possible, experimental-type researchers attempt to isolate the independent and dependent variables and then manipulate or change the condition of the inde-

pendent variable so that the cause-and-effect relationship between the variables can be examined.

The concept of manipulation is best understood within the context of a study testing the effects of an intervention, service, or program on a defined outcome or set of outcomes. For example, let's say you are interested in determining which types of interventions for families who are providing care to a frail older adult (e.g., skills training, social support, group counseling, education) promote positive well-being outcomes for the caregivers. One approach would be to use a randomized, two-group design. In this type of design, caregivers would be evaluated with regard to their well-being at baseline or before introducing the intervention. Study participants would then be randomly assigned (assigned on a chance-determined basis; see Chapter 13) to different intervention conditions (one group receives group counseling and the other group receives one-on-one skills training) and tested again after a specified time (e.g., 6 weeks, 3 months, or 12 months, depending upon the research question). Then caregivers switch groups and participate in the intervention group that they had not experienced. They would then be tested again to evaluate change in the dependent variable, "well-being." The interventions represent the independent variables being manipulated (received, not received). By manipulating the intervention timing and sequence, an investigator is able to examine the effect of each intervention and combinations on caregiver well-being.[6] •

Control

Control is defined as the set of action processes that direct or manipulate factors to achieve an outcome. Control plays a critical role in experimental-type design. By controlling not only the independent variable but also other aspects of the research context, such as how study participants are assigned to groups, or the timing with which data are collected, the relationships among the study variables can be observed. In experimental-type design, procedures to establish control are implemented to minimize the influences of extraneous variables on the outcome or dependent variable.

Various methods of control can be crafted to minimize bias, such as careful training of interviewers, using only standardized and well-validated measures, standardizing all procedures and ensuring adherence to the design, and controlling conditions in which data are collected or measures administered. Control is also implemented by clearly establishing inclusion and exclusion criteria for study participation. Without such criteria, a research team could, for example, choose only those participants believed to be cooperative or who are perceived to benefit from the program.

Control is particularly critical when conducting a randomized controlled trial. For this type of design, two basic methods of control are typically introduced: random group assignment and control group.

Let's consider random assignment (see Chapter 10 for a detailed discussion). Random assignment refers to a set of procedures that equalize the chance of assignment to any of the groups in a research study. By randomly assigning subjects to one group or the other using this systematic approach (discussed in Chapter 10), the investigator attempts to develop equivalence in the groups, which may not occur otherwise because of inherent differences that can occur if chances for assignment are not equivalent. Random assignment also eliminates sources of bias such as having participants choose their own group, or having the research team place participants in one group versus the other for "subjective" reasons (e.g., belief that the participant would do better in one group over the other or may comply with the program better).

In evaluating the outcome of interventions on caregivers' well-being, assume you do not use random assignment. Instead, you assign the first 10 volunteers to the first group, who receive the intervention involving group counseling, and the next 10 volunteers to the second group, who receive hands-on skills training. It is possible that the first 10 subjects know each other and agreed to participate in the study because they were highly motivated to seek help, and each person encouraged the other to join. In contrast, suppose the last 10 subjects were somewhat less motivated to participate or enrolled after a news article presented the benefits of joining a study for families. Familiarity with other subjects and high motivation to seek help (two factors inherent in the subjects assigned to the first group) may influence caregiver responses to the outcome measure of "well-being." Here the effects of history and personal motivations can act together to introduce sources of bias that can easily be controlled through random assignment. By not using random assignment, the investigator may risk developing groups that initially differ from one another. In turn, this initial difference may make it difficult to discern what effect, if any, the independent variable (intervention program) has on the outcome variable (well-being).   •

Another method to enhance control is the use of a control group. A control group is one in which the experimental or comparative condition is absent.

There are many different types of control groups. One type of group is referred to as "usual care" or the "do-nothing condition," in which participants assigned to this group do not receive any intervention, or receive what they usually would, independent of the study. Occasionally, the experimental treatment group is compared with an "attention" control group—that is, a group that receives some form of attention to control for its occurrence in the treatment group. By comparing caregiver scores in an attention control group to those in an intervention group, the investigator is able to determine whether changes in the dependent variable resulted from (1) the passage of time, (2) the attention factor inherent in an intervention involving interaction with a health or human service professional, or (3) the particular content of each group. Another way of creating a control group is through wait-listing participants for a designated period of time, during which they do not receive an intervention but are tested. Following a posttest, this group receives the treatment or tested program. In this type of design, the intervention is initially evaluated against a no-treatment condition. However, the researcher can also evaluate whether a delay in receiving treatment affects the magnitude of benefit received by comparing the wait-list control group's gains following treatment to those of the original intervention group. Yet another type of control group is a minimal control group in which participants receive some contact from the study team, mostly for the purposes of retention.   •

Validity

Validity is a concept that has numerous applications in experimental-type research. However, the concept as it applies to design refers to the extent to which your study answers the research questions and your findings are accurate or reflect the underlying purpose of the study. Although many classifications of validity have been developed, we discuss four fundamental types of validity, based on Campbell and Stanley's classic work.[7] These are internal validity, external validity, statistical conclusion validity, and construct validity.

Internal Validity   The ability of the research design to answer the research question accurately is known as *internal validity*. If a design has internal validity, the investigator can state with a degree of confidence that the reported outcomes are the consequence of the relationship between the independent variable and dependent variable and not the result of extraneous factors. Campbell and Stanley[7] identified seven major factors that pose a threat to the researcher's ability to determine whether the observable outcome is a function of the study or the result of external and unintended forces (Box 9-3).

To illustrate these threats to validity, consider a hypothetical example.

BOX 9-3   *Seven Threats to Internal Validity*

1. *History.* Effect of external events on study outcomes
2. *Testing.* Effect of being observed or tested on the study outcome
3. *Instrumentation.* Extent to which the instrument is accurate in its measurement and extent to which the instrument itself may be responsible for outcomes
4. *Maturation.* Effect of the passage of time
5. *Regression.* Effect of a statistical phenomenon in which extreme scores tend to regress or cluster around the mean (average) on repeated testing occasions
6. *Mortality.* Effect on outcome caused by subject attrition or dropping out of a study before its completion
7. *Interactive effects.* Extent to which each of these threats interacts with sample selection to influence the outcome of a study

From Campbell DT, Stanley JC: *Experimental and quasi-experimental design,* Chicago, 1963, Rand McNally.

Consider how each of the seven threats to internal validity affects your research outcomes.

Suppose you are conducting a study to determine the extent to which an acquired immunodeficiency syndrome (AIDS) prevention program has reduced behavior that increases the risk of developing AIDS in an adolescent population. This study is designed to answer the following research question: "To what extent is adolescent risk behavior reduced by the experimental preventive intervention?" Before the intervention, you evaluate the extent to which subjects exhibit risk behavior. You conduct a prevention program and then retest the participants. The retest shows an amazing reduction in risk behavior, and you claim that your program is a success. In doing so, you are making a claim that a relationship exists between your program (the independent variable) and risk behavior (the dependent variable). Furthermore, you are claiming that there is a causal relationship between the variables—that is, you claim that your program causes the reduction in behavior that increases the risk of developing AIDS. •

First, let us assume you have just learned that a celebrity has held a news conference in which he announced that he has tested positive for HIV. This announcement has come immediately after you first administered your test to your subjects but before the final testing occasion. It is possible that this historical event, rather than the independent variable, was the factor responsible for reducing risk behavior in your subjects.

However, assume that your subjects already knew about the celebrity before beginning the study. Now consider the threat of testing to the validity of your claims. As a sensitive researcher, you have decided to measure risk behavior by observing a discussion group about sexual behaviors among adolescents. Each time you hear a risk behavior, you score it as such without informing your subjects. In the first testing situation, the adolescents appear to discuss their sexual decision making openly. However, you note that they are aware of group norms and of being observed, and that they stay well within the boundaries tacitly set by the group when discussing their personal behavior and views. In the second test, you note a significant reduction in reported risk behaviors or in risky decision making.

Although the prevention program may be responsible for the reduction in risk behavior, there certainly are viable alternative explanations. In the first testing situation, the adolescents may have revealed what was normative and acceptable in the group rather than accurately representing their own risk potential. In the second test, the adolescents who underwent the intervention may have restricted their conversation to what they learned was desirable rather than revealing their own behavior. •

Another alternative for the observed reduction in risk behavior may be the result of the testing situation itself. Participants who are aware of what is being observed and recorded may answer more cautiously. In other words, the testing procedures may pose yet another threat to the internal validity of the design. The reduction in reported risk behaviors may be a function of participants actively changing or adjusting their behaviors or thoughts on the topic as a consequence of participating in a group discussion with peers. The test itself or mode of data collection may have influenced a change in behavior independent of the effect of participating in the intervention. Therefore, it is difficult to determine whether observed change is a consequence of the test, of the intervention, or both.

This example also illustrates the threat to validity posed by instrumentation. In this example, the instrumentation may not be measuring what was intended. Instead of measuring risk behavior, the instrumentation may be a more accurate indicator of group norms related to sexual decision making.

Another way in which instrumentation poses a threat to a study is through changes that may occur within interviewers over time or with the instrument itself. For example, if you are collecting data regarding weight or blood pressure, any deviation in the calibration of a scale or blood pressure cuff from one testing occasion to the next will pose a significant threat to the validity of the data that are obtained.

Further, interviewer influence or any change in the way interviewers pose questions may cause a

deviation in responses that will affect how the investigator interprets the findings.

 To illustrate the threat posed by maturation, assume that the AIDS prevention program is being conducted over a 1-year period. It is possible that the participants have matured in their thinking and have become more responsible in their decision making as a function of time rather than as a result of the prevention program. •

The threat of regression frequently occurs when subjects with extreme scores are selected to participate in a study.

 Assume that adolescents who are sexually active participate in the study and therefore tend to report extremely risky behaviors. Those who are high scorers at the beginning of the program tend to report lower scores at the end. •

This change in scores, however, may be a consequence of a statistical principle known as "statistical regression toward the mean," in which extreme scores tend to move toward the mean on repeated testing.

 Fifty participants began the AIDS prevention program, but only 10 remained by the final testing period. It is possible that as a result of "experimental mortality" (attrition of participants before a study's conclusion), those who remained in the study may be more committed to or had more immediate success in reducing risk behavior than those who dropped out. Alternatively, those who remained in the study may have had more social support from family and friends and that is what made the difference in their ability to remain in the study. •

Thus, experimental mortality poses a threat to the interpretation of study findings. Numerous interactive effects could also confound the accuracy of the findings.

🔍 Consider that the selected sample for the study was a population of adolescents on probation. This group was highly motivated to report a change in their risk behavior (a sampling bias) and was also sensitive to being tested because of their judiciary status. The interactive effect of the sample bias and the testing condition may wreak havoc on claims that the outcome was a result of the prevention program. •

The internal validity of the study is always the first priority of the researcher working in the experimental tradition.

External Validity *External validity* refers to the capacity to generalize findings and develop inferences from the sample to the study population stipulated in the research question. External validity answers the question of "generalizability."[8]

🔍 Remember our research question: "To what extent is adolescent risk behavior reduced by the experimental preventive intervention?" In this question, the population is stated as all adolescents. Now, assume that the investigator obtained a sample by asking for volunteers from a large group of adolescents between ages 12 and 18 years who were on probation in one large city. The potential to generalize the findings from the sample to all adolescents on probation is limited by several important factors. First, the sample was a volunteer sample, making them potentially different from adolescents who did not volunteer. Because the sample was voluntary, the researcher cannot know in what ways the sample may differ from the study population, which includes those who refused participation or did not have the opportunity to volunteer. Second, the experiences of adolescents who live in large cities may not necessarily represent the experiences of adolescents in rural or other geographic locations. Third, in selecting a volunteer urban sample on probation, the investigator should have limited generalizability to that select sample and will not be able to generalize the experiences of the research sample to all adolescents, such as those who are not on probation, who live in rural communities, or who may be sexually active and at risk. •

BOX 9-4 *Potential Threats to External Validity*

1. *Reactivity.* Extent to which the subjects are responding to the condition of being part of a study and thus do not represent the population from whom they are selected
2. *Realism.* Extent to which the experimental conditions simulate actual life situations to which the population is exposed

---

These factors represent some of the threats to external validity that may occur in a study. Although randomization decreases some of the threats to external validity, even when a sample is randomly selected, threats remain.[8,9] The two threats in Box 9-4 result from the experimental condition, not from the limitations of sample selection. Consider your own behavior when being watched in a simulated situation. Certainly you act differently than you would under similar but unobserved and nonsimulated conditions.

The internal and external validity of a study are interrelated. As an investigator attempts to increase the internal validity of a study, the ability to make broad generalizations and inferences to a larger population decreases. That is, as more controls are implemented and extraneous factors are eliminated from a study design, the population to whom findings can be generalized becomes more limited. Thus, although investigators try to enhance the internal validity of a study to ensure that valid and accurate conclusions can be drawn, these efforts may limit the scope of external validity of the findings. In balancing internal and external validity, it makes most sense to attend to internal validity first and external validity second. If a study lacks internal validity, there would be no purpose in generalizing what is not viable knowledge to the population from which the sample was selected. As you read further in this text, look for ways to reconcile internal validity and the scope of generalization that may be possible.

The tension between internal and external validity contributes in part to the gap between what we know from research and the evidence that is implemented in practice. For example, to ensure internal validity, the researcher may narrow study inclusion criteria to a select group who hypothetically could most benefit from a particular intervention or program. If a program is systematically supported as efficacious, practitioners may then find that the program does not work quite as well to accomplish its objectives with the broad population they encounter. However, if the researcher started with a broad set of eligibility criteria, he or she may have needed an unrealistic sample size to find treatment significance or may have run the risk of not showing efficacy. This is just one example of the delicate balance researchers need to consider in the design of their studies.

Statistical Conclusion Validity *Statistical conclusion validity* refers to the power of your study to draw statistical conclusions. One aim of experimental-type research is to find relationships among variables and ultimately to predict the nature and direction of these relationships. Support for relationships is contained in the action process of statistical analysis. However, selection of statistical techniques is based on many considerations. Even though the expectation of making errors in determining relationships is built into the theory and practice of statistical analysis (see Chapter 20), the accuracy and potential of the statistics to support or predict a relationship among variables must be considered as a potential threat to the validity of a design.

> Assume you want to ensure that you do not overestimate the effects of your AIDS prevention program on risk behavior. You select a statistic that will be less likely to find a relationship when there really is none. However, this decision increases the possibility that you may not find a significant relationship when, in fact, one exists. Thus, your statistical testing may lead you to believe that no relationship exists when there is one or, conversely, to believe that there is a relationship when it is absent. •

Construct Validity *Construct validity* addresses the fit between the constructs that are the focus of the study and the way in which these constructs are operationalized. As stated earlier, constructs are abstract representations of what humans observe and experience. The method used to define and measure constructs accurately is in large part a matter of opinion and consensus. It is possible for several factors related to construct validity to confound a study. First, a researcher may define a construct inappropriately.

> Although smiling may be one indication of happiness, if a researcher measured the level of happiness exclusively by observing the frequency of smiling behavior, the full construct of "happiness" would not be captured. Also, smiling has different meanings in different contexts and cultures. By merely observing frequency, one might not really know the meaning of what was measured. •

Poor or incomplete operational definitions can result from incomplete or vague conceptual (lexical) definitions or from inadequate translation of the construct into an observable one.

Second, when a cause-and-effect relationship between two constructs is determined, it may be difficult to define each construct exclusively (referring to both independent and dependent variables) and to isolate the effects of one on the other.

> Suppose you are a health and human service professional seeking to test a feeding program for persons with moderate to late-stage Alzheimer's disease. You design a program in which you choose certain foods and techniques to improve independent feeding. To ensure that your design can investigate a cause-and-effect relationship, you randomly select your sample and randomly assign them to the experimental group (which receives the program) and the control group (which does not receive the program). You measure feeding behavior by two methods: observation of independent feeding and volume of food consumed independently. You implement your feeding program with the experimental group and test all participants after the program to determine whether the experimental group scored higher on your measures of feeding than the group that did not receive the intervention. You conclude that your program was successful in improving independent feeding because the experimental group performed significantly better than the group without the intervention.

However, you begin to consider other confounding influences that cannot be separated from your two constructs—independent feeding and the experimental program. The attention of the experimenter may have influenced the improvement in the experimental group because eating is a social behavior and may change under different social conditions. Also, food preferences may have influenced the response of the groups to their respective conditions. Interactive effects of being observed and participating in an experiment (referred to as the "attention factor" or "Hawthorne effect"[9]) may also limit your capacity to isolate a causal relationship between the constructs. •

Reliability

Reliability refers to the stability of a research design. In experimental-type design, rigorous research is evaluated as well planned and properly executed when, if repeated under the similar circumstances, the design yields equivalent results. Investigators frequently replicate or repeat a study in the same population or in different groups to determine the extent to which the findings of one study are accurate in a broader scope. To replicate a study, the procedures, measures, and data analysis techniques must be consistent, well articulated, and appropriate to the research question. Reliability is threatened when a researcher is not consistent and changes a design in midstream, does not articulate procedures in sufficient detail for replication, or does not fully plan a sound design.

Summary of the Role of Design in Experimental-Type Inquiry

Design is a pivotal concept in experimental-type research that indicates both the structure and the plan of all action processes. Experimental-type designs are developed to eliminate bias and the intrusion of unwanted factors that could confound findings and make them less credible. Five primary considerations in the plan of a design are bias, control, manipulation, validity, and reliability. The four types of validity discussed are internal, external, statistical conclusion, and construct.

> **BOX 9-5** *Eight Elements of Naturalistic Design*
>
> 1. Purpose of research
> 2. Context of research
> 3. Pluralistic perspective of reality
> 4. Concern with transferability
> 5. Flexibility
> 6. Concern with language
> 7. Emic and etic perspectives
> 8. Interactive and analytical process

Experimental-type research is designed to minimize the threats posed by extraneous factors and bias by maximizing control over the research action process. In Chapter 10, we discuss how each type of design in the experimental-type tradition addresses these considerations through structuring and planning a design and using action processes to increase control.

Naturalistic Language and Thinking Processes

Let us now turn our attention to the attributes of naturalistic inquiry and the implications for design with these traditions. Eight elements are common to designs in the naturalistic tradition, as listed in Box 9-5. Recall that unlike experimental-type design, which aims to minimize or eliminate bias, naturalistic designs are underpinned by philosophies proposing that bias is inherent in human thinking and action and thus cannot be separated from any human process, including research.[10] The following discussion reflects this important distinction.

Purpose

Designs within the tradition of naturalistic research vary in purpose from developing descriptive knowledge to evolving full-fledged theories about observed or experienced phenomena. As discussed in earlier chapters, naturalistic designs tend to be preferred when no adequate theory exists to explain a human phenomenon or when the investigator believes that existing theory and explanations are not accurate, true, or complete. The flexible structure of naturalistic designs allows for exploration, enabling new insights and understandings to be revealed without the imposition of preconceived concepts, constructs, and principles.[11]

Although the specific purpose of a study may differ, all naturalistic designs seek to describe, understand, or interpret daily phenomena within the contexts in which they occur. Naturalistic inquiry has emerged through five phases of development to its current form of action-oriented social criticism, in which grand narratives are replaced by more local, small-scale theories fitted to specific problems and specific situations.[11] Thus, the importance of naturalistic inquiry is now widely recognized because of its usefulness in examining and revealing phenomena that can help guide health and human service practitioners to address specific problems that emerge in the clinical or community context or explain why or how particular programs or interventions benefit individuals.

For example, understanding how individuals experience a particular health condition or type of intervention by examining their lived experience within that state can help advance new professional and supportive approaches. Observing client and provider interactions or coding communication styles can yield essential information about how best to educate health and human service professionals and better prepare persons for a medical or therapeutic encounter. Identifying key themes in tweets and blog postings on health and social Internet sites can provide new insights as to how individuals who use the Web and engage in virtual interaction discuss personal health issues and for which types of problems they seek help. •

Context Specificity

In naturalistic inquiry, the investigator is interested in uncovering different realities rather than in imposing a particular frame of reference. Thus, the investigator typically seeks to become involved in the particular setting in which the human phenomenon of interest occurs. Alternatively, naturalistic investigators seek information from the perspective of individuals who experience the phenomenon of interest. Because of the revelatory potential of naturalistic research, this form of investigatory action is conducted in the natural context in which the phenomenon occurs (on a website, in a hospital setting, in a school system) or seeks explanations of the natural context from those who experience it. Naturalistic research is therefore context specific, and the "knowing" derived from this context is embedded in the context and does not extend beyond it. The designs in the tradition of naturalistic inquiry share this basic attribute of *context specificity* and development of knowledge that is grounded in or linked to the data that emerge from a particular surrounding.

Complexity and Pluralistic Perspective of Reality

As a result of its underlying epistemology and its inductive and abductive approaches to knowing, naturalistic research is founded on pluralism. Thus multiple realities, each with validity, are attributed to the phenomena under study.[11]

With inductive reasoning, principles emerge from seemingly unrelated information. One of the hallmarks of this logic structure is the capacity for identical information to be organized differently by each individual who thinks about it. The end result of induction is the development of a complex set of relationships that emerge from and thus link smaller pieces of information (not the reduction of principles to their parts, as in deductive reasoning). It is therefore possible that the same information may have different meanings depending on the lens through which the links are seen. Therefore, there may be multiple interpretations of the same experience and all of these interpretations then make up the complexity of what is being studied. Through abductive logic, the best fit can be determined from the multiple interpretations and theories that are all viable in explaining phenomena. Using abduction ensures that the information will be revisited and reanalyzed by the researcher at several points over the course of the study to determine goodness of fit between explanation and data, thereby sharpening and rendering the interpretation credible and trustworthy. Note that the rigor criteria, believable and trustable, differ from those of experimental-type design.

Let's say you are interested in understanding the experiences of cancer treatments. You choose to follow 20 individuals with different types of tumors and courses of treatment. The findings from each person, although yielding some similarities, indicated differences based on cultural background, access to resources, and locations and types of tumors. By observing and interviewing individuals as they move through treatments, the investigator is able to reveal the wide range of experiences while shedding light on the basic elements common to all, such as managing the trepidation and pain of chemotherapy treatments, secondary symptoms of chemotherapy such as hair loss, and fear of the unknown. •

Transferability of Findings

The findings from naturalistic design are specific to the research context and are not geared to generalizing findings from a small sample and applying this generalization to a larger group of persons with similar characteristics. Because the goal is not to generalize findings but to gain a more in-depth and nuanced understanding of a particular experience or phenomenon, you may ask, "Why bother doing a naturalistic study if you cannot use the research beyond the actual scope or context of the study?" The answer lies in one of the primary purposes of naturalistic research: generating theory. Naturalistic researchers use their methods and findings to generate or revise theory and to reveal the unique meanings of human experiences in human environments. Because the investigator assumes that current knowledge does not adequately explain the phenomenon under investigation, the outcome of naturalistic design is the emergence of explanations, principles, concepts, and theories.

A major purpose of naturalistic designs is highlighting the contextual contributions to knowledge while also yielding principles, concepts, and theories that may have relevance to a broader population or other arenas than that which was studied. Naturalistic inquiry generates knowledge that can be evaluated for relevance, or what Guba[12] named the "transferability of findings," to other similar populations and contexts.

Because phenomena are seen as context-bound and, according to naturalistic principles, may not be understandable apart from the spaces in which they occur, naturalistic inquiry is not concerned with the issue of generalizability or external validity as articulated in experimental-type inquiry. These terms do not have immediate relevance to designs operating out of naturalistic traditions. Rather, naturalistic researchers are concerned with understanding richness and depth in context, and thus with the capacity to retain unique meanings that are lost when generalization is a goal.[11] However, the development of "thick"[12] or in-depth descriptions and interpretations of different contexts leads to the ability to transfer, not generalize, meanings. Transferability refers to the potential relevance of knowledge across settings. Thus, although not aiming to generalize, the researcher is able to compare and contrast contexts and their elements to gain new insights within the research context as well as to suggest theory that may be pertinent to other domains. Note that we use the term "suggest" rather than "generalize," given the irrelevance of external validity to the naturalistic tradition.

Flexibility

The design of an experimental type of research provides the basic structure and plan for the thinking and action processes of the entire research endeavor before it is initiated. As we discussed earlier in this chapter, the design is followed as initially developed. In naturalistic research, however, there are alternatives; the study design is fluid and flexible. Design labels such as "ethnography," "life history," and "grounded theory" suggest a particular purpose of the inquiry and orientation of the investigator. These designs are not prescriptive, nor do they follow a fixed, a priori sequence of action processes. Naturalistic design designators do not refer to the specification of step-by-step procedures, a recipe or blueprint for action, or a predetermined structure to data-gathering and analytical efforts. These action processes unfold in the course of the conduct of this form of inquiry, not from a predetermined set of rules to which the study must conform.

Rather, a characteristic of naturalistic design is flexibility. An important and expected feature of a naturalistic study is that the procedures and plans for conducting it are apt to change as the research proceeds. Because data collection and analysis co-occur, the investigator may use the results of initial findings as guidance for planning or altering subsequent action processes. Not only do procedures change, but so may the nature of the research query, the scope of the study, and the manner by which information is obtained. These elements can be constantly reformulated and realigned to fit the emerging knowledge as it is discovered and obtained in the inquiry. This flexibility is illustrated more fully in Chapter 9.

Language

A major shared concern in many designs within naturalistic inquiry is understanding language and meanings. Focus on language is not only relevant to the etic or outsider ethnographer, who studies a cultural context in which the language is different from that of the investigator. Even within the same cultural or language context, people use and understand language differently. Thus, for some naturalistic investigators, language, symbols, and ways of expression provide the data through which the investigator comes to understand and derive meaning within each context.[13] Investigators proceeding from a postmodern philosophical foundation are particularly concerned with language itself. In contrast to previous philosophies that attribute meaning to symbols, postmodern thinkers suggest that language as a set of symbols is a grand narrative, or symbols without shared or substantive meaning.[14]

Depending on the philosophical approach, the investigator concerned with language may engage in a rigorous and active analytical process to "translate" the meaning and structure of the context of the studied group into meanings and language structures expressed in the investigator's world. In this type of inquiry, the investigator is careful to represent the meanings and intent of expression accurately in the reporting process. For example, different race and ethnic groups use various terms to express what is defined medically as clinical depression. From a medical perspective, depression is a series of symptoms (e.g., loss of interest, feelings of sadness that last for more than 2 weeks) that can be evaluated as to their frequency of occurrence and the severity

with which they interfere with daily function. As you will learn, this approach represents understanding depression from an outside "etic" perspective. However, the term "depression" can have diverse meanings and may be expressed as a complex web of feelings and actions that are part of a larger story about everyday life and its challenges. Understanding the meanings of "depression" and its various expressions from the person's (or "emic," described later) perspective can provide important insights about the context of this experience and how people label these feelings and can lead to new ways to detect and treat "depression" or suggest that it is simply a part of the continuum of human emotion not to be treated.

As mentioned, however, not all investigators concerned with language believe that naturalistic inquiry can reveal meaning. Postmodern inquiry aims to "deconstruct" language, or unravel it to illustrate its arbitrary structure and identify its political, economic, and purposive usage. For example, an investigator might examine the text of legislation designed to protect women against domestic violence to uncover the metaphors that help retain men's dominance and their fiscal and political power over women.

Throughout the full range of philosophical approaches that underpin the naturalistic tradition, the description and analysis of language are two of the primary concerns.

Emic and Etic Perspectives

As introduced earlier, design structures vary as to the extent to which they have an *emic* or *etic* orientation. An emic perspective refers to the insider's or informant's way of understanding and interpreting experience. This perspective is phenomenological in that experience is understood as only that which is perceived and expressed by informants.[15] Data gathering and analytical actions are designed to enable the investigator to bring forth and report the voices of individuals as they speak and interpret their unique perceptions of their reality. The concern with the emic perspective is often the motivator for naturalistic inquiry. For example, in her classic work,[16] Padilla explained why she decided to study head injury from a phenomenological perspective, highlighting the preference for an emic viewpoint shared by designs in this tradition, as follows:

A shift in view of life was noted in the participant as the reflective process of this study unfolded, suggesting a phenomenological collaboration between patient and therapist may engender a more genuine connection in which personal meaning is authentically the cornerstone of occupation-centered treatment. (p 413)

An etic orientation refers to those external to a group; that is, the etic perspective is held by nonmembers of the group being investigated (medical profession applying a diagnostic category such as depression). Unlike the emic perspective, in which individuals who have the "experience" are considered to be most knowledgeable about it, the etic perspective assumes that a phenomenon not only can be understood but is best understood through (1) structuring an investigation, (2) selecting a theoretical foundation that expands beyond the group being examined, and (3) through that lens, conducting the interpretation of data.[17] Many investigators integrate an emic with an etic perspective in the form of mixing methodologies. Investigators may start by using an emic perspective, or a focus on the voices of individuals. Further along the process, other pieces of information are collected and analyzed to place individual articulation and expression within a social structural or systemic framework.

Some designs, such as phenomenology and life history, favor only an emic orientation. In her classic study, Frank described her preference for an emic perspective and the purpose of her life history approach to a woman with severe impairment as follows:

The life history of Diane DeVries represents a collaborative effort, between the subject and researcher, to produce a holistic, qualitative account that would bear on theoretical issues, but that primarily and essentially would convey a sense of the personal experience of severe congenital disability. The life history, conceived in this way, emerged from a humanistic interest in presenting the voices of people often unheard, yet whose lives were otherwise studied, and acted upon, based on data that are decontextualized and fragmented from the standpoint of the individual.[18]

Because the investigator enters the inquiry having bracketed, suspended, or let go of any preconceived concepts, the naturalistic researcher defers to the informant or experiencer as the "knower." This abrogation of power by the investigator to the investigated is characteristic to a greater or lesser degree of naturalistic designs.

> An extreme example of relinquishing control over the research process is a study design in which informants themselves plan and conduct the research in its entirety (see Maruyama's classic prison study as an example).[19]

Where the investigator stands regarding an emic or etic perspective shapes the overall design that is chosen, as well as the specific data collection and analytical action processes that emerge within the context of the inquiry.

Gathering Information and Analysis

Although numeric data are captured in this tradition, analysis in naturalistic designs relies heavily on qualitative data and is an ongoing process throughout data-gathering activities. Thus, as we noted earlier, in the naturalistic tradition, data gathering and analysis are interdependent processes. In collecting information or data, the investigator engages in an active analytical process. In turn, the ongoing analytical activity frames the scope and direction of further data collection efforts. This interactive, iterative, and dynamic process is characteristic of designs within the tradition of naturalistic inquiry and is explored more fully later in this text.

Naturalistic Design Summary

The purpose of naturalistic inquiry and the nature of design in this tradition are vastly different from experimental-type research. The language and thinking processes that characterize naturalistic designs are based on the notion that knowing is pluralistic and that knowledge derives from understanding multiple experiences in context. Thus, the thinking process is inductive and abductive; the action processes are dynamic and changing; and these processes are carried out within the actual or theoretical context in which the phenomena of interest occur or are experienced. The outcome of these thinking and action processes is most often the generation of theory, principles, or concepts that explain human experience in human environments and capture its complexity and uniqueness.

Within any naturalistic design, the investigator can implement the 10 essentials in various ways. Designs vary from informant-driven with no structure to researcher-driven with more structure.

The nature of this form of inquiry has evolved in its forms, scope, and purposes[11] and is continuing to evolve in its standards, vocabulary, and criteria for design adequacy. It is a well-respected tradition in its own right, as it is increasingly being used to answer questions about health and human service practices, beliefs, and understandings.

Mixed Method Approaches

Studies that integrate experimental-type and naturalistic traditions have increased despite previous skepticism about philosophical inconsistencies. The mixed method approach for advancing knowledge has recently been referred to as the "third tradition"[10] with a foundation in pragmatism.

As quoted by Tashakkori and Teddlie,[10] Diesta explains pragmatism in this way:

> Pragmatism should not be considered as a philosophical position among others, but rather a set of philosophical tools that can be used to address problems—not in the least problems cared by other philosophical approaches and positions. One of the central ideas of pragmatism is the engagement in philosophical activity should be done in order to address problems, not to build systems.

Mixing methods is therefore a set of strategies that addresses the limitations of any one approach, and we therefore support its use whenever possible and appropriate. As discussed, however, both experimental-type and naturalistic traditions conform to diverse sets of rules, languages, and strategies for rigor. Therefore, the investigator who proceeds with an integrated approach heeds the important tenets of both traditions as well as the emerging rigor criteria of this third tradition. At this point in its development, mixed methods integrates experimental-type and naturalistic tools within a defined and purposive context and incorporates language and thinking processes from each of the other two traditions such that knowledge gained from one approach is integrated with knowledge gained from the other approach.

Summary

Experimental-type and naturalistic traditions have distinct language and thinking processes. Experimental-type researchers approach their studies with intact theory and a set of procedures. A plan is developed and followed to minimize the potential for factors other than those studied to be responsible for the findings. Dissimilarly, naturalistic language and thinking processes are flexible, fluid, and changing. As the investigator proceeds throughout the research design, the aim of capturing complexity from the perspective of the individuals or phenomena studied is actualized through systematic but dynamic interaction between collecting and analyzing information. Mixed method approaches combine the language and thinking processes of both traditions in purposive ways depending on the research queries posed and the approach to integrating the information obtained from different design elements.

EXERCISES

1. Select a research article from a journal that uses an experimental-type design. Identify the independent variable or variables, the dependent variable or variables, and any intervening variables that may be confounding the study.
2. Identify the conceptual definitions and the operational definitions in the article that you selected.
3. Using the same article, determine (a) threats to validity of the study, (b) how the investigator minimized bias and enhanced control and validity, and (c) ethical issues that shaped the design.
4. Select a research article that uses naturalistic inquiry. Identify and provide evidence of the following eight elements of the researcher's thinking process:

a. Purpose of research
b. Context of research
c. Pluralistic perspective of reality
d. Concern with transferability
e. Flexibility
f. Concern with language
g. Emic and etic perspectives
h. Interactive and analytical process

5. Using the same article, determine some of the ethical issues that shaped the investigator's behavior in the inquiry.

6. Find a mixed method study and identify strategies from both experimental-type and naturalistic traditions within the method.

....

References

1. Kerlinger FN: *Foundations of behavioral research*, ed 2, New York, 1973, Holt, Rinehart, & Winston, p 279.
2. Wilson J: *Thinking with concepts*, Cambridge, UK, 1966, Cambridge University Press, p 54.
3. Babbie E: *The practice of social research*, ed 13, Belmont, Calif, 2013, Wadsworth.
4. Roth DL, MacKinnon DP: Mediation analysis with longitudinal data. In Newsom JT, Jones RN, Hoefer SM, editors: *Longitudinal data analysis: a practical guide for researchers in aging, health and social sciences*, New York, 2012, Routledge, pp 181–216.
5. Gitlin LN, Roth DL, Huang J: Mediators of the impact of a home-based intervention (Beat the Blues) on depressive symptoms among older African Americans. *Psychol Aging* 29:601–611, doi:10.1037/a0036784.
6. Gitlin LN, Winter L, Corcoran M, et al: Effects of the home environmental skill-building program on the caregiver-care recipient dyad: six-month outcomes from the Philadelphia REACH Initiative. *Gerontologist* 43:532–546, 2003.
7. Campbell DT, Stanley JC: *Experimental and quasi-experimental design*, Chicago, 1963, Rand McNally.
8. Daniel J: *Sampling essentials: practical guidelines for making sampling choices*, Los Angeles, 2012, Sage.
9. Neuman WL: *Social research methods: qualitative and quantitative approaches*, ed 7, Boston, 2009, Allyn & Bacon.
10. Tashakkori A, Teddlie C: *Sage handbook of mixed methods in social and behavioral research*, ed 2, Thousand Oaks, Calif, 2010, Sage.
11. Denzin NK, Lincoln YS: *Sage handbook of qualitative research*, ed 3, Thousand Oaks, Calif, 2011, Sage.
12. Guba EG: Criteria for assessing the trustworthiness of naturalistic inquiries. *Educ Commun Technol J* 29:75–92, 1981.
13. Kress G: *Multimodality: a social semiotic approach to contemporary communication*, New York, 2010, Routledge.
14. Nealon J: *Post-postmodernism*, Stanford, Calif, 2012, Stanford University Press.
15. Detmer D: *Phenomenology explained: from experience to insight*, Chicago, 2013, Carus.
16. Padilla R: Clara: a phenomenology of disability. *Am J Occup Ther* 57:413–417, 2003.
17. Headland TN, Pike KL, Harris M: *Emics and etics: the insider/outsider debate*, Newbury Park, Calif, 1990, Sage.
18. Frank G: Life history model of adaptation to disability: the case of a congenital amputee. *Soc Sci Med* 19:639–645, 1984.
19. Maruyama M: Endogenous research: the prison project. In Reason P, Rowan J, editors: *Human inquiry: a sourcebook for new paradigm research*, New York, 1981, Wiley.

PART III Design Approaches

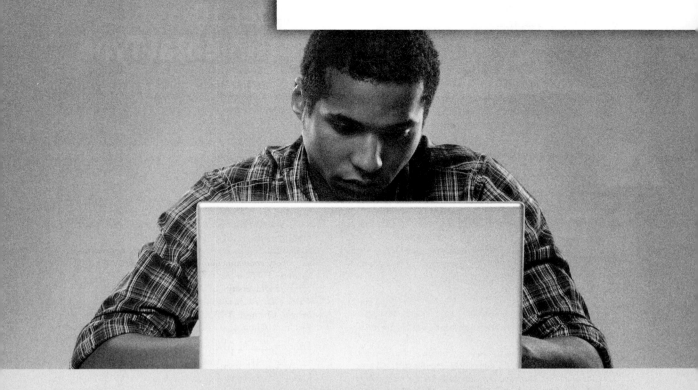

Now that we have delved into the thinking processes of research, we are ready to examine its structure. The structure of research refers to the design elements used by researchers to answer queries and questions. In Part III, we present diverse approaches to design that are used to conduct research in experimental-type, naturalistic, and integrated to mixed methods.

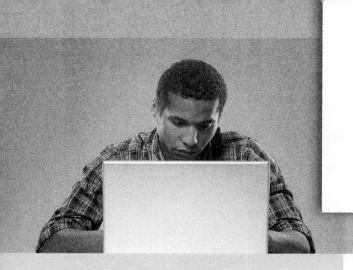

Chapter 10
Experimental-Type Designs

Using the language introduced in Chapter 9, we are ready to examine the characteristics of designs in the experimental-type research tradition. Experimental designs have traditionally been classified as true-experimental, quasi-experimental, pre-experimental, and nonexperimental. Within this tradition, the true experiment is the criterion by which all other methodological approaches are judged. Many people think that the only legitimate research or science is the experimental method. Of all the experimental-type designs, the true-experimental design offers the greatest degree of control and internal validity. It is this design and its variations that are used to reveal causal relationships between independent and dependent variables (Level 3 questioning). Also, within this tradition, this design is often upheld as the highest level of scientific evidence, particularly in evidence-based practice model research and ratings that are applied to studies for the development of clinical guidelines as we discuss subsequently.

Although the true-experimental design is repeatedly affirmed as the most "objective" and "true" scientific approach, we believe it is important to recognize that every design in the experimental-type tradition has merit and value. The merit of a design is based on how well the design answers the research question that is being posed and the level of rigor that the investigator brings to the plan and conduct of the inquiry. This view of research differs from the perspective of the many experimental-type researchers who present the true experiment as the gold standard and only design of choice, implying that other designs are deficient or limited.[1,2] We suggest that a design in the experimental-type tradition should be chosen purposively because it fits the question, level of theory development, and setting or environment in which the research will be conducted. True experimentation and variants that contain all the elements of this approach are the best designs to predict causal relationships, but they may be inappropriate for other forms of inquiry in health and human service settings. That is to say, not all research questions seek to predict causal relationships between independent and dependent variables. Recall our discussion on level of questioning in which inquiry within the experimental-type tradition begins with description and then proceeds to incrementally more abstract domains. True experimentation is not necessary or warranted for answering questions of description and association. Moreover, in some cases, using a true-experimental design may present major critical ethical dilemmas such that other design strategies may be more appropriate.

True-Experimental Designs

To express the structural relationships of *true-experimental designs,* we use Campbell and Stanley's classic, widely adopted notation system to diagram a design: *X* represents the independent variable, *O* the dependent variable, and *R* denotes random sample selection,[3] as follows:

$$R \quad O \quad X \quad O$$
$$R \quad O \qquad\quad O$$

We also find it helpful to use the symbol *r* to refer to random group assignment in the absence of random sample selection. It is often difficult and frequently inappropriate or unethical for health and human service professionals to select a sample from a larger, predefined population based on random selection (*R*); rather, subjects typically enter studies on a volunteer basis. Such a sample is one of convenience or purpose in which subjects are then randomly assigned to either the experimental or the control group. The addition of "*r*" denotes this important structural distinction. Designs in which samples are not randomly selected but are randomly assigned still meet the criteria for true experimentation and can answer predictive questions but, as we discuss later, are limited in their external validity—the degree to which the sample represents the population from which it was selected. Absence of random selection (*R*) also has implications for statistical choices (as we discuss in Chapter 14).

True-experimental designs are most commonly thought about when beginning researchers and laypersons hear the word "research." True-experimental design refers to the classic two-group design in which subjects are randomly selected (*R*) and randomly assigned to either an experimental or control group condition. Before the experimental condition, all subjects are pretested or observed on a dependent measure (*O*). In the experimental group the independent variable or experimental condition is imposed (*X*), and it is withheld in the control group. After the experimental condition, all subjects are posttested or observed on the dependent variable (*O*).

$$R \quad O \quad X \quad O$$
$$R \quad O \qquad\quad O$$

You are interested in enhancing shoulder range of motion in the affected upper extremity in persons with stroke. The dependent variable would be a measure of shoulder range of motion; the independent variable or experimental condition, a particular therapy protocol that is introduced; and the control condition,

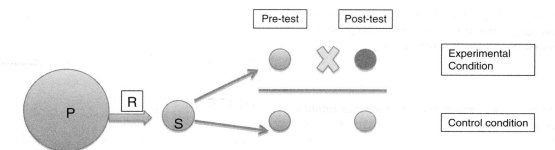

Figure 10-1 Logic—Both pre-test conditions and the control post-test condition remain unchanged from the sample and population. As a result of the experimental condition, the post-test following "X" is changed and logically can only be a result of X.

a control group that receives usual care. Subjects in a rehabilitation facility who meet specific criteria for study participation would be pretested on the measure of shoulder range of motion, randomly assigned to receive the experimental condition or usual care, and then retested using the same range-of-motion measure. •

> **BOX 10-1** *Three Characteristics of True-Experimental Design*
>
> • Randomization
> • Control group
> • Manipulation of an independent variable

Figure 10-1 denotes the logic of this structure.

In this design, the investigator expects to observe no difference between the experimental and control groups on the dependent measure at pretest. In other words, subjects are chosen randomly from a larger pool of potential subjects and then assigned to a group on a "chance-determined" basis; therefore, subjects in both groups are expected to perform similarly. In the example, we would expect that subjects in experimental and control group conditions would have similar shoulder range-of-motion scores at the first baseline or pretest assessment. However, because the experimental group is exposed to only one condition (*X*) that the control group does not experience, the investigator anticipates or hypothesizes that differences will occur between experimental and control group subjects on the posttest scores. In other words, as a result of the introduction of an independent variable, the experimental condition, the members in the experimental group have been changed and thus no longer belong to the sample from which they were selected and the population from which they were recruited. This expectation is expressed as a null hypothesis, which states that no difference is expected. In a true-experimental design,

the investigator always states a null hypothesis that forms the basis for statistical testing. Usually in research reports, however, the alternative (working) hypothesis is stated (i.e., an expected difference). If the investigator's data analytical procedures reveal a significant difference (one that does not occur by chance) between experimental and control group scores at posttest, the investigator can fail to accept the null hypothesis with a reasonable degree of certainty. In failing to accept the null hypothesis, the investigator accepts with a certain level of confidence that the independent variable or experimental condition (*X*) caused the outcome observed at posttest time in the experimental group. In other words, the investigator infers that the difference at posttest time is not the result of chance but is caused by participation in the experimental condition.

Three major characteristics of the true-experimental design allow this causal claim to be made (Box 10-1).

Randomization

Randomization occurs at the sample selection phase, the group assignment phase, or both. If random sample selection is accomplished, the design notation appears as presented earlier (R). If randomization occurs only at the group assignment phase, we represent the design accordingly (r):

$$r\ O \quad X \quad O$$
$$r\ O \qquad\quad O$$

As we noted earlier, this variation has implications for external validity. Remember that a true-experimental design that does not use random sample selection is limited in the extent to which conclusions can be generalized to the population from which the sample is selected. Because subjects are not drawn by chance from a larger identified pool, the generalizability or external validity of findings is limited. However, such a design variation is common in experimental research and can still be used to reveal causal relationships within the sample (or the population if the entire population is tested) itself. The choice to call the participants a sample or a population has implications for statistical choice as we discuss in Chapter 14.

Although random sample selection is often impossible to achieve, random assignment of subjects to group conditions based on chance is essential in true experimentation. It enhances the probability that subjects in experimental and control groups will be theoretically equivalent on all major dependent variables at the pretest occasion. Randomization, in principle, equalizes subjects or provides a high degree of assurance that subjects in both experimental and control groups will be comparable at pretest or the initial, baseline measure. How is this possible? By randomizing, people are assigned by chance, and therefore the researcher does not introduce any systematic order to the selection and assignment of the sample. Thus, any influence on one group theoretically will similarly affect the other group as well. In the absence of any other differences that could influence outcome, an observed change in the experimental group at posttest then can be attributed with a reasonable degree of certainty to the experimental condition.

Randomization is a powerful technique that is designed to increase control and eliminate bias by neutralizing the effects of extraneous influences on the outcome of a study. For example, the threats to internal validity by historical events and maturation

are theoretically neutralized and thus eliminated because, based on probability theory, such influences should affect subjects equally. Without randomization of subjects, you will not have a true-experimental design.[4]

Control Group

We now extend the concept of control introduced in Chapter 9 to refer to the inclusion of a control group in a study. The control group allows the investigator to see what the sample would be without the influence of the experimental condition or independent variable. Recall Figure 10-1. The control group theoretically performs or remains the same relative to the independent variable at pretest and posttest, because the control group has not had the chance to be exposed to the experimental (or planned change) condition and thus has not been changed. Therefore, the control group represents the characteristics of the experimental group before being changed by participation in the experimental condition.

The control group is also a mechanism that allows the investigator to examine what has been referred to as the "attention factor," "Hawthorne effect," or "halo effect."[5] These three terms all refer to the phenomenon of the subject experiencing change as a result of simply participating in a research project. For example, being the recipient of personal attention from an interviewer during pretesting and posttesting may influence how a subject feels and responds to interview questions. A change in scores in the experimental group may then occur, independent of the effect of the experimental condition. Without a control group, investigators are not able to observe the presence or absence of this phenomenon and are unable to judge the extent to which differences on posttest scores of the experimental group reflect the experimental effect, not additional attention.

Interestingly, this attention phenomenon was discovered in the process of conducting research. In 1934, a group of investigators were examining productivity in the Hawthorne automobile plant in Chicago. The research involved interviewing workers. To improve productivity, the investigators recommended that the lighting of the facility be brightened. The researchers noted week after week that productivity increased after each subsequent increase in illumination. To confirm the success of their amazing findings, the researchers then dimmed the light. To their surprise, productivity continued to increase even under this circumstance. In reexamining the research process, they concluded that it was the additional attention given to the workers through the ongoing interview process and their inclusion in the research itself, not the lighting, that caused an increased work effort.[6]

Manipulation

In a true-experimental design, the independent variable is manipulated either by having it present (in the experimental group) or absent (in the control group). *Manipulation* is defined as the ability to provide and withhold the independent variable that is unique to the true experiment.

According to the classic work of Campbell and Stanley,[3] true experimentation theoretically controls for each of the seven major threats to internal validity (see Chapter 9). However, when such a true-experimental design is implemented in the health care or human service environment, certain influences may remain as internal threats, thereby decreasing the potential for the investigator to support a cause-and-effect relationship. For example, the selection of a data-collection instrument with a learning effect based on repeated testing could pose a significant threat to a study, regardless of how well the experiment is structured. It is also possible for experimental "mortality" (withdrawal of participation) to affect outcome, particularly if the groups become nonequivalent as a result of attrition from the experiment. The health or human service environment is complex and does not offer the same degree of control as a laboratory setting. Therefore, in applying the true-experimental design to the health or human service environment, the researcher must carefully examine the particular threats to internal validity and how each can be resolved.

True-Experimental Design Variations

Many design variations of the true experiment have been developed to enhance its internal validity. For example, to assess the effect of the attention factor,

a researcher may develop a three-group design. In this structure, subjects are randomly assigned to (1) an experimental condition, (2) an attention control group that receives an activity designed to equalize the attention that subjects receive in the experimental group, or (3) a silent control group that receives no attention other than that obtained naturally during data-collection efforts. The term "silent control group" can also refer to the situation in which information is collected on subjects who have no knowledge of their own participation, ostensibly eliminating any influence whatsoever that would change the group.

 For example, extracting information from medical records on a group that remains unaware may provide the researcher with an understanding of how subjects in the study compare with those with similar demographic and medical characteristics who are not included in the study.

Let us examine four basic design variations of the true experiment.

Posttest-Only Designs

Posttest-only designs conform to the norms of experimentation in that they contain the three elements of random assignment, control group, and manipulation. The difference between classic true-experimental design and this variation is the absence of a pretest. The basic design notation for a posttest-only experiment follows for randomly selected and randomly assigned samples:

$$R \quad X \quad O$$
$$R \qquad\quad O$$

In a posttest-only design, groups are considered equivalent before the experimental condition as a result of random assignment. Theoretically, randomization should yield equivalent groups. However, the absence of the pretest makes it impossible to determine whether random assignment successfully achieved equivalence between the experimental and control groups on the major dependent variables of the study. Some researchers assume that the control group posttest scores are equivalent to pretest scores for both control and experimental groups. However, caution is advised, especially considering the influence of attention on subjects that we discussed earlier. There are a number of variations of this basic design. For example, the researcher may add other posttest occasions or different types of experimental or control groups.

Posttest-only designs are most valuable when pretesting is not possible or appropriate but the research purpose aims to examine causal relationships. Also, a posttest-only design might be chosen if the threat to learning is highly likely with repeated testing using the same measure of the dependent variable.

Solomon Four-Group Designs

More complex experimental structures than those previously discussed, *Solomon four-group designs* combine the true-experiment and posttest-only designs into one design structure. The strength of this design is that it provides the opportunity to test the potential influence of the test-retest learning phenomenon by adding the posttest-only two-group design to the true-experimental design. This design is noted as follows if random selection occurs:

$$
\begin{array}{cccc}
R & O & X & O \\
R & O &   & O \\
R &   & X & O \\
R &   &   & O
\end{array}
$$

If random assignment without random selection occurs, the notation *r* would be noted in lowercase.

As shown in this notation, Group 3 does not receive the pretest but participates in the experimental condition. Group 4 also does not receive the pretest but serves as a control group. By comparing the posttest scores of all groups, the investigator can evaluate the effect of testing on scores on the posttest and interaction between the test and the experimental condition. The key benefit of this design is its ability to detect interaction effects. An interaction effect refers to changes that occur in the dependent variable as a consequence of the combined influence or interaction of taking the pretest and participating in the experimental condition.

The following example illustrates the power of the Solomon four-group design and the nature of interaction effects.

You want to assess the effects of an informational training program (independent variable) about acquired immunodeficiency syndrome (AIDS) on the sexual risk-taking behaviors (dependent variable) of adolescents. You can pretest groups by asking questions about sexual activities and levels of knowledge regarding behavioral risks of developing AIDS. You can expose one group to the experimental condition, which involves attending an educational forum led by peers. On posttesting, you discover that levels of knowledge increased and that risk behaviors decreased in subjects who received the experimental program. However, you cannot determine the effect of the pretest itself on the outcome. By adding Group 3 (experimental condition without pretest), you can determine whether the change in scores is as strong as when the pretest is administered (Group 1). If Group 2 (control) and Group 3 (experimental) show no change but experimental Group 1 does, you can be relatively certain that this change is a consequence of an interaction effect of the pretest and the intervention. If there is a change in experimental Groups 1 and 3 and some change in control Group 2, but none in control Group 4, there may be a direct effect of the intervention or experimental condition plus an interaction effect. •

This design allows the investigator to determine the strength of the independent effects of the intervention and the strength of the effect of pretesting on outcomes. If the groups that have been pretested show a testing effect, statistical procedures can be used to correct it, if necessary.

As you can see, the Solomon four-group design offers increased control and the possibility of understanding complex outcomes. Because it requires the addition of two groups, however, it is a costly, time-consuming alternative to the true-experimental design and infrequently used in health and human service inquiry.

Factorial Designs

These designs offer even more opportunities for multiple comparisons and complexities in analysis. In *factorial designs,* the investigator evaluates the

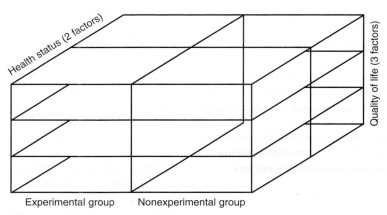

Figure 10-2 Factorial design (2 × 2 × 3) used to investigate quality of life in elder participants in an experimental exercise program.

effects of two or more independent variables (*X1* and *X2*) or the effects of an intervention on different factors or levels of a sample or study variables. The interaction of these parts, as well as the direct relationship of one part to another, is examined.

> You are interested in examining the effects of an organized group exercise program on older adults. Specifically, you want to determine the extent to which two levels of "health status" (good and poor) influence three "quality of life" areas for participants. In this case, the first independent variable that is manipulated assumes two values: participation in the exercise experimental group or participation in a nonexercise control group. The other independent variable that is not manipulated (health) also has two values (good and poor). The dependent variable or outcome measure (quality of life) is composed of three factors (activity level, overall satisfaction, sense of well-being). This study represents a factorial design in which the independent variables have two factors or levels and the dependent variable has three levels. This structure is referred to as a "2 × 2 × 3" factorial design (Fig. 10-2). This design allows you to examine the relationship between different levels of health and specific quality-of-life indicators for two conditions, subjects exercising and subjects participating in a nonexercise control group. •

The factorial design enables you to examine not only direct relationships but interactive relationships as well. You can determine the combined effects of

two or more variables that may be quite different from each direct effect. For example, you may want to examine whether the less healthy exerciser scores higher on a life satisfaction assessment than the less healthy nonexerciser. To statistically evaluate all the possible configurations in this design, you need to have a large sample size to ensure that each cell or block (see Fig. 10-2) contains an adequate number of scores for analysis.

Of course, you can develop more complex factorial designs in which both independent and dependent variables have more than two values or levels. With more complexity, however, increasingly large sample sizes are necessary to ensure sufficient numbers in each variation to permit analysis.

Counterbalance Designs

When more than one intervention is being tested and when the order of participation is manipulated, *counterbalance designs* are often used. This design allows the investigator to determine the combined effects of two or more interventions and the effect of order on study outcomes. Although there are many variations, the basic design (with random sample selection) is as follows:

$$R\ O^1 \quad X \quad O^2 \quad X \quad O$$
$$R\ O^2 \quad X \quad O^1 \quad X \quad O$$

Again, lowercase *r* would denote random assignment and would still qualify for this true-experimental design.

Note the superscript numbers on the independent variables. The reversal of the conditions is characteristic of counterbalance designs in which both groups experience both conditions but in different orders. This reversal is called "crossover." In a crossover study, one group is assigned to the experimental group first and to the control condition later; the reverse order is assigned for the other group. Measurements occur before the first set of conditions, before the second set, and after the experiment. Such a study allows you to eliminate the threats to internal validity caused by the interaction of the experimental variable and other aspects of the study.

> Suppose you were interested in the psychosocial effects of two interventions for women whose husbands had been killed in military service in Afghanistan. You randomly assign your sample to one of two conditions, on-site support group only and peer virtual support, and then reverse their assignment. Testing would occur at three intervals: just before the experiment, after participation in condition 1, and after the experiment. By structuring your research with this design, you would be able not only to ascertain the effects of each program on a single group but also to compare groups over time in each of the conditions. •

True-Experimental Design Summary

True-experimental designs must contain three essential characteristics: random assignment, control group, and manipulation. The classic true experiment and its variations all contain these elements and thus are capable of producing knowledge about causal relationships among independent and dependent variables. The four design strategies in the true-experimental classification are appropriate for an experimental-type Level 3 research question in which the intent is to predict and reveal a cause. Each true-experimental-type design controls the influences of the basic threats to internal validity and theoretically eliminates unwanted or extraneous phenomena that can confound a causal study and invalidate causal claims. The three criteria for using a true-experimental design or its variation are (1) sufficient theory to examine causality, (2) a Level 3 causal question, and (3) conditions and ethics that permit randomization, use of a control group, and manipulation.

Developing even the most straightforward experimental design, such as the two-group randomized trial, involves many other considerations. In the early stages and even throughout your research career, consulting with a statistician can help you determine the best approach to randomizing subjects based on your study design and the basic characteristics of the subjects that you plan to enroll. There are many ways to randomize to ensure that subjects are assigned to groups by chance. In complex designs or large clinical trials, a statistician is usually responsible for setting up a randomization scheme and placing group assignments in sealed, opaque envelopes so that the investigators or research team members cannot influence the group assignment.

Quasi-experimental Designs

Although true experiments have been upheld as the ideal or prototype in research and the gold standard for evidence-based practice,[1] such designs may not be appropriate for many reasons, as we have indicated throughout this book. First, in health and human service research, it may not be possible, appropriate, or ethical to use randomization or to manipulate the introduction and withholding of an experimental intervention. Second, and perhaps most important, not all inquiries ask causal questions, and the true experimental design is not appropriate for questions that do not seek answers about cause-and-effect relationships. So what can you do when it is not possible or appropriate to use randomization, manipulation, or a control group?

You can select other design options that do not contain the three elements of true experimentation to generate valuable knowledge. Even though the language of the experimental-type tradition implies that these designs resemble true experimentation but are missing one or more of its essential features, we suggest that these designs are not "inferior" or even comparative but rather parallel in value in that they produce different knowledge, interpretations, and uses than true experimentation.

As in all design decisions, the decision to use quasi-experimental designs should be based on the

BOX 10-2 *Quasi-experimental Designs*

- Nonequivalent control group
- Interrupted time series

level of theory, type of research question asked, and constraints of the research environment. Cook and Campbell,[7] who wrote the seminal classical work on quasi-experimentation, defined these designs as

> experiments that have treatments, outcome measures, and experimental units, but do not use random assignment to create comparison from which treatment-caused change is inferred. Instead, the comparisons depend on nonequivalent groups that differ from each other in many ways other than the presence of the treatment whose effects are being tested.[7]

The key to the efficacious use of quasi-experimental designs lies in the claims made by the researcher about the findings. Because random assignment is absent in quasi-experimentation, the researcher can (1) suggest causal claims while acknowledging the alternative explanations for these claims and design limitations or (2) avoid making causal inferences when they are unjustified by the design.[6]

Designs in the quasi-experimental category have two of the three true-experimental elements: control group and manipulation. Two basic design types fit the criteria for quasi-experimentation (Box 10-2).

Nonequivalent Control Group Designs

There are at least two comparison groups in non-equivalent control group designs, but subjects are not randomly assigned to these groups. The basic design is structured as a pretest and posttest comparison group, as in the following notation:

$$O \quad X \quad O$$
$$O \quad \quad O$$

It is also possible to add comparison groups or to alter the testing sequence. This design can answer the basic question, "What changed after being exposed to the experimental condition compared to nonexposure?"

Consider this example. You want to test the effectiveness of an innovative mental health program designed to alleviate depression, but it is not possible to use randomization. You arrange for a community mental health center to use the experimental intervention for 1 month. You find another community mental health center in which the population is comparable and assign the comparison condition (conventional intervention) to that group. As with true-experimental design, you pretest and posttest all subjects, then compare group scores both within group and between groups. If the group scores for the experimental condition are significantly different on posttest than pretest and between group posttests, there is strong support for the value of the innovative program. Once again, however, because of the multiple threats to internal validity, most likely you will not use this design to support cause but to explain the comparative changes in each of the study groups. That is, you can indicate that the changes after the intervention in the experimental group were significantly greater than the changes in the comparison group. •

As an example, suppose you wanted to test the change in fitness after a new exercise program in a population of individuals who had sustained mild stroke. However, you cannot institute random assignment because the exercise program is only offered at one facility for all outpatients who meet the diagnostic criteria. So you decide to compare groups in two facilities, the one offering the program and one that does not. A nonequivalent control group design would be appropriate for the context and to answer the following Level 2 question:

> Compared to the group that did not undergo the experimental exercise program, what changes in fitness occurred in the group that participated in this program?

You might even hypothesize that the experimental group scores would improve compared with the control condition. However, because the groups were not randomly assigned to experimental and control groups, it would not be possible to isolate, theoretically, the experimental condition (the fitness program) and examine its effect on fitness improvement. However, you can look at comparative change, providing important knowledge for further inquiry and clinical guidance.

Interrupted Time Series Designs

Interrupted time series designs involve repeated measurement of the dependent variable both before and after the introduction of the independent variable. There is no control or comparison group in this design. The multiple measures before the independent variable control for the threat to internal validity based on maturation and other time-related changes. A typical time series design is depicted as follows:

$$O_1 \quad O_2 \quad O_3 \quad X \quad O_4 \quad O_5 \quad O_6$$

Although the number of observations may vary, it is suggested that no fewer than three occur before and three after the independent variable is introduced. The investigator is particularly interested in evaluating the change in scores between the observation that occurs immediately before the introduction of the intervention (O_3) and the observation that follows the intervention (O_4). Any sharp change in score compared with the other measures may suggest that the intervention had an effect (note that we say "suggest" because this design cannot produce a causal claim). The investigator must evaluate changes in scores in terms of the scoring patterns that occurred both before and after intervention. For example, if there is a trend for scores to increase at each testing occasion, even a sharp difference between O_3 and O_4 may not reflect a change resulting from the intervention. Rather, the pattern of ascending scores would be observed as a natural occurrence without influence from the introduction of the intervention.

Because of the absence of the control group and randomization, the interrupted time series design cannot strongly support a causal relationship between the independent and dependent variables. In this type of design, however, the series of premeasures theoretically controls threats to internal validity, except for the threat of history. Maturation, testing, instrumentation, regression, and attrition are considered threats that may occur among all measures and thus are detectable and controlled by repeated measurements. In this design, however, it is extremely important to choose a form of measurement in which there is no learning effect or threat of testing. In the health and human service context, researchers often use an interrupted time series design when they may not be able to manipulate the experimental intervention but they have knowledge of its introduction. In other words, the intervention or experimental program may be a naturally occurring event in which it is possible to document performance of the dependent variable before and after the event's occurrence.

Consider the fitness example described earlier. You might choose this configuration if you do not have or choose to use a control condition. Using an interrupted time series design, you would ask the following questions:

How did fitness scores change immediately following the intervention? How consistent were fitness scores over time following the intervention?

Now consider this example. A hospital announces a plan to implement a new employee benefits program to enhance job satisfaction. The effects of this program on job satisfaction can be determined by taking a quarterly survey of employees for 1 year before the introduction of the new program. The same survey can be used quarterly after employee participation in the new benefits program. In this way, the hospital will have four data points regarding employee satisfaction before the program's introduction that can be compared with four data points after its implementation. This strategy will allow for such extraneous factors as staff turnover and fluctuations in patient census to be tracked over time to account for their effect on job satisfaction. •

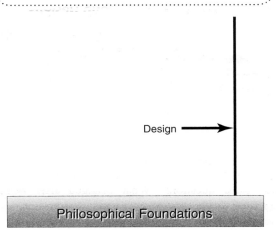

Design ⟶

Philosophical Foundations

The interrupted times series design is extremely useful in answering questions about the nature of change over time.

Combined Design

A combination of nonequivalent groups and interrupted time series is a quasi-experimental design that can be considered appropriate for answering causal questions, albeit with limitations. In this combination, some of the potential bias attributable to nonequivalent groups is limited by multiple measures, whereas the time series design is strengthened by the addition of a comparison group.

Suppose you instituted a combined design to test the outcome of your fitness program. If scores were relatively stable in both groups before the intervention and there was a significant increase in scores only in the experimental group immediately following the intervention and then at the remainder of the testing intervals, you could surmise that the program achieved its outcome.

Quasi-experimental Design Summary

Quasi-experimental designs are characterized by the presence of some type of comparison group and manipulation, but they do not contain random group assignment. Although there is no control group in time series and single-subject designs, control is exercised through multiple observations of the same phenomenon both before and after the introduction of the experimental condition. In nonequivalent group designs, the control is built in through the use of one or more comparison groups.

We suggest that quasi-experimentation is most valuable in three instances: (1) when the investigator is attempting to search for change over time; (2) when causal attribution is not the aim of the study; or (3) when a comparison between groups and the constraints of the health or human service environment are such that random assignment is not appropriate, ethical, or feasible.

Pre-experimental Designs

In *pre-experimental designs,* two of the three criteria for true experimentation are absent. In pre-experiments, it is possible to describe phenomena or

---

BOX 10-3   *Pre-experimental Designs*
....

- One-shot case study
- Pretest-posttest design
- Static group comparison

---

relationships. However, the outcomes of the study do not support claims for a causal relationship because of inadequate control and the potential of bias. Pre-experimental designs can be of value to answer descriptive Level 1 questions or Level 2 relational questions, or to generate pilot, exploratory evidence, but the investigator using these designs cannot answer predictive questions or support causal claims. The numerous pre-experimental designs are all variations on three designs (Box 10-3).

One-Shot Case Study

In the one-shot case study, the independent variable is introduced, then the dependent variable is measured in only one group, as follows:

$$X\ O$$

Without a pretest or a comparison group, the investigator can answer the question, "How did the group score on the dependent variable after the intervention?" As you can see, a cause-and-effect relationship between the two variables cannot be supported because of the seven threats to internal validity (see Box 9-3). In this design, the value is chronological, examining what happened following the introduction of the independent variable. Everyone recalls midterms and finals in courses. Assuming that good scores on a midterm resulted from learning in a class is an example of a misinterpretation of the one-shot case study. We discuss this point next.

Suppose you want to know whether your online cardiac health education program for elders (*X*) is meeting its aim of improving their knowledge about diet and exercise strategies (*O*). You decide to pilot the program at a senior center and recruit a sample of healthy elders to view the site and then take an online test to determine their knowledge. The subjects score relatively high on the test, and thus you conclude that it is likely they learned from the site.

From this study, you can answer the following question:

How did elders in the senior center score after participating the online education program?

Adding a comparison group to the one-shot case study strengthens the design, but not enough to allow Level 3 questions to be answered. This configuration is referred to as a static group comparison.

Static Group Comparison

In static group comparison, a comparison group is added to the one-shot case study design, as follows:

$$X \; O$$
$$O$$

This design, as in other pre-experimental structures, can answer descriptive questions about phenomena or relationships but is not considered a desirable choice for causal studies.

Some researchers consider the comparison group score as a pretest measure, because the group that did not receive intervention could approximate the pretest condition of the group receiving the intervention.

Introducing a static comparison group offers more control over extraneous factors than the one-shot case and pretest-posttest designs. However, we caution against its use to make statements on causal relationships between the independent and dependent variables.

Consider the cardiac education program. To institute a static comparison group design, you would provide the program to your subjects as we described in the one-shot case study design and recruit a similar sample from another senior center that would not participate in the online program. Both groups would receive the posttest at the same time. If the group that participated in the educational program scored significantly better than the group that did not participate, you could conclude that those who participated had more knowledge than those who did not. However, once again, you cannot conclude that the program influenced knowledge acquisition without random assignment or pretesting.

Here is another example. Suppose researchers want to test an intervention designed to reduce depression in young adults. The investigator who uses the static group comparison will select two nonequivalent groups, such as two groups of persons with depression receiving treatment in two different community mental health centers. One group will receive the intervention and one will not. A posttest measuring the level of depression will be administered to both groups and then compared. This design can answer the following question with a fair degree of certainty: "How did the experimental group compare with the comparison group on the measure of depression following the intervention?" Because random assignment did not occur, it is difficult to infer cause. Furthermore, there is minimal control in that the level of depression in either group was unknown before the introduction of the experimental condition. Yet, such a design adds compelling knowledge to guide further research and practice.

One-shot case study and static group comparisons are most useful in answering descriptive questions such as "What happened after a phenomenon occurred (e.g., an intervention, or the introduction of a new or revised approach to promoting health, education, and wellness) or "Compared to the control group, what happened after a phenomenon occurred?" For example, as introduced earlier, many university courses use a one-shot case study design to test student learning. Typically, no pretest is given when students enroll in a class. The course (*X*) proceeds and then an exam (*O*) is given. Student scores on the exam can only tell what they learned; their learning cannot be attributed to the course.

As demonstrated in the examples just given for both the one-shot case study and the static group comparison design, there is insufficient control and a lack of the randomization necessary to support or infer a causal relationship between the independent and dependent variables.

Pretest-Posttest Design

The pretest-posttest design is also valuable in describing what occurs after the introduction of the independent variable, as follows:

$$O \qquad X \qquad O$$

This design can answer questions about change following exposure to the independent variable in that the pretest is given before its introduction. If subjects are tested before and after the intervention, a change in scores on the dependent variable can be reported but, again, cannot be attributed to the influence of the independent variable. Threats to internal validity, if one were to attempt to infer cause using this design, include maturation, history, testing, instrumentation, experimental mortality, and interactive effects.

Returning to students in a university course, suppose the instructor wanted to know whether knowledge changed over the course of the semester. In this case, the instructor would choose to test students on day 1 before any reading, in-class lecture or activity, or assignments. If student scores improved by the midterm, the instructor can claim that improvement occurred in knowledge but cannot attribute this to the course.

If you want to test change in knowledge in the cardiac education program for elders, you would similarly give a pretest before any participation and examine the change in scores. A significant difference would indicate learning, but without attribution to your program because the absence of random assignment and the limited control would not support a causal claim.

Pre-experimental Design Summary

Pre-experimental designs may be valuable in answering a descriptive question. You may want to consider using a pre-experimental design for the specific purpose of pilot testing an intervention protocol or particular measurement approach. However, the absence of two of the three major conditions for true experimentation makes these designs an inappropriate choice if your pursuit is prediction and causal inference. If you attempt to answer predictive or causal questions with these designs, the seven basic threats to internal validity limit effective checks against bias.

At this point, you may be asking why an investigator would choose a design that cannot attribute an outcome to a cause. As we noted earlier, not all questions are causal. Think back to the chapters on theory

---

BOX 10-4 *Nonexperimental Designs*
• Surveys • Passive observation • Ex post facto designs

and literature. Remember we said that theory is incrementally built and tested. Descriptive findings support the conduct of more complex research. Without sound description, relational and causal studies may not be indicated. Knowing "what" must precede knowing "why."

Nonexperimental Designs

Nonexperimental designs primarily rely on statistical manipulation of data rather than mechanical manipulation and sequencing. By definition, nonexperimental designs are those in which none of the three criteria for true experimentation exists in the structure of sample selection and assignment, exposure to an experimental condition, and data collection. These designs are most useful when testing a concept or construct or set of relationships among constructs that naturally occur. Any manipulation of variables is done post hoc through statistical analysis. Three nonexperimental designs are frequently used in health and human service research (Box 10-4).
— no manipulation or no treatment

Survey Designs

Survey designs are primarily used to measure characteristics or attributes of a population. Through survey designs, it is possible to describe population parameters and features as well as to predict relationships among these phenomena. Typically, surveys are conducted with large samples. Questions are posed either through online or mailed questionnaires or through telecommunications or face-to-face interviews. Perhaps the most well-known survey is the U.S. Census, in which the federal government administers mailed surveys and conducts selected face-to-face interviews to develop a descriptive picture of the characteristics of the U.S. population. The census qualifies as a data collection project rather than a full inquiry because it does not have an articulated theory base. However, an excellent example of a large-scale survey inquiry of interest to health and human service providers is the recent analysis of well-being in America.[8] On the basis of human development and capability theory[9,10] and relying on secondary data, the American Human Development Index measured the main and interactive effects of three primary variables: a long and healthy life, access to knowledge, and a decent standard of living.[8] In addition, gender, geographic, and race/ethnicity correlates were included in the analysis.

> Applying this approach, suppose you are interested in examining and predicting job satisfaction of health and human service faculty who are teaching in distance education programs. You create and host a survey on the Internet and email program directors of diverse health and human service programs with distance education components to ask them to elicit participation from faculty who are teaching in distance courses. After receiving 500 faculty responses containing demographic characteristics and job satisfaction scores, you conduct statistical analysis of the data and are able to develop descriptive and predictive conclusions. •

The advantages of survey design are that (1) the investigator can reach a large number of respondents with relatively minimal expenditure and time, (2) numerous variables can be measured by a single instrument, and (3) statistical manipulation during the data analytical phase can permit multiple uses of the data set. Disadvantages may result from the survey structure.[11] For example, the use of mailed or online questionnaires may yield a low response rate, compromising the external validity of the design. Face-to-face interviews are time-consuming and may pose reliability problems.

Online surveys are gaining in popularity and use. There are many online survey options, some of which are free to the investigator. Using online surveys has both advantages and disadvantages. Online survey methods are inexpensive in that they do not require postage, they are password protected, and they control for multiple responses from one computer. Many formats have automated data entry, eliminating manual entry of data into a spreadsheet. Distribution is instantaneous, and surveys can be accessed around the globe. However, online methods eliminate those who do not have or choose to have

access to computers. Email lists to recruit respondents are often expensive, and caution must be taken to ensure that respondents cannot answer multiple times. For example, suppose you are interested in studying the relationship of health provider attitudes toward obesity and planned quality of health care treatment. Using an online survey program, you create a survey of planned health care for a fictitious patient. You recruit a sample of health providers and randomly assign each to one of two groups. Group 1 receives the survey and case information with a photo of the "case" at a typical weight, and Group 2 receives identical information with a photograph of an obese patient. Because you are using online survey methods, you are able to reach a wide audience and use automated data entry. In a relatively short period of time, this type of online survey design allows you to answer Level 1 and 2 questioning because you can recruit, conduct your survey, receive immediate responses, and enter and analyze data in a short time.

Many books and online resources can guide you in designing a survey study on the Internet, by mail, by telephone, or in person. For more detailed discussion of how to structure surveys, these resources should be consulted.

Passive Observation Designs

Passive observation designs are used to examine phenomena as they naturally occur and to discern the relationship between two or more variables. Often referred to as "correlational designs," passive observation can be as simple as examining the relationship between two variables (e.g., height and weight) or it can be as complex as predicting scores on one or more variables from knowledge of scores on other variables. As in the survey, variables are not manipulated but are measured and then examined for relationships and patterns of prediction.

> In the survey on job satisfaction of health and human service faculty, you would be able to examine the relationships among multiple variables and to predict the degree of job satisfaction with respondent scores on other variables such as professional discipline or respondent age. •

Ex Post Facto Designs

Ex post facto designs are considered to be one type of passive observation design. In ex post facto ("after the fact") designs, however, the phenomena of interest have already occurred and cannot be manipulated in any way. Ex post facto designs are frequently used to examine relationships between naturally occurring population parameters and specific variables.

You are interested in understanding the effects of coronary bypass surgery on morale and resumption of former roles for men and women. Coronary bypass surgery is an event that the researcher cannot manipulate, but it can be examined for its effects after its occurrence. Additional examples include ex post facto survey designs used to examine phenomena such as career patterns of graduates of professional curricula, recovery process, and differences in job satisfaction between male and female professionals.

Nonexperimental Design Summary

Nonexperimental designs have a wide range of uses. The value in these designs lies in their ability to examine and quantify naturally occurring phenomena so that statistical analysis can be accomplished. Therefore, the investigator does not manipulate the independent variable but rather examines it in relation to one or more variables for descriptive or predictive purposes. These designs have the capacity to include a large number of subjects and to examine events or phenomena that have already occurred. Because random selection, manipulation, and control group are not present in these designs, investigators must use caution when making causal claims from the findings.

As in the quasi-experimental and true-experimental situations, the researcher is still concerned with potential biases that may limit the internal validity of the nonexperimental design. The researcher tries to control the influence of external or extraneous influences on the study variables through the implementation of systematic data collection procedures, the use of reliable and valid instrumentation, and other techniques including statistical manipulation. The researcher also increases the generalizability of a study or its external validity by using random sample selection procedures, when appropriate and feasible, to ensure representation and minimize systematic sampling bias.

Experimental-Type Meta-analysis

A review of the literature is the core action process in meta-analysis (see Chapter 6).

Meta-analysis is a methodology in the experimental-type tradition that can be understood as a form of survey research. In meta-analysis, however, research reports, rather than real people, are surveyed and become the unit of analysis.[12] In using reports as a form of survey research, first a specific research question must be posed, followed by boundary setting, development of a coding scheme, and implementation of analytical action processes. Box 10-5 outlines the basic steps in the meta-analysis research approach.

The purpose of experimental-type meta-analysis is to summarize, integrate, and interpret an empirical body of research or studies in which the outcomes are quantitative. In meta-analysis the findings of more than one study can be combined and averaged. As with all methodologies, there are certain limitations with a meta-analysis. Because you are

---

BOX 10-5 *Basic Steps in a Meta-analysis*

1. Specify a topic.
2. Specify the type of research finding of importance.
   a. Treatment outcomes
   b. Covariation
3. Establish "bounding criteria" (inclusion/exclusion criteria for selecting studies).
4. Identify, locate, and retrieve studies that meet study criteria.
5. Establish a systematic approach to organizing research records.
   a. Consider using a computer database program
   b. Entries include bibliographic information, descriptive study information (e.g., type of sample, intervention, and study design)
6. Derive numerical value or index representing "effect size" for each study.

delimiting your "sample" of reports by both content and method, meta-analysis is only applicable to one tradition at a time and thus cannot be used with mixed methods. Also, it can be used only with studies using similar constructs or reporting specific statistical analyses (e.g., inferential statistics) that can be meaningfully compared.

The strength of meta-analysis lies in its ability to synthesize a body of research that focuses on a specific topic (e.g., treatment for stroke) and to derive interpretations of the degree of effect of similar treatments. Meta-analysis provides a systematic and structured way of summarizing and analyzing research findings from more than one study in a specified area of inquiry. It can be applied to an area of inquiry with few studies or one with many studies. In essence, meta-analysis can expand the scope and application of small-sample studies to broad populations.[13]

The key concept in experimental-type meta-analysis is *effect size*, a statistic that codes the magnitude of the effect (or outcome) as a result of being exposed to the independent variable (e.g., treatment, intervention, experimental condition). Different statistics to derive an effect size are used, depending on the type of data and specific research question and hypotheses being tested. The calculation of effect size is beyond the scope of this text, but it is important to understand that experimental-type meta-analysis focuses specifically on statistical outcome of an intervention or experimental condition.[12,13]

Meta-analysis is important in health and human service research. It enables the researcher to derive a systematic interpretation rather than a critical review of the literature as to the state of knowledge in a particular area. With the increasing popularity of evidence-based practice, as discussed in Chapter 24, meta-analysis provides a methodology through which to combine and integrate studies to identify "the best intervention."

Geographic Techniques

Geographic analysis is a set of techniques in which data are geographically referenced. That is to say, information including economics, population parameters, epidemiology, natural and built resources, and policy, among many others, is geographically situated. Grounding information through its location provides a powerful tool for analysis, with particular attention to global, national, and local community comparisons.[14] Although geographic methods are not a specific design and employ multiple experimental-type approaches to answer Level 1, 2, and 3 questions, we discuss this genre of inquiry here because of its increasing use and importance to health and human service professions in generating location-based knowledge.

There is a wide range of applications and complexity in geographic analysis, from static, slice-in-time snapshots to temporally changing dynamic modeling.[14] What all have in common is the use of visual-spatial locations as delimiters of information and analysis. Further, whereas static, hand-drawn maps can be used for rudimentary examination, the development of computerized technology applications has resulted in the increasing use and scope of geographic analysis in research, planning, and theory building, with the geographic information system (GIS) becoming a valued analytic tool in diverse health and human service academic and professional arenas.

A GIS comprises the hardware and software used to input, organize, store, retrieve, and depict geographically situated information.[15] Although the technical details of GIS are beyond the scope of our book, we bring to your attention several important concepts that are critical for understanding the power of GIS.

First, GIS is a computer-assisted system and thus has the capacity to handle and analyze multiple sources of data, providing that they are relevant to spatial depiction. Second, GIS relies on two overarching spatial paradigms, raster and vector. Raster GIS carves geography into mutually exclusive spaces and then examines the attributes of these. Thus, the attributes of one space can be represented and compared with the attributes of another. For example, consider infant mortality. Knowing geographic variation could assist providers in targeting specific locations for further inquiry and prevention of infant death.

Vector GIS relies on location points. This approach locates points and identifies spaces and the attributes delimited inside of them by the lines that connect the points. This technique allows an in-depth look at local phenomena, such as the health and welfare of neighborhood youth.

Each approach has its strengths and limitations, but both have valuable applications. To compare approaches, suppose you are interested in the causes of underage drinking and you ascertain that incidence in various geographic areas differ. To look at the attributes from the raster approach, you would obtain a frequency count of the number of establishments that sell alcoholic beverages in delimited areas and then depict by color the number of establishments in that area. However, from the vector approach, you would identify the addresses or geographic coordinates of each alcohol sales establishment and plot it on your map.[14]

Finally, because GIS has the capacity to represent multiple data layers on a single map, the ability to analyze multivariate relationships is one of its most powerful functions. Consider the earlier example once again. In addition to examining the density or location of alcohol sales outlets, you also hypothesize that the availability of money to purchase alcohol and the freedom to do so without parental interference are important predictors of underage drinking.

To test the hypothesis, you map and depict the socioeconomic status of each location, the youth ages, the percentage of youth working, and the working hours of parents. Using geographic software, each variable can be translated into spatial data, located on a single map layer, and then aggregated into a complex map that depicts the relationship among two or more of the variables (Fig. 10-3).

Geographic analysis is a powerful tool in itself, but when coupled with statistical analysis, it can be an even more potent strategy for association and prediction. Both tell the same story but through different means, and thus the strength of multiple communication formats and evidentiary bases can be brought to bear on dissemination to diverse audiences.[1] Furthermore, because geographic analysis programs base maps on data tables, and because the software allows the importation of data from frequently used spreadsheets and databases

such as Excel, Access, and even SPSS, combining visual and statistical analytic techniques is relatively simple.

Epidemiology

Epidemiology is a genre of research that examines the distribution of disease in populations and seeks to reveal the factors that influence population-based illness and disease as the basis for prevention, optimizing health services, tracing historical trends and risks, and influencing health policy.[16] Although not a single design, we discuss epidemiology in this chapter because of its centrality to public health and the professions concerned with disease prevention and health promotion. Epidemiological studies focus on the body and the environment as well as their interactions as the basis for investigation and application of knowledge.

Epidemiological methods are complex, and thus a detailed discussion of them is beyond the scope of this text. Here we introduce you to concepts and general approaches to investigation that are central to the field. Epidemiologists conduct research to describe disease distribution, measure the severity of disease through morbidity and mortality (incidence and prevalence), and uncover the etiology (risk factors that are associated with or causative of disease). Incidence refers to the number of new occurrences of a disease, and prevalence denotes the number or proportion of disease in a specified population.

Epidemiologists use large-scale surveillance methods, such as survey, secondary analysis of hospital data, and birth and death certificates, to answer Level 1, 2, and 3 questions. Of particular importance are the techniques of complex statistical modeling and geographic analysis to describe and predict the occurrences and causative factors of disease distribution. As an example, an epidemiological study might measure (surveillance) the occurrence of birth defects in populations living near nuclear power plants and then conduct complex modeling that can statistically create conditions, based on current descriptors, that would indicate high risk. Models can serve as the basis for prevention, intervention, and policy responses and can be evaluated

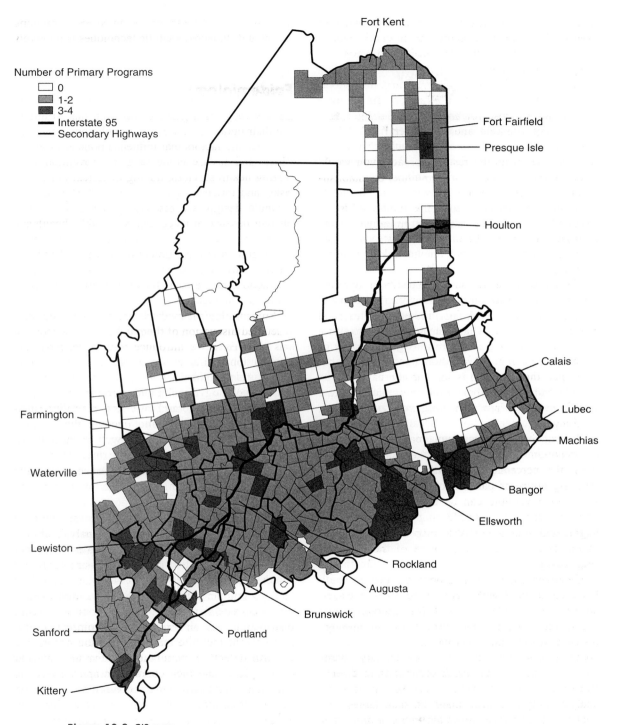

Figure 10-3 GIS map.

after they are enacted to determine their success in preventing illness and promoting health.

Clinical Trial Methodology

Most quantitative investigators and scientific journals consider the true-experimental design, also referred to as the *randomized clinical trial* (or RCT), as the design of choice to answer specific questions related to the efficacy of behavioral or biomedical interventions, including drugs, treatments, service programs, and devices. Also within the world of evidence-based practice, the RCT is upheld as the most important design structure from which "best" evidence can be deduced. Thus, we now focus on the application of the true-experimental design to clinical practice.[17]

Although seemingly straightforward, as we discussed earlier, the traditional two-group randomized controlled design is actually rather complex, and many action processes have been developed to structure this study design and ensure rigor. Because of its importance in health and human service research and its prominence in scientific journals, let us examine some key critical issues in implementing a clinical trial in an applied setting, such as the clinic, community center, or home. Because it is not possible to cover every aspect of the RCT in this text, we highlight here the key language that sets clear rules and expectations for the adequacy of the RCT design and research procedures.

Phases of Clinical Trials

Clinical trials are designed to address three levels of development for interventions. A Phase I clinical trial is the first type of randomized design that is usually conducted. The purpose of the Phase I study is to test a new behavioral or biomedical intervention not previously evaluated in a small group of people (20 to 80) to determine its acceptability, feasibility of implementation, and safety (e.g., side effects, safe dosage range for drugs). The next step, a Phase II clinical trial, is conducted to study the intervention in a larger group of people (several hundred) to determine efficacy and further evaluate safety. The final step, a Phase III clinical trial, may have a three-fold purpose: (1) to evaluate effectiveness further in a much larger group of persons (several hundred to

thousands), (2) to compare the intervention to other standard or experimental interventions to determine its added value or significance, and (3) to evaluate how the intervention can be implemented safely in a larger community.

Each clinical trial phase may use randomization procedures and strict adherence to various protocols, but their goals differ. For Phase I the goal is "proof of concept," for Phase II it is "efficacy," and for Phase III it is "effectiveness and safety" related to clinical implementation. These phases tend to fit best with classic pharmacological drug trial research, for which many of the procedures discussed in relation to *clinical trial methodology* have been developed. Nevertheless, these terms continue to be applied to behavioral and other clinical-type interventions and are noted here because they are used frequently by the experimentalist and lauded as the knowledge basis for evidence-based practice.

An additional phase is specific to behavioral interventions most relevant to health and human service and involves the "translation" of an evidence-based intervention into a service or clinical setting. Most intervention protocols that are tested using clinical trial methodology require additional modification or translation to fit into and be effective in an applied setting or with a different target population than those involved in the initial testing. The translational phase may or may not involve a randomized two-group design, but it does require an evaluative approach to determine acceptability and benefit. In this translational phase, it is important to ensure that the core components of a well-supported intervention remain intact. However, small changes that may have a large impact in the new setting or with a different target population may be necessary to ensure contextual appropriateness and fit.

For example, suppose you want to implement a well-supported group-exercise conditioning program. However, the population you want to target does not typically engage in formal exercise programs. Thus, you may need to modify specific aspects of the program to enhance its acceptability and preserve its effectiveness in achieving its outcomes. A small change that would not affect the fidelity of the tested program might involve naming and framing the program differently or offering a wider range of exercise options. However, changing the frequency of the exercise regimen or offering it as a private versus group activity would alter the integrity of the intervention and possibly its outcomes.

Now, let us examine how you might enact each phase of your clinical trial. You have an idea for a new therapeutic regimen to enhance community reintegration for persons with traumatic head injury. You first conduct a Phase I study with a small group of clients, approximately 30 people, who fit highly specified inclusion and exclusion criteria. In this first phase, your goal is to evaluate whether your intervention approach is acceptable to clients, the extent to which participants comply with the innovative regimen, and the initial impact on treatment outcome (magnitude of change). Your main outcome is "life satisfaction," as measured by self-report, and the "ability to live alone safely," as measured by professional observation of daily self-care. You decide to use a two-group design and randomly assign 15 persons to receive the experimental intervention program and 15 persons to a "usual care" control group who receive a traditional rehabilitation program.

Assume this first phase is successful in achieving its outcomes. You have evidence of treatment effect; 10 of the 15 persons randomized to treatment are able to perform self-care independently and safely, compared with 5 of 15 persons in the control group. Also, persons who received the treatment seemed to enjoy the therapeutic regimen and attended all skill classes and one-on-one sessions such that compliance was close to 95%. On the basis of this evidence, you design a Phase II trial involving many more persons, perhaps more than 150, recruited from two rehabilitation facilities. In Phase II, you seek to achieve statistically significant treatment effects and continue to monitor acceptability and participation, as well as safety (e.g., unsafe incidents from attending classes, living alone). Again, you find that your results from this phase are promising, with small to medium treatment effects, high compliance, and no adverse or unsafe events related to treatment.

Your next step is to develop a Phase III study, which might involve participation by numerous rehabilitation centers across the country and an attempt to implement the intervention in multiple sites. With the success of the intervention at each stage, there is great interest in using your intervention in rehabilitation.

However, another translational step is necessary to integrate your treatment into the current structure of rehabilitation. The intervention, as tested, is too labor intensive, and third-party intermediaries may not reimburse every component. Thus, you develop a translational phase in which you modify aspects of the intervention while preserving its essential elements, to integrate it successfully into clinical practice and obtain reimbursement for at least some of its therapeutic components.[18,19]

Blinding (Masking)

Another key language structure of clinical trials is blinding or masking techniques. Remember that the procedures put into place in RCTs are designed to reduce bias. This point is important for the RCT structure because its main intent is to determine the impact or effect of a specific treatment regimen or intervention on a set of outcomes. Thus, critical to this design is the minimization of any competing reasons (e.g., Type I and II errors) that could explain a particular outcome.[17] Potential sources of bias are the tester, investigator, or interventionist.

Consider this example. You are an interviewer in a large study that is testing the efficacy of social support groups for persons undergoing cancer treatments. You are responsible for conducting both the pretest and the posttest interviews to evaluate whether group support affects a person's well-being. However, you are aware of a person's assignment to intervention or control as you interview. You may be favorably predisposed to observing positive changes in the intervention group. Or, because of your enthusiasm and investment in the intervention, you may inadvertently set a tone or ask questions that introduce a source of bias.

Thus, to minimize partiality or the possibility of introducing any form of bias, most clinical trials implement some types of blinding procedures. One simple approach to blinding, or masking, is to minimize who among the research team in contact with study participants is informed of group assignment. It is usually possible to mask interviewers to group assignments.

Blinding works best in medical trials. A single-blind trial means that the persons enrolled in the study do not know to which group or treatment they have been assigned, but the investigative team does know. In a double-blind trial, neither study participants nor investigators (nor anyone else on the research team) are aware of group assignments. As you can see, this level of blinding is difficult to achieve in behavioral-oriented treatments that are being evaluated in an RCT.

Randomization Scheme

The language of randomization is also essential to the clinical trial design structure. The way in which study participants are randomized to the experimental and control group conditions can take different forms and is scrutinized by institutional review boards, data and safety monitoring boards, and scientific journals (see Chapter 14).

There are many ways to randomize in order to ensure that subjects are assigned to experimental and control groups by chance. In complex designs or large clinical trials, a statistician is usually responsible for establishing a randomization scheme. After a randomization format has been developed, assignments are typed up on single sheets of paper, and each is sealed in opaque double envelopes so that the investigators or research team members cannot see the paper until it is opened and cannot influence the group assignment.[4]

A related consideration is whether simple randomization alone is sufficient to ensure comparability between the experimental and control groups. Suppose you are testing a mental health intervention involving counseling and activity engagement for persons with functional limitations. The dependent or outcome variable is a measure of depressive symptoms. You know that gender is highly related to depressive symptoms, with women reporting higher scores than men. Given the strong association between gender and your treatment outcome, you might want to consider a method of randomization to ensure that an equal number of men and women will be assigned to both the experimental and the control condition.

One approach would be to "stratify" randomization by gender (male, female) to ensure that the two groups will be balanced with respect to this factor. This process involves setting up a separate or

independent randomization scheme for both males and females. Within each stratum (male and female), randomization would occur by the method of "random permuted blocks" to control for possible changes over time in the subject mix. A blocking number is usually developed by a statistician and is not disclosed to the investigators or members of the project team. The statistician generates randomization lists for each of the two strata and then prepares two sets of randomization envelopes (double-enveloped), one set for males and the other for females. Each subject is randomized by opening the next envelope with the appropriate stratum.

Criteria for Selecting Appropriate and Adequate Experimental-Type Designs

As discussed, some researchers believe that the true-experimental design represents the only structure that is appropriate and adequate for generating legitimate professional knowledge. However, each design in the experimental-type tradition has its strengths and limitations. The true experiment is the best design for testing theory, making causal statements, and determining the efficacy of treatments. If causality is not your purpose, however, or if the design structure does not fit the particular environment in which the research is to be conducted, true-experimental design is not an appropriate or adequate choice.

It is often difficult to apply strict experimental conditions to a field setting. For example, although subjects may be randomly assigned to a group, it may not be possible to obtain the initial list of subjects for a random sampling process, or it may be unethical to withhold a type of treatment (or experimental intervention) from a consumer in a service setting. Although clinical drug trials or testing of new technologies can often obtain the degree of control necessary for true-experimental conditions, research on the social and psychological dimensions of health and human service work often poses a different set of issues and challenges for the researcher. These challenges make it essential for the investigator to be flexible in the use of design so that a research strategy appropriate to the question and to the level of theory, purpose, and practical constraints can be selected and rigorously applied.

To illustrate the value of each type of research design within the experimental-type tradition, apply the concepts in this chapter to the following example that you could encounter in your practice.

> You are employed in a hospital in the rehabilitation unit. You have just read about a new computer intervention that seems to enhance the cognitive recovery of persons with traumatic brain injury. You order the program and recruit a group of patients to use it. To determine the extent to which the program works (which you have defined as "significant improvement in cognitive function"), you select an instrument to measure cognitive function (operationalizing your concept of cognitive improvement), and then you test a sample of 10 patients with the same instrument after their use of the computer intervention. •

This type of inquiry is an *XO* design (preexperimental) in which the computer program is the independent variable and cognitive performance is the dependent variable. The mean score for your sample was within normal limits, with a normal dispersion of scores around the mean. From this design, you have answered the question, "How did subjects score on a test of cognitive performance after their participation in a computer intervention?" Although these data are valuable to you in describing your sample, you still have not answered the question about whether the program "works." Multiple threats to internal validity interfere with your ability to make a causal inference between variables with any degree of assuredness. You therefore decide to build on this study by adding a pretest.

> In the next study, you pretest your new sample, introduce the computer intervention, and then posttest the sample. •

This type of study is an *OXO* design (also preexperimental). Because the subjects have greatly improved from the pretest to the posttest, you conclude that your program has "worked." However, can you really come to this conclusion? What about

the effects of sampling bias, maturation, and history on your sample? You realize that even though you have stronger evidence for the value of the program, the design that you have selected has answered the question, "To what extent did the subjects change in cognitive function after participating in the experimental condition?"

> For your next sample, you add a control group so that your research structure is now a quasi-experimental design. •

Your design now appears as follows:

$$O \ X \quad O$$
$$O \qquad O$$

When the experimental group improves more than the control group, you now are convinced that your program "works." However, can you make that claim? What about sampling bias and other interactive effects that might confound your study? From this design, you can answer the question, "Which group made more progress?" This type of design provides fairly strong support for the value of your program, but it cannot be used yet to make causal claims.

> For your next project, you add random group assignment to your design so that you are conducting a true experiment. •

Your design looks like the following:

$$r \ O \quad X \quad O$$
$$r \ O \qquad O$$

> Because your experimental group has improved significantly more than the control group, you can now make the claim, with reasonable certainty, that the program works to attain the tested outcomes. You have used true experimentation to test the efficacy of the computer intervention in producing cognitive improvement in your sample. However, can you advise your colleague to use this intervention for his or her clients? The answer is a resounding "maybe." •

Because you did not randomly select your sample, the capacity to generalize your findings beyond your own experiment is limited. We are often faced with the desire to generalize, but practical restraints of conducting practice research will not allow us to select our sample randomly, as discussed later in the text. You might select experimental-type meta-analysis to expand your scope of knowledge beyond a single study if studies have used similar methods about the same constructs in your study.

> 🔍 Now, suppose you are interested in examining the extent to which the cognitive intervention produced client outcomes that were satisfactory to family members after a client's discharge. You may then select a nonexperimental survey design to examine the level of satisfaction. You also may include predictor variables, such as length of time in treatment and degree of family support, to inform the future use and success with this intervention. •

Each research design has strengths and limitations related to claims about the knowledge generated as well as practical and ethical issues. The key to doing rigorous and valued research with experimental-type designs is to (1) state your question clearly; (2) select a design that can best answer the question given the level of theory development, the practical considerations, and the purpose in conducting the study; and (3) report accurate conclusions.

Now that you are aware of experimental-type designs and techniques for enhancing the strength of these designs, you still may wonder how to select a design to fit your particular study question. Begin by asking yourself five guiding questions (Box 10-6).

What does each of these questions really ask you to consider? Question 1 raises the issues of validity. When a design is selected, the project must be internally consistent, construct valid, and the research capable of providing the level of answers that the question seeks. Question 2 also addresses validity but issues of control and structure as well. The researcher must consider what extraneous influences could confound the study and in what ways maximum control can be built into the design. Question 3

> **BOX 10-6** *Guiding Questions in Selecting a Research Design*
>
> 1. Does the design answer the research question? Is there congruence between the research question(s) and hypotheses and the design?
> 2. Does the design adequately control independent variables? Are other extraneous independent variables present that may confound the study?
> 3. Does the design maximize control and minimize bias?
> 4. To what extent does the design enhance the generalizability of results to other subjects, other groups, and other conditions?
> 5. What are some of the ethical and field limitations of the research question that influence the research design?

summarizes the previous issues raised by guiding the researcher to be most rigorous in planning control and minimizing bias. Question 4 addresses external validity and sampling. The researcher must develop a design that allows as broad a generalization as possible without threatening internal validity. Question 5 reminds the researcher of practical and ethical concerns that shape the design.

If these questions are answered successfully, the criteria for adequacy of experimental-type designs have been addressed. However, keep in mind that design considerations within the experimental-type tradition are more than just knowing the definitions of design characteristics. Knowledge of these design possibilities is your "set of tools," which you can then apply and modify to fit the specific conditions of the setting in which you are conducting research. Developing a design within the tradition of experimental-type research in the health and human service field is a creative process. Use your knowledge of the language and thinking processes, the basic elements of design, and the issues of internal and external validity to develop a study that fits the particular environment and question that you are asking.

Summary

Experimental-type research designs range from true-experimental to nonexperimental, and each design

TABLE 10-1   *Summary of Design Characteristics in Experimental-Type Research*

True-Experimental	Quasi-experimental	Nonexperimental	Pre-experimental
Randomization	Yes	No	No	No
Control group	No	Maybe	Maybe	No
Manipulation	Yes	Maybe	No	Yes

varies in its level of control, randomization, and manipulation of variables (Table 10-1). Also, field conditions and other practicalities influence the implementation of any type of design. The basic elements of design structure in the experimental-type tradition have many variations, and new applications of experimental designs are being advanced with the advent of meta-analysis and field-based intervention studies.

EXERCISES

1. Select an experimental-type research article and identify the dependent and independent variables. Diagram the design using *XO* notation.
2. Develop research questions and designs using the *XO* notation to illustrate (a) true-experimental design, (b) quasi-experimental design, (c) pre-experimental design, and (d) nonexperimental design.
3. Identify up to three potential ethical and field limitations of each research design developed in Exercise 2.

References

1. Creswell J: *Research design*, Los Angeles, 2014, Sage.
2. DePoy E, Gilson SF: *Theories of human behavior*, Los Angeles, 2012, Sage.
3. Campbell DT, Stanley JC: *Experimental and quasi-experimental designs for research*, Chicago, 1963, Rand McNally.
4. Alferes V: *Methods of randomization in experimental design*, Thousand Oaks, Calif, 2012, Sage.
5. Hatch M: *Organization theory: modern, symbolic, and post-modern perspectives*, New York, 2013, Oxford University Press.
6. Roethlisberger FJ, Dickson WJ: *Management and the worker*, Cambridge, Mass, 1947, Harvard University Press.
7. Cook TD, Campbell DT: *Quasi-experimentation: design and analysis for field settings*, Boston, 1979, Houghton Mifflin.
8. Burd-Sharps S, Lewis K: *The measure of America 2013–2014*, 2014. Available at http://ssrc-static.s3.amazonaws.com/moa/MOA-III-June-18-FINAL.pdf.
9. Nussbaum MC: *Frontiers of justice: disability*, Boston, 2006, President & Fellows of Harvard College.
10. Sen A: *The idea of justice*, New York, 2009, Columbia Press.
11. Fowler J: *Survey research methods*, Los Angeles, 2014, Sage.
12. Cooper HM: *Research synthesis and meta-analysis: a step-by-step approach*, ed 4, Los Angeles, 2009, Sage.
13. Borenstein M, Hedges L, Higgins J, et al: *Introduction to meta-analysis*, West Sussex, UK, 2009, Wiley.
14. Gilson SF, DePoy E: Geographic analysis for the social sciences. *Int J Interdisciplinary Social Sci* 1:86–96, 2007.
15. Ormsby T, Napoleon E, Burke R, et al: *Getting to know ArcGIS desktop*, ed 2, Redlands, Calif, 2004, ESRI Press.
16. Gordis L: *Epidemiology*, ed 5, Philadelphia, 2014, Saunders.
17. Guest G, Namey E: *Public health research methods*, Thousand Oaks, Calif, 2015, Sage.
18. Gitlin LN: Introducing a new intervention: An overview of research phases and common challenges. *Am J Occup Ther* 67(2):177–184. doi: 10.5014/ajot.2013.006742, 2013.
19. Gitlin LN, Czaja SJ: *Behavioral Intervention Research: Designing, Testing and Implementing*, in press, Springer Publishing Company.

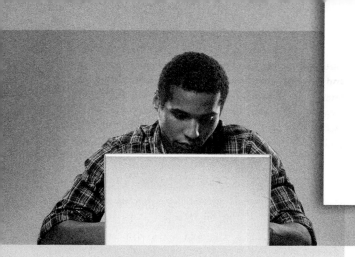

Chapter 11
Naturalistic Designs

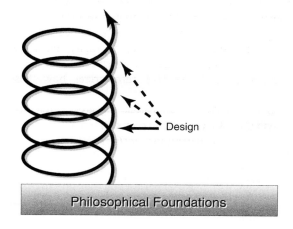

Philosophical Foundations

traditions organize the "10 essentials" of the research process are presented in this chapter (see Chapter 2 for a refresher on the 10 essentials). Although there are other naturalistic inquiry approaches that could be discussed, examining these 11 designs provides the foundational knowledge necessary to become familiar with naturalistic inquiry and its use in health and human service research.

First, let us reflect a bit on naturalistic inquiry and what we have learned thus far. You may recall our discussions in previous chapters about context-embeddedness, a fundamental principle of all naturalistic designs. That is to say, within this tradition phenomena are seen as occurring or are embedded in a context and cannot be objectively separated from it. Second, recall that naturalistic thinking processes tend to rely on inductive and abductive thinking and

Using the language and thinking processes you learned in Chapter 9, we are now ready to explore naturalistic inquiry in more detail. This chapter highlights 11 specific designs of relevance to health and human service research. Wide variation in the naturalistic tradition, the different ways in which complex social phenomena are tackled, and how researchers working out of different naturalistic logic. As such, these designs are initially implemented in the identified context and as they unfold may move to other environments throughout the course of conducting the study. The investigator enters an identified conceptual, virtual, or physical setting to experience and understand it without artificially altering or manipulating conditions other than his/her presence. Third, although the designs in this tradition share basic language and thinking processes discussed in Chapter 9, each is also based in its own distinct philosophical tradition. Therefore, designs differ in some purposes, sequencing, and investigator involvement (Box 11-1).

This chapter provides the basic framework of the designs that we believe have greatest methodological value for health and human service research: endogenous, participatory action, critical theory, phenomenology, heuristic, ethnography, narrative, life history, object reading, grounded theory, and meta-analysis. Table 11-1 summarizes how these

naturalistic designs compare in purpose, sequence, and investigator involvement. Remember as you read that these designs do not prescribe a fixed sequence for the conduct of the 10 essential thinking and action processes. Therefore, how each study unfolds is unique.

Endogenous Research

Endogenous inquiry represents the most open-ended approach in the naturalistic tradition.[1] This research is conceptualized, designed, and conducted by researchers who are emic, or considered members of a group or culture that is the subject of the inquiry. What is unique about this infrequently used design is the relinquishment of all parts of knowledge generation on the part of the researcher who is initially asking the research question. Thus, the "subjects" do not simply respond to interview or become the subjects for observation but design an inquiry themselves in a manner that they believe will generate knowledge about the group. In this type of design, the subjects are truly leaders in the process.

Endogenous research can be organized in a variety of ways and may include the use of any strategy and technique in the naturalistic or experimental-type tradition or an integrated design. What makes endogenous inquiry naturalistic is not its action processes

---

> **BOX 11-1** *Three Differences in Naturalistic Designs*
>
> - Purpose of the research
> - Sequence and use of the 10 essentials
> - Nature of investigator involvement

TABLE 11-1 *Basic Framework of 11 Designs in Naturalistic Inquiry*

Design Strategy	Purpose	Sequence	Investigator Involvement
Endogenous	To yield insider perspective through involvement of subject as researcher	Variable	Determined by subjects/informants
Participatory action	To generate knowledge to inform action	Variable	Inclusive team of investigators and participants
Critical theory	To understand experiences for social change	Variable	Investigator directed
Phenomenology	To discover meaning of lived experience	Narrative	Listener/reporter
Heuristic	To reveal personal and lived experience	Variable	Investigator and informant
Ethnography	To understand culture	Prescribed	Investigator directed
Narrative	To understand stories of marginalized individuals	Can be embedded in other designs; analytical strategy	Investigator directed
Object reading	To understand the meaning of artifacts	Variable	Investigator directed
Life history	To yield biographical experience	Narrative	Investigator directed
Grounded theory	To generate theory	Prescribed	Investigator directed
Meta-analysis	To synthesize body of knowledge	Prescribed	Investigator directed

structure but rather its framework; that is, the investigator views knowledge as emerging from individuals who know the best way to obtain it. Endogenous design is consistent with the contemporary notion of "emancipatory research," a relatively recent approach to investigations of the needs of marginalized and oppressed groups who do not often get a chance to reflect their perspectives outside of knowledge driven by professionals.[2] This strategy is also consistent with community-based participatory research and participatory action research described later in the chapter,[3] both of which emphasize the importance of involving members in the community of interest in all 10 research essentials.

The endogenous approach is based on a classic proposition developed by the social psychologist Kurt Lewin,[4] as Argyris and Schon[5] explained:

> *Causal inferences about the behavior of human beings are more likely to be valid and enactable when the human beings in question participate in building and testing them. Hence it aims at creating an environment in which participants give and get valid information, make free and informed choices (including the choice to participate), and generate internal commitment to the results of their inquiry.*

Different from any other inquiry structure in any of the traditions, this design gives "knowing power" exclusively to the persons who are the participants of the inquiry. Also, because the researcher's involvement in the knowledge generation enterprise is determined by the individuals who are the "subjects" of the investigation, the role of the researcher is variable from participation as an equal partner to not at all or somewhere between these two levels.

Because endogenous research is not used frequently, we turn back the clock to Maruyama,[1] who conducted a classic study. However, we include this design in the book to illustrate its power in revealing knowledge about need without influence from the researcher in any way with the exception of asking for the knowledge at the outset. Maruyama[1] was interested in understanding the nature of violence among prison inmates. He therefore entered the prison environment as a collaborator and participant observer rather than as leader, an important characteristic of endogenous

research. As a collaborator, Maruyama deferred to the subjects of the investigation to determine the degree of investigator involvement. Two teams, composed of prisoners who had no formal education in research methods, held a series of group meetings and created purposes and plans of action that were important and meaningful to each group. Maruyama described the research in this way:

> *A team of endogenous researchers was formed in each of the two prisons. The overall objective of the project was to study interpersonal physical violence (fights) in the prison culture, with as little contamination as possible from academic theories and methodologies. The details of the research were left to be developed by the inmate researchers.[1]*

The inmates themselves chose both experimental-type interview techniques and a form of qualitative data analysis to characterize the violence in the environments in which they were insiders. Even without any formal education in research methods, the inmates were able not only to collect extensive and meaningful data but also to conduct sophisticated conceptual analyses of their data. As illustrated in this classic example, the findings from a study "owned" and conducted by insiders, particularly in sensitive circumstances, are likely to produce very different results from knowledge developed by a researcher who enters the environment as a stranger. From Maruyama's study, violence was explained in the language of the inmates, and the findings clearly displayed the culturally specific nature of violence in each prison setting. Consider how different the findings might have been if an investigator went to a group of inmates and asked questions about the reasons prison violence occurs. The endogenous methodology not only gave the inmates a voice, but also revealed insights that might not have been obtained by techniques in which the investigator would have taken an authoritative position in the project. •

As you can surmise from this example, the investigator's concerns in the endogenous research design include how to build and work with a team, how to relinquish control over process and outcome, and how to shape the group process to move the research team along in the study of themselves. These considerations arise from the nature of endogenous research and are distinct from other approaches.

Participatory Action Research

Participatory action research broadly refers to different types of action research approaches. The varied approaches to action research each reflect a different epistemological assumption and methodological strategy. However, all are "participative, grounded in experience, action-oriented"[3] and are founded in the principle that those who experience a phenomenon are the most qualified to investigate it. Similar to endogenous research, participatory action research involves individuals as first-person, second-person, and third-person[3] participants in designing, conducting, and reporting research. By "first-person research," we mean that individuals who experience the phenomenon of interest systematically reflect on their own lives to crate data for analysis. "Second-person research" refers to the initiation of an inquiry by a researcher who then branches out to collaborate directly with individuals and communities about a shared problem. In "third-person research" the collaborative nature is still present but indirect. Communication takes place through other venues, such as written formats and reports.[6] Consistent with others, we believe that the ideal participatory action inquiry includes all three perspectives and approaches.

The purpose of action research is to generate knowledge to inform responsive action. Researchers using a participatory framework usually work with groups or community members experiencing issues and needs related to health and welfare, disparities in health and access to health care, elimination of oppression and discrimination, equal opportunity, and social justice.[7]

The concept of action research was first developed in the 1940s by Kurt Lewin,[4] who blended experimental-type approaches to research with programs that addressed critical social problems. These problems served as the basis for formulating a research purpose, question, and methodology. Therefore, each research step was connected to or involved with the particular organization, social group, or community that was the focus of inquiry and that was affected in some way by the identified problem or issue. More recently, others have expanded this approach to inquiry. The action research design is now used in planning and enacting

---

> **BOX 11-2** *Four Principles of Action Research*
>
> - Democracy
> - Equity
> - Liberation
> - Life enhancement

---

solutions to community problems and service dilemmas.[4-6,8]

Action research is based on four principles or values (Box 11-2). The principle of democracy means that action research is participatory; that is, all individuals who are stakeholders in a problem or issue and its resolution are included in the research process. Equity ensures that all participants are equally valued in the research process, regardless of previous experience in research. Liberation proposes that action research is a design aimed at giving the power of inquiry to participants themselves, decreasing oppression, exclusion, and/or discrimination.[3] Life enhancement positions action research as a systematic strategy that promotes growth, development, and fulfillment of participants in the process and the community they represent.

Participatory action research may use the thinking and action processes from the experimental-type, naturalistic tradition or a combination of the two. Similar to endogenous design, there is no prescribed or uniform set of systematic strategies. Nevertheless, action research is consistent with naturalistic forms of inquiry in that all research occurs within its natural context or where the phenomenon of interest resides. Also, most action research relies on action processes that are characteristically interpretive in nature or a combination of interpretative and quantitative work.[6]

Let us examine the sequence in which the 10 research essentials are followed in a participatory action research study. Action research is best characterized as cyclical, beginning with the identification of a problem or dilemma that calls for action, moving to a form of systematic inquiry, and culminating in planning and using the findings of the inquiry. Each step is informed or shaped by the participants of the study. The purpose of the following participatory action study was to establish community programs to enhance the transition of adolescents with special health care needs from high school to work or higher education.[10]

> Using the principles of action research and first-, second-, and third-person approaches, the investigators first identified the stakeholders involved in this issue. They included adolescents and their parents, educators, health care providers, employers, and policy makers. To ensure that the research plan reflected the underlying principles of democracy and equity, the investigators convened a group made up of representatives from each of the stakeholder groups. This group became the core participatory researchers. These participatory researchers and the two investigators discussed the research problem and collaboratively negotiated and structured the research method. Focus groups were identified as the primary data collection method, so all team members were trained in this approach. Focus groups of each of the stakeholder groups examined the service needs perceived by each group. Each focus group was facilitated by two members of the participatory team. Data were collected and analyzed by the participatory team. The team reported the findings to planning groups consisting of the same stakeholder groups. A comprehensive service plan was developed, implemented, and evaluated by the participatory action team.[10] •

Note that all members of the team were valued and contributed equally to the design, implementation, analysis, and application of the research.

Participatory action research is now used for many purposes, often involving advocacy for underserved groups. For example look at this study description by Sweitzer who conducted a investigation of runaway and homeless youth (RHY):

> *By employing participatory **action research** methods, this **study** privileges youth voice and asks two **research** questions: 1) what are current program models doing right with regards to RHY services, and 2) what can be learned by employing youth analysts in **research**? Findings indicate that how services are offered is as important as what services are offered. Additionally, by privileging youth and providing meaningful participation, youth are exceptionally capable to develop and evaluate services, programs*

and policy. The pragmatic foundation combined with its democratic values render action research a useful tool for identifying, empirically supporting, and assessing needed change with targeted individuals, groups or communities. Also, the approach involves a flexible stance towards methodology making it ideal for combining or mixing experimental-type and naturalistic forms of inquiry.

Critical Theory

Critical theory is not a research method but a "worldview" that suggests both an epistemology and a purpose for conducting research. The debate continues on whether critical theory is a philosophical, political, or sociological school of thought. In essence, critical theory is a response to post-Enlightenment philosophies and positivism in particular. Critical theorists "deconstruct" the notion that there is a unitary truth that can be known by using one way or method.

Critical theory is a movement best understood by philosophers. Because critical theory is inspired by diverse schools of thought, including those informed by Marx, Hegel, Kant, Foucault, Derrida, and Kristeva, it is not a unitary approach. Rather, critical theory represents a complex set of strategies that are united by the commonality of sociopolitical purpose.[10]

Critical theorists seek to understand human experience as a means to change the world.[10] The common purpose of researchers who approach investigation through critical theory is to come to know about social justice and human experience as a means to promote local change through global social change.

Critical theory was born in the Social Institute at the Frankfurt School in the 1920s. As the Nazi party gained power in Germany, critical theorists moved to Columbia University and developed their notions of power and justice, particularly in response to the hegemony of positivism in the United States. With a focus on social change, critical theorists came to view knowledge as power and the production of knowledge as "socially and historically determined."[10] Derived from this view is an epistemology that upheld pluralism, or a coming to know about phenomena in multiple ways. Furthermore, "knowing" is considered to be a dynamic process that changes (is not static) and that is embedded in the sociopolitical context of the times. According to critical theorists, no one objective reality can be uncovered through systematic investigation. Critical theorists and those who build on their work are frequently concerned with language and symbol as the vehicle through which to uncover multiple meanings and to examine power structures and their interactions.[14]

Critical theory is consistent with fundamental principles that bind naturalistic strategies together in one grand category, such as a view of informant as knower, the dynamic and qualitative nature of knowing, and a complex and pluralistic worldview. Furthermore, critical theorists suggest that research crosses disciplinary boundaries and challenges current knowledge generated by experimental-type methods. Because of the radical view posited by critical theorists, the essential step of literature review in the research process is primarily used as a means to understand the status quo. Thus, the action process of literature review may occur before the research, but the theory derived is criticized, deconstructed, and taken apart to its core assumptions. The hallmark of critical theory, however, is its purpose of social change and empowerment of marginalized and oppressed groups. Critical theory relies heavily on interview and observation as methods through which data are collected. Strategies of qualitative data analysis are the primary analytical tools used in critical research agendas (as discussed in Chapter 21).

A researcher is interested in understanding the relationship between clients who are substance abusers and formal service providers and the influence of this relationship on the outcome of therapeutic interventions. First, using a critical theory perspective, the researcher would review the literature critically. Of particular importance for the critical theorist would be an examination of the underlying assumptions in the language and textual symbols that reflect a power imbalance based on disparities in resources, and between client and practitioner. In critical theory, this imbalance is presumed to have an effect of oppressing the client while elevating the status, control, and power of the service provider. Second, the researcher would use a range of strategies based in naturalistic inquiry to observe and explore the relationship of client and service provider from the perspectives of both parties. Third, the understandings derived from the research would be used to promote social change, with a particular focus on advancing social justice and equality for clients.[10]

Phenomenology

The specific focus of phenomenological research is the explication, narrative presentation, and understanding of the meaning of lived experiences. *Phenomenology* differs from other forms of naturalistic inquiry in that phenomenologists believe that meaning can be explained and interpreted only by those who experience it. In many other forms of naturalistic inquiry, the researcher attributes meaning to experience in the analytical phases of the inquiry. In contrast, phenomenologists do not impose an interpretive framework on data but look for it to emerge from the information they obtain from their informants. Phenomenological research is further anchored in the principle that the methods by which we share and communicate experience are limited. Listen to Darroch's classic description[15]:

The phenomenon we study is ostensibly the presence of the other, but it can only be the way in which the experience of the other is made available to us. (p 4)

The singular focus on how individuals experience the phenomenon of interest is what sets this approach from other forms of naturalistic inquiry.

The primary data collection strategy used in this design is the telling of a biographical story or narrative with emphasis on eliciting experience as it relates to time, body, conceptual, and physical and virtual space, as well as to other persons. For example, in eliciting experience, the phenomenologist will ask such questions as, "What is it like to have been diagnosed with breast cancer?" "What was the day like when you learned of your diagnosis?" "What is it like for you to live with breast cancer?" and "What does it mean to you to tell others about your diagnosis?" The elicitation of the ways in which people experience a particular phenomenon differs from other approaches, such as life history. In phenomenology, it is the informant who interjects the primary interpretation and analysis of experience into the interview rather than, as in life history research, for instance, the investigator, who imposes an interpretative structure.

How do phenomenologists use literature review? Literature review is framed by the phenomenological principle of the "limits of communication." Thus, the literature may be used to illustrate the constraints of our understanding of human experience or to corroborate the communication of the other.[15] It may also support the experiences that emerge from informants.

> To understand how this approach works, suppose you plan to conduct a phenomenological study on the experience of aging among urban poor older African-American men. This group is of particular interest because they have lower life expectancy than their white counterparts and have faced multiple social and economic jeopardies. You seek study participation from a small number of individuals, maybe 10 to 15 persons. Then you engage in lengthy discourse with each about his life experiences and the meanings that each person attributes to his lived experience. You also examine previous published research and clinical literature on aging to ascertain the commonalities of what is being communicated. In addition, you use the literature to suggest a rationale for using phenomenological methodology, and then abductively draw on diverse theoretical perspectives to inform yourself of the context of the experiences that emerge. •

In phenomenological research, involvement by the researcher is limited to eliciting life experiences and hearing and reporting the narrative perspective of the informant. Active interpretive involvement during data collection is not typically part of the investigator's role.[16]

Heuristic Research

Heuristic research is another important design in the naturalistic tradition. According to Moustakas, heuristic research is an "approach which encourages an individual to discover, and methods which enable him to investigate further by himself."[17]

The heuristic design strategy involves complete immersion of the investigator into the phenomenon of interest, including the use of self-reflection of the investigator's personal experiences as primary data. The investigator engages in intensive observation of and listening to individuals who have experienced the phenomenon of interest, recording their individual experiences. Then the researcher using this approach interprets and reports the meanings of these experiences.

The premise of the heuristic approach is that knowledge emerges from personal experience and is revealed or known to the investigator through his or her own experience of the phenomenon being studied. In contrast to the phenomenological approach, researchers working within the heuristic tradition seek opportunities to become immersed in the actual experience of interest. Thus, investigator involvement in heuristic design is extensive and pervades all areas of inquiry, from the formulation of the query to the collection of data from the investigator as an informant.

Moustakas's classic work provides an excellent example of heuristic research.

> When his daughter became ill, Moustakas experienced his own loneliness and realized that health care professionals, revealed by their behavior, did not understand the nature of loneliness in persons who were sick. Moustakas therefore engaged in an extensive study in which he examined his own loneliness, listened to the stories of hospitalized children, and critically engaged with the literature on loneliness to further reveal the meaning of the concept. In this design, the literature served as another form of data. It was not used as a source for defining the concept of loneliness before the field was entered.[15] •

This example illustrates how heuristic research is conducted by an individual for the purpose of discovery and understanding of the meaning of human experience. The research involves total immersion in the domain being targeted (e.g., loneliness in illness), including that of the investigator, as a way to understand their perspectives. The experiences of the researcher and the information derived from a literature review are considered primary and critical sources of data. Note the sequence and blurring of the 10 essentials in which the literature review is a source of data and is synthesized with other data sources. The term "heuristic" suggests that this form of inquiry serves as a foundation for further inquiry into the human experience it describes.

Ethnography

Ethnography, a primary method used in the discipline of anthropology, is a systematic approach to understanding the beliefs, rituals, patterns, and institutions that define a culture. Classic ethnography was conducted by etic researchers in previously unexplored remote geographies of the globe with the aim of using knowledge of isolated cultures to reveal the universal commonalities of all cultures.[18]

There are numerous definitions the culture. Fundamental to the construct is the set of patterns that characterize and thus define a group and its membership.[19] Ethnography is thus the accepted method for coming to understand culture. Classic systematic ethnographic methods relied on the investigator becoming immersed in a distant culture for extended periods of time, during which observation, interview, and artifact review were conducted as methods to obtain information for subsequent analysis. The term "informant" emerged from this systematic approach. "Informant" refers to membership in the culture of study and the attribution that this insider status was the only criterion that constituted expert and legitimate knowledge of the culture.[20]

Contemporary ethnography retains some of the tenets and practices of classical methods but is enacted in diverse groups with essential characteristics that no longer are defined by geography. Given the ubiquity of the Internet and virtual worlds, it is not surprising that many investigators activate ethnographic methods to discover interactive constructions of electronic, social media, and gaming cultures among others located online.[21]

Ethnographic methods begin by using a range of techniques to gain access to a context or cultural group. Initial research activity involves observation to characterize the context and to begin describing a culture. Equipped with this understanding, the researcher uses participant and nonparticipant observation, interview, and examination of materials, texts, or artifacts to obtain data. Recording may occur in multiple narrative, text, voice, and video formats. Analysis of the data is concurrent with their collection, and thus is continuous, moving from description to explanation. The knowledge generated therefore begins with description and then expands to meaning and theory.

To ensure rigor, you would conduct specific methods to verify that interpretive analysis and thus the theory derived is endorsed as accurate by those emic to the group. Reflexive analysis, or the analysis of the extent to which the researcher influences the results of the study, is one of the most important strategies and involves the researcher examining the influence of his/her thinking and action on the knowledge generated (see Chapter 20).

We classify ethnography as a naturalistic design because of its reliance on qualitative data collection and analysis, the assumption that the researcher is not the knower, and the absence of a priori hypothesis derived from theory, or a theory imposed before entering the setting. However, ethnographers may draw on various theories to inform their query. It is the investigator who makes the decisions regarding the "who, what, when, and where" of each observation and interview experience. The belief that knowledge can be generated about the "other" without the viewpoint of the investigator influencing the study is a different philosophical approach from heuristic and endogenous designs. Furthermore, ethnography is a design that is capable of moving beyond description to reveal complex relationships, patterns, and theory.

Classical ethnography upheld the belief that through reflexivity, the researcher could remove personal bias from any interpretation and thus understand and analyze the "reality" of a culture. More contemporary forms of ethnography challenge some of those basic assumptions such as investigator objectivity and the presence of an objective social setting apart from its ongoing construction and reinvention through human agency.[18] Current ethnographers aim to represent the participants' own views and ways of explaining their lives. The researcher therefore focuses on the interpretive practices of group members themselves, or how people make sense of their lives in context as reflected in their own words, stories, objects, and narratives. These concerns are similar to those of the phenomenological and life history approaches.

Ethnography has changed from its classic roots in other ways as well. Recall the discussion of critical theory earlier. If ethnography is used within a critical theory framework, its purposes and action processes become diverse and designed to develop and apply knowledge for the social change. In any case, one key element is essential to all forms of ethnography: the examination of cultural and social groups and underlying patterns and ways of experiencing context.[22,23]

Health and human service investigators increasingly turn to ethnography to obtain an insider's perspective on the meaning of health and social issues as a basis from which to develop meaningful health care and social service interventions or to promote policy and social change. Ethnography has also been used to understand various service environments. One example is the classic ethnography of a nursing home conducted by Savishinsky.[24] Several data collection strategies, including interview and participant observation, were used to describe the culture of the nursing home and the meaning of life in that setting. Through analysis and synthesis of the perspectives of residents and staff, Savishinsky was able to identify ways to change that environment to improve the quality of life of the residents.

Narrative Inquiry

The many definitions of and approaches to *narrative inquiry* all have the common element of "storytelling."[18,25] The storytelling may be autobiographical, biographical, testimonial, or in another form. Thus, narrative is a spoken, written, or visual story[24,25] that can be presented in various discursive formats, serves multiple purposes, and can be approached in diverse analytical and interpretive ways.[9] Narrative inquiry is frequently used to illuminate the voices and experiences of marginalized or excluded populations and individuals, although this is not its only

---

BOX 11-3   Guidelines in Applying Narrative Inquiry to Clinical Work

1. Avoid jargon.
2. Specify the purpose of your inquiry.
3. Detail method and the boundaries of this approach.
4. Make your research credible.
5. Help your audience make the connections between the meaning in the story and professional practice.
6. Highlight what can be learned from this approach that cannot be learned from nomothetic approaches.

From Miller WL, Crabtree BF: Clinical research. In Denzin NK, Lincoln YS, editors: *Sage Handbook of qualitative research,* ed 3, Thousand Oaks, Calif, 2011, Sage.

---

purpose. Because of the complexity and extensive detail, narrative data provide rich description and reveal meanings embedded not only in the content of the story but also in the words and images (symbols) used to tell the story Box 11-3.[26]

Remember the primacy of language, communication, text, and image in contemporary naturalistic traditions. Narrative has become one of the most popular postmodern methods because it yields a contextually embedded text or set of images that can be subjected to multiple interpretations and discursive analysis. The view of language as a dynamic, embedded human phenomenon drives the analysis of multiple and reciprocal meanings that can be ascertained through examining the symbolic, tacit, deconstructive, and non-neutral nature of the data.[27]

Let's say you are interested in influencing state policy so that students with limited financial resources can be recruited and supported to study in health and human service programs at your university. You have decided that one of the most compelling ways to provide evidence of need is to obtain narrative stories from community members who wanted to enter these professions but did not have the opportunity. You select several informants and conduct in-depth interviews with them about their experiences and perspectives. From analyzing the transcripts, you find not only that your informants had to settle for available work but that embedded in their images, symbols, and stories were unfulfilled lives because of ongoing questions from informants and their families about "what could have been." You then use the narrative findings and the words of your informants to provide a strong and compelling rationale for policy change and establishing student financial support programs. •

Narrative has also been used for clinical purposes, such as therapeutic use of autobiography and biography. The power of story in healing has been highlighted in numerous scholarly works.[28,29]

The methods to obtain narrative data are diverse. Interviewing and recording (audio or video) are among the information-gathering strategies used most frequently in health and human services to collect narrative data.[29] Photography,[30] drawing, painting, creative nonfiction, autobiography, object reading,[24] and co-constructed narrative[16] are other methods used to tell and present the "story."[34] Yet another method to obtain narrative data is through the use of email, text, or other online venues.[35] These data collection modalities may be particularly appropriate for gathering the experiences and personal stories of vulnerable populations who use these media, such as young adults, and for sensitive topics such as mental illness, sexual activity among individuals with sexually transmitted diseases, or drug use, in which a face-to-face encounter may be viewed as too threatening, stigmatizing, or objectionable by participants.[25]

Selecting the methods for collecting narrative information is first purposive[36] and then practical in nature. Each method will have strengths and limitations; there are tradeoffs for any methodological decision made. In the previous example, interview provided the forum through which to hear the voices of the informants. But what if you were interested in examining the discursive power in the client-provider relationship? You might turn to video and audio recording, because discursive analysis would be focused on the tacit rules already established in relationships and social activity. In the recordings, you would then look for how these unspoken rules of communication and behavior were illustrated in the interaction between those observed.

In Chapter 21, we discuss the basic analytical action processes used in the naturalistic tradition. These same strategies are used for narrative analysis.[37] From a data set, inductive analysis is used to reveal the themes, patterns, and meanings that emerge from storytelling.

It is important to keep in mind that many health and human service professionals and those who influence policy, funding, education, and practice have typically been educated to value knowledge that has been generated from experimental-type inquiry. Therefore, investigators who choose narrative strategies for inquiry must be sure to explain adequately its value and purpose and report their narrative in a compelling way that is relevant to the health and human service contexts[35] (see Box 10-3).

Although narrative can generate theory,[34] we do not view this purpose as its primary aim. Narrative strategies typically employ small numbers of informants in the creation of stories that illuminate underlying processes and meanings of experiences.

Life History

Life history, another important design in naturalistic inquiry, uses a narrative strategy. Life history, also called "biography of life narrative" or "memoir," is an approach that can stand by itself as a legitimate type of research study, or it can be an integral part of other forms of naturalistic inquiry, such as ethnography.[38] The life history approach is a part of the naturalistic tradition because of its focus on examining the social, cultural, and political context of individual lives. Similar to other designs such as phenomenology, the investigator is primarily concerned with eliciting life experiences and with how individuals themselves interpret and attribute meanings to these experiences.

The aim of life history research is to reveal the nature of the "life process traversed over time."[38] The assumption is that individual lives are unique. These unique life processes are important to examine to understand the context in which people live their lives. Researchers who use a life history approach therefore focus on one individual at a time. A study may be composed of just one individual or a few individuals.

There are many diverse purposes for using a life history approach. A life history might be used to explicate the impact of major sociopolitical events on individual lives,[39] the processes of developing an identity growing up with a physical impairment, or the unfolding of self-esteem as women age. Depending on the aim of inquiry, life history researchers sequence the essential action processes and use literature in diverse ways. Investigators who attempt to abductively analyze the value of different theories for explaining the complexity of a human life may begin with literature review and use it as an organizing framework. Researchers who seek new theoretical understandings, however, may conduct literature review at different junctures in the research thinking and action processes.

Life history research involves a particular methodological approach in which the sequence of life events is elicited and the meaning of those events examined from the perspective of the informant within a particular sociopolitical and historical context.[39] In eliciting events, the researcher seeks to uncover and characterize marker events, or "turnings," defined as specific occurrences that shape and change the direction of individual lives.[40] Typically, researchers rely heavily on unstructured interviewing techniques. The research may begin with asking an informant to describe the sequence of life events from childhood to adulthood. On the basis of a time line of events, the investigator may ask questions to elicit the meanings of these events.[40] Participatory and nonparticipatory observation may also be combined with the interview as data collection strategies to examine meanings and understand how life is experienced.

Although life history relies mostly on the person who tells his or her story, the investigator shapes the story in part by the types of questions asked. For example, the researcher may ask for more detail about a particular life event than is initially offered by the participant. This probing by the researcher structures, in effect, the telling of the story to fit the interests or concerns of the researcher. Also, the researcher may impose an analytic framework, identifying and isolating key events or turning points that the person who is telling the story may or may not identify him/herself.

Consider how you might use life history to understand the process of developing a disability identity among disability rights activists. First, you would identify an individual or several individuals who are involved in disability rights activities, such as leaders of ADAPT or disabled scholar-activists. For each individual, you would aim to create a narrative or biography by conducting in-depth interviews, to uncover the chronology of life events as well as the symbolic and practical meanings of these events to your informant. Analysis of "turnings" would allow you to examine the types of experiences that were most influential in determining the future direction of the informant's life, identity development, and call to action. The experience of several individuals who provide narrative would illuminate invaluable insights into the sociocultural world of this group of individuals who have disability and a call to civil action. •

Life history studies can be retrospective or prospective. In health and human service research, it is not surprising, in light of practical constraints, that the majority of life history studies are retrospective in their approach; that is, informants are asked to reconstruct their lives and reflect on the meaning of past events. Prospective life histories would rely on the investigator's ability to devote significant time to the observation and analysis of meaning as an individual traveled through chronological time.

Object Reading

Object reading is a relatively contemporary approach within naturalistic inquiry but of great use to health and human service researchers.[26] Let us consider why. Rehabilitation, health interventions and treatment, and counseling often involve adaptive devices, medical equipment, and architectural spaces, respectively, all of which hold diverse meanings to clients. Understanding, for example, the meaning of a walker or crutch design to a client can make the difference between acceptance and abandonment.[41] Although objects have been considered to be the research domain of archeology over several centuries, the recent emergence of the field of material culture has brought life, interactivity, and interpretation to objects in their contexts. "Object" is broadly defined here as tangible artifacts and structures but may also include visual, text, or oral images.[42] "Reading" refers to the interpretation of meaning of an object, similar to the analysis of narrative in which texts are inductively analyzed not only for their description but for meanings embedded within them. Object reading involves both description and analysis of meaning.

Let's return to the example of mobility device abandonment. Although Bateni and Maki[43] found that people who were prescribed mobility devices tended to abandon them because of the inadequate function of these objects, you realize that people who need them are not using them at home, regardless of improvements in function or safety that this equipment can provide. So you set out to find alternative explanations. The systematic inquiry involved interviewing elders about the meaning of these objects to them. To analyze the meanings for observers and prescribers of these objects, you take photos of typical walkers, crutches, and canes, show them to informants, and then ask the views to tell a story about people who might be likely to be seen using these objects. This object reading technique leads to how the devices are interpreted as stigmatizing and ascribing dependency and shame to people who need them. Object reading belongs under the naturalistic umbrella because of its inductive, open-ended search for meanings. The sequence of the essentials in this design is not fixed, as the researcher can consult literature before, during, or after obtaining information. Investigator involvement is extensive in this design, as the researcher chooses the objects and their presentation to purposively selected informants.

Grounded Theory

Grounded theory is defined as "the systematic discovery of theory from the data of social research."[44] It is a more structured and investigator-directed strategy than the previous naturalistic designs that we have thus far discussed. Developed by Glaser and Strauss,[44] grounded theory represents the integration of a quantitative and qualitative perspective in thinking and action processes. The primary purpose of this design strategy is to evolve or "ground" a theory in the context in which the phenomenon under study occurs. The theory that emerges is intimately linked to each datum of daily life experience that it seeks to explain.

This strategy is similar to other naturalistic designs in its use of an inductive process to derive concepts, constructs, relationships, and principles to understand and explain a phenomenon. However, grounded theory is distinguished from other naturalistic designs by its use of a structured data-gathering and analytical process called the constant comparative method.[45] In this approach, each datum is compared with others to determine similarities and differences. Researchers have developed an elaborate scheme by which to code, analyze, recode, and produce a theory from narratives obtained through a range of data collection strategies.[45]

Let us briefly consider how you might use grounded theory.

> Let's say you are interested in characterizing single, head-of-household mothers receiving public assistance who have returned to college to understand their experiences and parenting styles. After identifying the contextual boundaries of your study, you would interview the women and then, using constant comparison, analyze the narratives. Using this method, you would first read and reread the entire data set to induce categories of data that were repeated throughout the experiences of the women who served as your informants. Then you would return to the transcripts to analyze each datum, an experience, articulation, or observation, and compare it with the data in the existing categories to determine similarities and differences between new data and previous information. If it did fit, you would code the datum with an existing code. If it did not fit, a new category or subcategory would be developed and used as a basis for comparing subsequent data analysis. •

The purpose of the constant comparative method is not only to reveal categories but also to explore the diversity of experience within categories, as well as to identify links among categories. Grounded-theory strategies can also be used to generate and verify theory.[45] A query using a grounded-theory approach begins with broad descriptive interests and then, through data collection and analysis, moves to discover and verify relationships and principles.

Naturalistic Meta-analysis

Now we turn to another approach, *naturalistic meta-analysis,* which seeks to aggregate small and disparate data sets from which to derive a global synthesis.[46] *Meta-analysis* is a research approach in which multiple independently conducted studies are synthesized and analyzed as a single data set to answer a research question or query. Naturalistic meta-analysis is the application of naturalistic methods to the analysis of many studies. Interestingly, naturalistic meta-analysis is not restricted to the analysis of naturalistic studies. Rather, this approach to meta-analysis is characterized by the philosophical perspective that underpins naturalistic inquiry and the use of inductive methods of analysis applied to multiple studies, literature, and theory.[12]

If you are interested in understanding the experiences and turning points in the lives of people living with acquired immunodeficiency syndrome (AIDS) or, for that matter, any other challenging and enduring condition such as dementia or multiple sclerosis, you could aggregate written literature and look for themes throughout narratives, theory, and even experimental-type studies that focus on the particular population of interest. •

There are many purposes of naturalistic meta-analysis.[46] Similar to experimental-type meta-analysis (see Chapter 10), some naturalistic meta-analyses seek to identify and summarize a universe of studies on a particular topic. In anthropology, however, meta-ethnography[47,48] has been used interpretively to reveal global themes and patterns. The Qual-Quan Evidence Synthesis Group[49] seeks to establish "rigor" standards for naturalistic meta-analysis to contribute to evidence-based practice in health care. This group suggests that meta-analytic approaches are valuable in reviewing diverse perspectives and findings as the basis for deriving single definitions and understandings of complex constructs (e.g., quality, satisfaction).[49]

The thinking and action processes of naturalistic meta-analysis follow the processes that you would use in any naturalistic study. The difference, however, is that your data set comprises studies already conducted and existing sources of literature, theory, and other data sources. Thus, you are aggregating and conducting a secondary analysis of existing knowledge from the perspective of naturalistic inquiry.

If we apply the elements of naturalistic inquiry to existing sources, we begin to see how meta-analysis might be approached within this tradition. First, we specify a query or queries that conceptually "bound" a study and provide guidance for seeking sources for analysis. Remember that after the queries are articulated, they can undergo modification as the data sources are initially reviewed and analyzed. In meta-analysis, the step analogous to gaining access to a physical or virtual research setting is deciding which sources to access first. In concert with the thinking and action processes of naturalistic inquiry, data collection and analysis are concurrent and ongoing, and the investigator modifies the inquiry in response to the analysis and emerging findings. Final analysis and reporting to audiences occur after saturation occurs with the data set. Let us consider the investigator who is interested in characterizing the experience of AIDS.

Because there are such diverse findings and accounts of living with a disease such as cancer or AIDS, naturalistic meta-analysis is an excellent method to choose to determine whether any global themes characterize the current knowledge base. But where do you start? You make a decision based on purpose and practicality. You gain access to the literature by entering keywords such as "living with AIDS," "story," and "life history" into a search engine. You search dissertation abstracts for any work done on living with AIDS, regardless of the methodology used. The decision to stop collecting sources is based on saturation and such practical factors as the amount of time and resources that are available to conduct your study. •

Naturalistic meta-analysis can be an extremely valuable methodology for health and human service researchers. This approach not only allows the researcher to use data already generated by others, but also provides the tools to reveal consensus on competing theories and research, to arrive at single definitions of complex constructs, and to illuminate important themes and patterns across large bodies of literature.

Summary

The 11 design strategies discussed in this chapter differ in their purpose, the sequencing of the essentials of research, and the nature of the investigator's involvement. Naturalistic designs are flexible in the degree to which the investigator participates in the formulation of the design, data collection, and interpretive analysis. Moreover, the sequences of the 10 essential thinking and action processes vary, and boundaries between these processes, such as data collection and analysis, which are clearly delineated in experimental-type designs, may be blurred in naturalistic inquiry.

With this introduction to 11 frequently used designs in the naturalistic tradition, you may want to explore each in greater depth by following up with the references to this chapter.

EXERCISES

1. To understand the different purposes of naturalistic designs, identify a broad topic or problem area. Formulate at least four distinct research queries that lead to four designs discussed in this chapter.
2. Go to a public place and determine how you would conduct a study using classic ethnography to determine public behavior patterns. Determine how you would conduct the study using heuristic research. Now think of how you might conduct object reading in the setting to answer your queries.
3. Plan a study using a naturalistic design to discover the health beliefs of an older Asian population living in an urban community. Plan a study using a naturalistic design with Asian children who are chronically ill and living with their families. How would your strategies differ?
4. Identify an area of your practice in which participatory action research would be useful for defining and guiding necessary change. How would

you design your study to ensure that you upheld the four values that underpin all action research?
5. Find, compare, and contrast narrative formats on a single topic. Which presentation do you prefer? Why? Which is most compelling and clinically convincing, and why?
6. Pose a broad query and select four sources of data for your analysis. Look for themes that unify your four sources. After conducting this exercise, identify the strengths and limitations of the approach you have chosen to answer your query.

References

1. Maruyama M: Endogenous research: the prison project. In Reason P, Rowan J, editors: *Human inquiry: a sourcebook of new paradigm research*, New York, 1981, Wiley & Sons, p 270.
2. Torres MN, Reyes LV: *Research as praxis: democratizing education epistemologies*, New York, 2011, Peter Lang.
3. Chevalier JM, Buckles DJ: *Participatory action research: theory and methods for engaged inquiry*, London, 2013, Routledge.
4. Lewin K: *Field theory in social science*, New York, 1951, Harper and Row.
5. Argyris C, Schon DA: Participatory action research and action science compared: a commentary. In Whyte WF, editor: *Participatory action research*, Newbury Park, Calif, 1991, Sage, p 433.
6. Reason P, Bradbury H, editors: *Handbook of action research: participative inquiry and practice*, ed 2, Thousand Oaks, Calif, 2008, Sage, p xxiv.
7. Fortune AE, Reid WJ, Miller RL: *Qualitative research in social work*, ed 2, New York, 2013, Columbia University Press.
8. Whyte WF, editor: *Participatory action research*, Newbury Park, Calif, 1991, Sage.
9. Stringer ET: *Action research: a handbook for practitioners*, Thousand Oaks, Calif, 1996, Sage.
10. DePoy E, Gilmer D, Martzial E: Adolescents with disabilities and chronic illness in transition: a community action needs assessment. *Disability Stud Q* 20:34–57, 2000.
11. Schweitzer DD: *2011, Runaway and homeless youth: changing the discourse by legitimizing youth voice*, 2011, dissertation, Pacific University.
12. Denzin NK, Lincoln YS: *Sage handbook of qualitative research*, ed 4, Thousand Oaks, Calif, 2011, Sage.
13. MacKinnon ST: Social work intellectuals in the twenty-first century: critical social theory, critical social work and public engagement. *Social Work Educ* 28:512–527, 2009.
14. Macey D: *Penguin dictionary of critical theory*, 2002, Penguin Books.

15. Darroch V, Silvers RJ, editors: *Interpretive human studies: an introduction to phenomenological research*, Washington, DC, 1982, University Press of America, p 4.

16. Van Manen M: *Phenomenology of practice: meaning-giving methods in phenomenological research and writing*, Walnut Creek, Calif, 2014, Left Coast Press.

17. Moustakas C: *Heuristic research: design, methodology, and applications*, Thousand Oaks, Calif, 1990, Sage.

18. Salkind N: *Encyclopedia of research design*, Los Angeles, Calif, 2010, Sage.

19. DePoy E, Gilson SF: *Human behavior theory and applications: a critical thinking approach*, Thousand Oaks, Calif, 2012, Sage.

20. Sperber D: *On anthropological knowledge*, Cambridge, UK, 1987, Cambridge University Press.

21. Kozinets R: *Netnography: doing ethnographic research online*, Thousand Oaks, Calif, 2012, Sage.

22. Agar M: *An ethnography by any other name*, 2006. http://www.qualitative-research.net/index.php/fqs/article/view/177/395.

23. Lofland J, Snow D, Anderson L, et al: *Analyzing social settings*, ed 4, Belmont, Calif, 2006, Wadsworth.

24. Savishinsky JS: *The ends of time: life and work in a nursing home*, New York, 1991, Bergen & Garvey.

25. Silverman D: *Doing qualitative research*, ed 4, Thousand Oaks, Calif, 2013, Sage.

26. Berger A: *What objects mean*, Walnut Creek, Calif, 2009, Left Coast Press.

27. The Centre for Narrative Research: http://www.uel.ac.uk/cnr/index.htm. Accessed April 1, 2010.

28. Abell J, Stokoe E, Billig M: Narrative and the discursive (re) construction of events. In Andrews M, Sclater SD, Squire C, et al, editors: *Lines of narrative*, London, 2000, Routledge.

29. Seale C: Resurrective practice and narrative. In Andrews M, Sclater SD, Squire C, et al, editors: *Lines of narrative*, London, 2000, Routledge.

30. Lister M: *The photographic image in digital culture*, ed 2, London, 2013, Routledge.

31. Squire C: *Centre for narrative research, school of social sciences*, 2004, University of East London. Available at www.uel.ac.uk/cnr/documents/Newsletter5April2004.doc.

32. Bell S: Photo images: Jo Spence's narratives of living with illness. *Health* 6:5–30, 2002.

33. Silverman D: *Doing qualitative research: a practical handbook*, ed 2, Thousand Oaks, Calif, 2004, Sage.

34. Pagnucci G, Mauriello N: *Re-mapping narrative: technology's impact on the way we write*, New York, 2008, Hampton Press.

35. Riessman CK: *Narrative methods for the human sciences*, Thousand Oaks, Calif, 2008, Sage.

36. Gubrium JF, Holstein JA, Marvasti AB, et al: *Sage handbook of interview research*, Thousand Oaks, Calif, 2012, Sage.

37. Schwandt TA: *The SAGE dictionary of qualitative inquiry*. Los Angeles, Calif, 2007, Sage 7.

38. Goodwin John: *SAGE Biographical Research*, Los Angeles, CA, 2012, Sage.

39. Mkhonza S: Life histories as social texts of personal experiences in sociolinguistic studies: a look at the lives of domestic workers in Swaziland. In Josselson R, Lieblich A, editors: *Interpreting experience: the narrative study of lives*, Newbury Park, Calif, 1995, Sage.

40. Verd JM, López M: *The rewards of a qualitative approach to life-course research*, 2011. http://nbn-resolving.de/urn:nbn:de:0114-fqs1103152.

41. DePoy E, Gilson SF: *Branding and designing disability: reconceptualizing disability studies*, London, 2015, Routledge.

42. Harper D: *Visual sociology*, New York, 2012, Routledge.

43. Bateni H, Maki B: Assistive devices for balance and mobility: benefits, demands, and adverse consequences. *Arch Phys Med Rehabil* 86:134–145, 2005.

44. Glaser B, Strauss A: *The discovery of grounded theory*, New York, 1967, Aldine.

45. Creswell J: *Research design*, Los Angeles, 2014, Sage.

46. Flick U: *The SAGE handbook of qualitative data analysis*, Los Angeles, 2013, Sage.

47. Fauzan N: *Reviewing research evidences in psychological research: using meta-ethnography and meta-analysis*, 2010, Lambert Academic Publishing.

48. Noblitt GW, Hare RD: *Meta-ethnography: synthesizing qualitative studies*, Newbury Park, Calif, 1988, Sage.

49. Qual-Quan Evidence Synthesis Group: http://www.prw.le.ac.uk/research/qualquan/publications.htm. Accessed April 1, 2010.

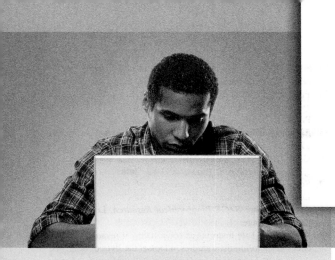

Chapter 12
Mixed Method Designs

You should now be familiar with the language, thinking processes, and designs of experimental-type and naturalistic traditions. Because researchers who use mixed method designs draw from both traditions, it is important to have a good understanding of designs from both traditions before reading this chapter. If you need to review, revisit Chapters 10 and 11. As you probably can guess by now, the ways in which researchers approach mixing methods are limited only by imagination, purpose, and the constraints imposed by settings and resources.

Remember that we discussed mixed methods previously, indicating that this tradition transcends the debates about which type of design, experimental-type or naturalistic, produces legitimate and accurate knowledge for use in health and human services. Rather than viewing mixing methods as a philosophical snafu, Tashakkori and Teddlie[1] located mixed methods within pragmatism, therefore allowing researchers to pick and choose methods and strategies from diverse designs and traditions to accomplish the purposes of conducting a study. Through mixing and integrating strategies, investigators can account for the limitations of each design tradition. Johnson and Onwuegbuzie[2] remind us about the purpose of all research:

> *Regardless of paradigmatic orientation, all research in the social sciences represents an attempt to provide warranted assertions about human beings (or specific groups of human beings) and the environments in which they live and evolve. (p 15)*

Approaches to Mixing Methods

Building on these commonalities of purpose, researchers integrate experimental and naturalistic research strategies in a number of ways depending on the nature of the research questions and query depending, and the level of knowledge development within the particular area of study. These fall into four categories (Box 12-1).

BOX 12-1 *Four Approaches to Using Mixed Methods*

Convergent or concurrent designs
Sequential designs
    Naturalistic to experimental
    Experimental to naturalistic
Embedded or nested designs
Multi-phase designs

Designs can be integrated in various ways as suggested by Box 12-1. Let us look at how you might proceed with each of these approaches.

A convergent or concurrent design involves merging both experimental-type and naturalistic forms of data that have been collected to address a specific research question/query. For example, let's say you conduct a focus group to derive qualitative feedback about a group's perceptions of their experiences using assistive devices. You could also have the group complete a questionnaire to examine the relationship between assistive device use and affective well-being. The data from both sources would be combined to more fully understand experiences with assistive devices.

A sequential or stepwise process can begin first with naturalistic inquiry followed by an experimental approach or the other way. An approach in which the researcher starts with naturalistic inquiry is often used to develop new theory and then test its accuracy. Suppose you were interested in developing a program to improve aging in place for rural elders who were not fully independent in self-care. In light of the shortage of home health aids,[3] you believe that robotic assistants would be one way of providing in home help for this population. However, you have not found any programs that have used and tested this strategy or theorized about the extent to which these elders would accept robotic devices in their homes. You therefore set out to develop theory, using naturalistic inquiry to answer your query about robotic assistant acceptance and comfort with use. Your findings lead you to knowledge about elders in one community who would accept assistants for moving objects and virtually communicating with their families but not for helping with more intimate tasks. Given this finding, you then proceed to use experimental-type design to test your theory in a large group of rural elders. You decide to conduct closed-ended interviews and quantify acceptance of robotic assistance for numerous self-care tasks.

Now, let's move in the other direction, from experimental-type to naturalistic design. Proceeding from experimental to naturalistic strategies offers the opportunity to test theory first and then fill gaps in knowledge through an inductive process. Continuing with the example above, you have tested a large sample of elders by randomly selecting them from a population of elders with self-care limitations. You interview them and find that they are not similar in their acceptance scores. So you decide to conduct open-ended interviews to discover concepts that might be related to acceptance.

A third way to mix methods is to use different strategies in a single study in one or more of the essentials. This has been referred to also as a "nested" design. For example, let's say you are testing an intervention to improve heart patients' engagement in an exercise program. The intervention is being tested in a randomized clinical trial. In addition to determining the intervention's efficacy, it would be important to also understand how participants experience the program. Do they find it too difficult, too time consuming or does it require too much energy? Collecting qualitative data could be introduced during the trial and after, or any combination.

Let's also consider our example above concerning assistive devices. Suppose you now find that familiarity and experience with technology is an important element of robotic acceptance but you are not satisfied that these two concepts are the only ones to consider. So you conduct an interview which contains both closed and open-ended questions to verify technology experience and familiarity as variables related to acceptance and then ask what else might be important to consider.

Integrating strategies in one or more of the essentials, suppose you now find that familiarity and experience with technology are important elements of robotic acceptance, but you are not satisfied that these two concepts are the only ones to consider. So you conduct an interview that contains both closed- and open-ended questions to verify technology experience and familiarity as variables related to acceptance, and then ask what else might be important to consider.

> Let us consider another example. Suppose you are interested in developing a smoking prevention program for new immigrants in your suburban area. You know the parameters of the population and therefore select a purposive sample (see Chapter 14 for discussion of sampling). However, you do not know what would be important to include for content and how this content should be delivered. So you conduct a focus group using inductive methods to develop an understanding of what would be important for this sample. In this example, you have mixed experimental-type boundary setting with naturalistic data-collection techniques. •

A fully integrated design applies naturalistic and experimental strategies throughout the research process so each informs the other. You might decide to consult the literature on smoking prevention for immigrant populations first. But what if you find that you do not know about the linguistic parameters of your population? You may know something else about the population, so you use sampling along with naturalistic boundary setting to further understand who is part of the population that you should involve in your study. In your data collection, you proceed to mix both deductive and inductive methods and also do so in your analysis. This approach to mixed methods provides a rich understanding that may even be generalized to other immigrant populations if that is your aim.

The fourth way to mix methods is to merge data from multiple projects that have been conducted over time that are linked to address a particular research question or query. This approach can be used to develop an intervention in which a series of studies are conducted, some qualitative and some quantitative to derive a treatment approach.[4]

Of particular importance within the mixed method tradition is case study design. We now turn to this category of research.

Case Study

Case study design is one of the most frequently used mixed method research approaches in social work. The following two-part definition is derived from the work of Yin.[5]

Case study is an empirical inquiry that:

1. "Investigates a contemporary phenomenon within its real life context; especially when the boundaries between phenomenon and context are not clearly evident"; and an inquiry that
2. "Copes with the technically distinctive situation in which there will be many more variables of interest than data points, and as one result, relies on multiple sources of evidence, with data needing to converge in a triangulating fashion, and as another result, benefits from the prior development of theoretical propositions to guide data collection and analysis."[5]

Yin's definition clarifies why we classify case study design as mixed method. Case study is particularly useful when it is not possible or desirable to randomize, when it is not possible or desirable to study a particular population as a group with similar characteristics, when you seek to assess outcomes or change in a single unit of analysis, and when you want to obtain pilot information in a cost-efficient way. Moreover, case study is an excellent theory-generating tool because the findings of a single case can be theoretically explained and then tested through other types of design strategies.

Structure of Case Study Designs

There are many variations of case study designs that are also referred to as single-subject, single-system, or "N of 1" single-case experimental trial (N refers to the size of the sample; see Chapter 14).

Case studies can be treated as holistic or embedded (Table 12-1). Holistic studies are those that investigate a unit as single global phenomenon, whereas embedded approaches treat a single unit as a sum of its parts.[4] For example, suppose you are looking at implementing an exercise program in a large corporate environment and decide to conduct a study to determine what type of program to implement and for whom. If you treated the workplace as

TABLE 12-1	*Four Types of Case Studies*	
	Single	**Multiple**
Holistic	One case, global	Multiple cases, global
Embedded	One case, multiple elements	Multiple cases, multiple elements

a single unit of analysis because you are only interested in developing a single intervention, you would be treating the unit of analysis as a holistic case. However, if you were considering the work environment as composed of different segments (e.g., employees who exercise regularly and those who do not; different ages, job functions, and schedules), you would be treating your unit of analysis still as a case but embedded with different parts. From an embedded design approach, the single workplace would still be your case but would be considered the sum of its parts. When considering holistic versus embedded designs, the investigator must examine the nature of the phenomenon that is of interest as the basis for deciding how to proceed. Does the unit of analysis have natural parts that will reveal relevant information? If "yes," then an embedded approach would be used. Does the "whole" provide the most informative approach? If "yes," then a holistic approach is used.

A second design consideration in case study is the determination of the number of cases to be included in the research (see Table 12-1). In a single-case design, only one study of a single unit of analysis is conducted. In a multiple-case design, more than one study of single units of analysis is conducted. Therefore, if you conducted your study in a single workplace, you would be using single-case design, but if you expanded your study to a number of separate work environments and did not see them as part of the same case, you would be conducting a multiple-case study design.

The decision to conduct a single-case or multiple-case study depends on several considerations. First, the aim of the research must fit the structure that is selected. Multiple-case studies enable the investigator to examine the same phenomenon across several different cases. It is somewhat analogous to the concept of "replication" in group (or nomothetic)

designs. Thus, if an investigator wants to repeat a study to strengthen theory or test the findings of a single case on other cases, a multiple-case study approach is preferred. However, if the purpose of the research is to generate theory, explicate an atypical phenomenon, or describe the progress of an individual over time, a single-case study approach is warranted.

It logically follows, therefore, that the holistic single-case study is conducted only once on one case. The holistic multiple-case study examines several global units of analysis more than once. An embedded single-case study focuses on multiple parts of a single case using only one case whereas an embedded multiple-case study examines more than one case in which each case contains many subparts.[5,6]

Because the methods for boundary setting in case study design are not consistent with experimental-type boundary setting (see Chapter 14), using multiple studies to make up a sample or a population is not appropriate or legitimate. The purpose of selecting a multiple-case study design instead of a more traditional experimental-type design lies in the definition of case study designs. Case study, whether single or multiple, is ideal for health and human service researchers who are describing a single unit in depth.

Design Sequence

Assume you plan to conduct a case study and have decided on its basic structure and size; that is, you have determined whether you will use a holistic or embedded, single-case or multiple-case approach. Deciding on basic structure and size is one of the first thinking processes involved in implementing a case study design. The second thinking process involves determining the sequence of the design.

Many types of case study design sequences can be used, depending on the purpose of the study and the questions and queries posed. Each design sequence has specific strengths and weaknesses. Some design sequences are more flexible and fluid and thus lean more toward the naturalistic tradition. Alternatively, the design sequence may be linear and fixed, similar to experimental-type designs. We discuss these now but remind you that regardless of the design sequence, case study design lies within mixed methods, at minimum because it relies on multiple methods of integrated data collection.

AB Design

Single-subject case studies that follow experimental-type structuring have their own notation system similar to experimental-type design. However, different symbols are used. Rather than denoting the phases with X and O, case study uses A and B; A depicts the observation, and B indicates the intervention or independent variable. The most basic design is called the "AB design," in which A represents the baseline phase and B represents the intervention phase. Although this type of design cannot predict, it can explain what happens during an intervention.

During the baseline period (A), repeated measures using diverse approaches are obtained on specified variables. For numeric data, the investigator obtains as many measurements as possible and feasible, typically from six to nine observation points, to establish a stable baseline. Of course, the number of measurements may vary depending on whether the observed behavior is stable or in response to contextual constraints. If, for example, observed scores are highly variable, many repeated measures may be necessary to detect a baseline pattern of behavior. Yet, if the intervention cannot ethically be delayed, multiple measures may not be possible despite the research importance.

After a baseline pattern has been established, the intervention is introduced, followed by repeated measurement. The A phase forms the "control." The B phase measures are obtained after intervention. A and B phase measures are compared to examine changes ostensibly resulting from the intervention. It is recommended that a similar number of observations be obtained in both the A phase and the B phase to monitor the stability of change over time.

Because case studies examine a single unit of analysis, they often rely on visual techniques and multiple methods of analysis[5] to display and ascertain change. This line denotes the "best fit" of the baseline data points. The same line is then drawn along the data points in phase B to determine whether there is a difference in the direction and placement of scores and is referred to as the celeration line. Figure 12-1A shows a case in which no change

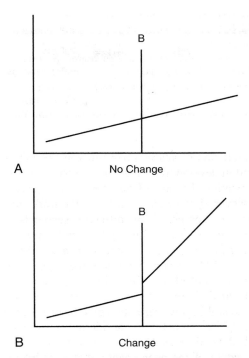

Figure 12-1 Celeration lines for no change and change in case study analysis.

occurs whereas Fig. 12-1B denotes a change in direction.

Structural Variations

There are many variations on the AB design, such as the ABA and $ABAB$ designs. In the "ABA design" a baseline period (A) is followed by an intervention period (B), which is then followed by the withdrawal of the intervention (A). In the "$ABAB$ design" the previous sequence is followed, and then the intervention is reapplied.

Many more options can be introduced into designs that use phases A and B. For example, there may be multiple B phases in which each B phase may involve different strategies. The structure of the ABA design is stronger than a simple AB sequence when there are questions regarding the extent to which change is produced as an outcome of an intervention.

Time Series Design

The *time series design,* another type of single-subject design, is used to follow one subject over time. Consider the following example.

You want to determine whether an innovative intervention with a chronically depressed population decreases levels of depression. Because you want to look at individuals instead of groups, you select a single-subject design. For the first three sessions, you administer a depression inventory. You then conduct the intervention and follow up with three administrations of the same instrument. If, on the basis of visual inspection, you observe a difference between the observed scores immediately preceding and after the intervention, you can surmise that a change occurred and that this change may be a consequence of the intervention. With this type of design, you cannot claim that the intervention is the cause of the improvement. However, you have demonstrated that a change occurred with credible evidence to support the need for further investigation. •

Data Collection and Analysis

Now that we have discussed the basics of structure, size, and sequence, let us further explore the nature of data collection in single-case designs. As suggested by Yin,[4] even when your study leans toward the experimental-type tradition in its structure, multiple data-collection strategies strengthen the credibility of findings. Ideally, several methods of data collection should be used at both baseline and follow-up phases.

Consider this example. Because of the omnipotence of social networking sites and their use by this population, you are aware that employers often look online to see what potential employees have posted about themselves. You therefore develop a "personal branding" intervention to improve the online posting awareness of young adults who are about to graduate from undergraduate education and are facing a difficult job market. You select an embedded single-case study. The unit of analysis is the group in whom the subparts are the participants. You establish an interview protocol to test awareness before the initiation of the group. You complete this interview several times prior to the implementation of the project to obtain a baseline. In addition, you monitor online posts of your participants and score them for positive to negative self-branding. You continue data collection using the two strategies

throughout the intervention and after its termination. Your results therefore provide several points before, during, and after the program to inform you about change. •

A major concern in case study research for studies relying on experimental-type structures is "generalizability." Although generalization of findings is not viable nor the aim of case study, this limitation is in part overcome by the ability to generate and theory to be evaluated through replication and expansion to other designs.

Naturalistic Structure

Now let us look at case studies that are structured more in line with the naturalistic tradition. As you would expect, these studies are flexible in size and sequence. For example, it is possible to move between holistic and embedded designs or from single to multiple cases, depending on the emergence of insights as the study proceeds. What characterizes naturalistic case study structure and distinguishes it from other naturalistic designs is its logic—that is, the identification of a "case" as the phenomenon of interest. Let us consider the example of personal branding again.

Suppose you not only wanted to know changes in awareness that your intervention produced but were also interested in the nature of the awareness as well. In a naturalistic case study, you might observe participant postings at various times, evaluate their meaning, and proceed inductively to search for patterns and meanings that would provide more insight into how college-age youth use social networking and thus could still accomplish their communication aims without risking negative results on a job interview.

Summary

In this chapter, we discussed mixed method designs. These research approaches are based on pragmatism as their philosophical foundation and thus are purposively used by researchers. We then explored case study research as an example of mixing methods through structure, data collection, and analysis.

EXERCISES

1. Find a mixed method research article and identify the purpose and both the experimental-type and naturalistic parts of the design.
2. Find an example of each of the four types of case studies depicted in Table 12-1.
3. In each case study article, determine if it leans toward a naturalistic or experimental-type structure.

· ·

References

1. Tashakkori A, Teddlie C: *Sage handbook of mixed methods in social and behavioral research*, ed 2, Thousand Oaks, Calif, 2010, Sage.
2. Johnson RB, Onwuegbuzie AJ: Mixed methods research: a research paradigm whose time has come. *Educ Researcher* 33:14–26, 2004.
3. 2012 Health Care Personnel Shortage Task Force: *Annual report*, 2012. www.wtb.wa.gov/Documents/HealthCareReport 2012.pdf.
4. Creswell JW, Klassen AC, Clark VL, et al: *Best practices for mixed methods research in the health sciences*, National Institutes of Health, 2011, Data retrieved. http://obssr.od.nih.gov/mixed_methods_research.
5. Yin R: *Case study research: design and methods*, ed 5, Los Angeles, 2014, Sage.
6. Riley-Tillman TC, Burns MK: *Evaluating educational interventions: single-case design for measuring response to intervention*, New York, 2009, Guilford.

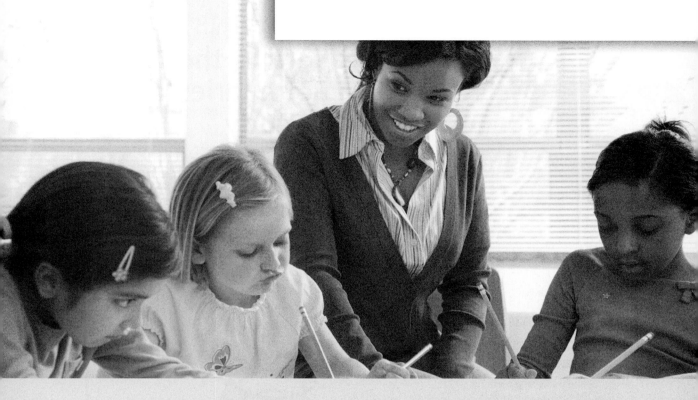

PART IV Action Processes

Now that you have grasped the vocabulary and general thinking processes across the research traditions, we are ready for action. In Part IV, we focus on the way in which researchers implement, or put into action, their design strategies. Each chapter introduces specific research action processes of naturalistic inquiry and experimental-type research. You will learn diverse and varied ways to put into action the following four processes:

1. Bounding your study and obtaining individuals, concepts, or other phenomena to study (Chapters 13 through 16)
2. Collecting information or data using a range of strategies (Chapters 17 to 19)
3. Analyzing and interpreting information or data (Chapters 20 to 22)
4. Reporting and using information and conclusions (Chapters 23 and 24)

As you read about each action process, keep in mind that five factors affect the selection of an action process, as follows:

1. Philosophical or epistemological framework of the research
2. Investigator's specific research purpose
3. Nature of the research question or query
4. Particular type of design
5. Resources available and practical limitations or challenges of the environment in which the research occurs

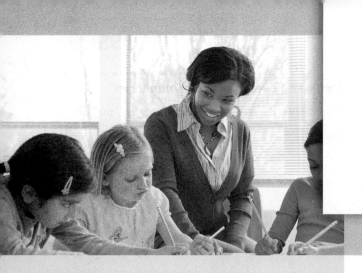

Chapter 13
Setting the Boundaries of a Study

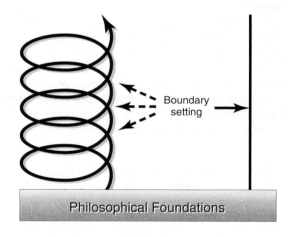

Philosophical Foundations

Mixing Boundary Setting Methods

Assume that you have a research problem and an appropriate design that matches your research purpose and question or query. You are now ready to consider how individuals, concepts, or locations will be selected for your study and how particular phenomena will be defined and identified. Selecting

research participants, whether they are human or not, and identifying concepts and phenomena represent one of the first action processes that set or establish the boundaries or limitations of a study.

Setting boundaries is inextricably linked to important ethical considerations, such as how people or nonhuman units of analysis are selected for study participation, how they are informed of study procedures (in the case of human participants), how the information humans share or that is shared about humans is managed and treated confidentially, and to whom or what the study results are applied. Because of the significance of the ethical component of *boundary setting*, we have examined protection of human subjects in depth in Chapter 3. This chapter provides an introduction to this action essential and concludes with words about mixed methods. The two chapters that follow detail boundary setting in the experimental-type and naturalistic traditions. We do not include a chapter on mixing boundary setting from both traditions, as the methods used will be drawn from what we have already discussed in the tradition-specific chapters. However, at the end of this chapter, we will address mixed methods so that, when using mixed methods designs, you can select and integrate strategies from both traditions in a purposive fashion.

Why Set Boundaries to a Study?

Setting limits or boundaries as to what and who will be in a study is an action that occurs in every type of research design, whether in the experimental-type, naturalistic, or mixed method tradition. A researcher sets boundaries that limit the scope of the investigation to a specified group of individuals, phenomena, geography, or set of conceptual dimensions (Box 13-1). The following example demonstrates why it is important to set boundaries or limitations.

> Consider a study that uses a survey design to describe the health and social service needs of "parents of children with intellectual impairments." It would be impossible to interview every person who falls into this category in the United States. As the researcher, you need to make some decisions about whom you should specifically interview and how. One consideration may be to limit the survey to one or more particular geographic locations. Another way to limit the study may be to consider only certain types of conditions that fall under the rubric of intellectual impairment. Another may be delimiting the study by the age of the children, and so forth. Limiting the number of parents of children with intellectual impairments who are selected for study participation is an example of setting a boundary by restricting the characteristics of the persons who will be studied. •

Studies are also necessarily limited or bounded by identifying particular data collection strategies and concepts that will be considered.

BOX 13-1 *Reasons to Set Boundaries*

1. Delimit the scope of units of study (e.g., subjects, geographies, concepts)
2. Delimit the scope of data collection
3. Determine to whom and/or what the study results apply and how

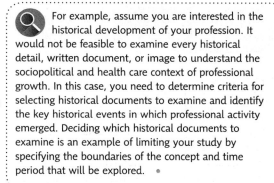

> For example, assume you are interested in the historical development of your profession. It would not be feasible to examine every historical detail, written document, or image to understand the sociopolitical and health care context of professional growth. In this case, you need to determine criteria for selecting historical documents to examine and identify the key historical events in which professional activity emerged. Deciding which historical documents to examine is an example of limiting your study by specifying the boundaries of the concept and time period that will be explored. •

Now consider an example from material culture methods of object reading. As the basis for examining the history of mobility device design to understand current design trends, we recently were funded to study the meaning and aesthetics of mobility aids in the Gilded Age in the United States. Given the largess of potential data sources, we have delimited the study by identifying specific museum collections that showcase historical adaptive devices, such as the Library of Medicine.

There are numerous ways to limit the scope of a study. As discussed in previous chapters on the thinking processes of research, an investigator actively bounds a study on the basis of five interrelated considerations (Box 13-2).

Your philosophical approach or the particular research tradition you are using to develop your study will set the backdrop from which all action decisions will be made. A deductive, experimental-type study tightly bounds the study to pre-identified concepts and a highly specified population. The purpose of the study, the particular research question, and the design will also shape the extent to which concepts, phenomena, and populations are delimited.

> ### BOX 13-2 *Considerations in Setting Study Boundaries*
>
> 1. Researcher's philosophical framework
> 2. Study purpose
> 3. Research question/query
> 4. Research design
> 5. Access to the object(s) of inquiry (participants, locations), investigator's time frame, and monetary limitations

For example, an intervention study that tests the effectiveness of a particular home care service in producing a specified outcome must carefully match the intent of the intervention with specific characteristics of the subject group or individuals who will be targeted and recruited for the study. Thus, identifying highly specified criteria as to who is eligible and who is not eligible to participate is a required action process. These criteria are referred to as *"inclusion and exclusion criteria,"* as discussed later in subsequent chapters.

On the other hand, a broad inquiry designed to investigate the experiences of persons with acquired immunodeficiency syndrome (AIDS) may set few restrictions, except diagnostic condition, as to who can participate in the study and thus cast a wide net for participant enrollment. An investigator might even delimit a study by virtual location such as a listserv or virtual chat room for persons with AIDS. Or consider the historical mobility device study, which was delimited by both time period and location of objects to be included.

Finally, your ability to access the population of interest or the phenomenon to be studied is another consideration in how a study is bounded. Limits on resources such as money and time will likely yield a study design that is tightly delimited or bounded.

Thus, there are both practical and theoretical considerations in how researchers bound the context of an experimental-type, naturalistic, or mixed method form of inquiry. In practical terms, it would be impossible to observe every speech event, personal interaction, image, or activity in a particular natural setting. Studies are therefore bounded by making purposeful selections as to what will be observed,

where and when it will be observed, and who will be interviewed.[1,2]

In experimental-type designs, boundary setting is a process that occurs before initiating or beginning the study. Boundaries are set in three ways: (1) specifying the concepts that will be operationally defined, (2) establishing inclusion and exclusion criteria that define the population that will be studied, and (3) developing a sampling plan.

Boundary-setting action processes in naturalistic designs differ from those in the experimental-type tradition. Naturalistic boundary setting may occur throughout the research endeavor, depending on how the dynamic design unfolds. Initial boundaries are set by the investigator through defining the particular domain of interest and the point of access from which to enter that domain.

 This domain may be (1) place-based, as in the selection of an urban community in which to study health behaviors of low-income families or an on-line community for veterans with posttraumatic stress disorder; (2) a group of individuals, such as the selection of persons with a particular health condition (e.g., stroke, diabetes, traumatic brain injury), living in an identified community; (3) a particular experience, such as trauma, dialysis, caregiving, pain, or chronic health problems; (4) a set of images or objects that may be analyzed for material and visual cultural meaning; and (5) concepts such as stigma, health healing that are explicated in narrative, image, and object. •

Next, within the context of the defined domain, a selection process then occurs as to who should be interviewed and when; what scenes, images, or events to observe; and which materials, texts, or artifacts to review. This selection process occurs or unfolds in the course of conducting the study and comprises important boundary-making decisions. Setting boundaries in most forms of naturalistic inquiry can therefore be an ongoing process that moves the researcher from a broad stance to a more narrow focus and perhaps then broadens once again. The actions of data collection, analysis, and further data collection (see Chapters 18 and 19) can be understood as a process of redefining and refining the boundaries of the phenomenon being studied.

In mixed methods, boundary setting can use a unitary boundary-setting strategy from either naturalistic or experimental-type design, or the boundary-setting essential itself can integrate methods from both traditions. Consider this example of integrated boundary setting. In a study of the meaning of independence to youth with chronic health conditions as they transition to adulthood, specific populations were identified and sampled: youth between the ages of 17 and 21 with chronic health conditions; parents or guardians of these youth; teachers; and health care providers. Because population parameters were known for each group, sampling was possible. However, when the sample groups were convened and the initial data collection completed, insufficient findings led to a second data-collection session in which open participation was enacted. Flyers and online announcements were disseminated so that diverse informants with an interest and/or experience in transition and independence were recruited. As you can see, the first boundary-setting approach was linear and followed the rules of experimental-type sampling, whereas the second was flexible.[3]

Implications of Boundary Setting

Bounding a study is a purposeful action process in all research traditions. That is, boundary setting involves making conscious decisions based on a sound rationale that can be documented or articulated to the larger scientific, professional, and scholarly communities. The inclusion or exclusion of people, concepts, events, objects, or other phenomena has considerable implications for knowledge development and its translation or use in professional practice. As you make decisions about how to bound your study and then actively set limits, you reflect on your actions and understand the implications of each boundary-making decision.

One of the most important consequences of researchers' bounding actions is what can ultimately be concluded (or not) about the phenomenon of interest and then applied to whom or what. Within the experimental-type tradition, the ability to generalize from a study sample to the population from which the sample was derived is referred to as *external validity*.

Suppose you are interested in studying the adaptive mechanisms used by geographically diverse groups of adults to manage chronic illness. You need to bound your study to one geographic community—in this case, an urban community in the northeastern United States. Your findings and interpretations will necessarily be limited to this particular group and may not be valid for the full range of diversity of groups living in rural and southern communities, where the cultural context and access to health care may differ significantly from that of the study participants. •

Assume an investigator is interested in symptom reporting among older men and women. The exclusion of a particular group of individuals, such as Asian or Hispanic elder persons, or other ethnic groups from study participation may limit the researcher's ability to relate or generalize findings from the study to these other groups. This limitation may therefore be a consequence of the way in which the researcher sets the boundaries of the study population at the start of the project. •

The same principles hold for defining and operationalizing major constructs.

If a study focuses on mental health outcomes narrowly operationalized as "depressive symptoms," the results are specific to this single dimension and how it is measured in the study. The study results cannot be generalized to other aspects of mental health. •

The consequences of boundary setting are often described in an experimental-type proposal or a research report as "limitations" of the study. As you read research articles in professional journals, take a close look at how authors describe their recruitment process, the inclusion and exclusion criteria, and other methods that they follow to enroll and engage *subjects,* participants, or other elements (e.g., research reports for meta-analysis, secondary data) into the study and how they define and operationalize primary concepts. Also, carefully read how researchers describe the limitations of their study. Finally, look closely at the discussion section of a published article, where the researcher should be precise and transparent in interpreting the findings as they relate to specific populations and concepts. Sometimes you will find that researchers overstate their case or stretch their results to include a broader population or set of constructs than was actually studied or warranted. Critically evaluate reports to ascertain if the researcher exceeded the boundaries by asserting or implying in the conclusion that the findings are applicable beyond the studied population or delimited phenomena.

The ways in which studies are bounded have particular significance for translating research findings into the professional arena, particularly for evidence-based practice models, as we describe in Chapter 24. For example, in the clinic setting, it is important to know whether a particular technique, intervention modality, or teaching approach is effective in producing a desired outcome for a specific client. If you search the literature to identify the evidence for using a specific practice approach, you may find that the published studies involve study participants who may or may not match your clients. You should carefully decide how best to interpret and translate such findings for your particular group. The first step in this translational effort is to recognize the ways in which the studies you have identified as relevant to your own work are bounded. The second step is to evaluate whether specific characteristics of your group would determine the extent to which the results of the studies are applicable to the group members.

Another implication of bounding studies relates to building programs of research or what is referred to as "research agendas." Remember that research involves the incremental construction of knowledge. Each study answers a specified question or query and in turn generates the next steps toward understanding a particular phenomenon. The way in which a study is bounded will have implications for building knowledge and for identifying the direction for subsequent research steps.

Conclusion

Consider this example. Substantial evidence suggests that case management helps decrease depression in caregivers of persons with dementia. These studies are bounded in the scope of the intervention and the target population. Considering the boundaries of the current literature, future research to build on existing knowledge may include expanding or adding other components to a case management intervention or evaluating the same intervention with another group of caregivers, such as persons caring for individuals who have had stroke. Changing the boundaries therefore expands the reach and incrementally enlarges the initial studies over time such that the body of knowledge becomes useful in a broader arena than that informed by the initial studies. •

Implications of boundary setting in naturalistic studies is just as profound as in the experimental-type tradition. Because of its inductive or abductive nature, the well-known adage "Where one stands is dependent on where one was sitting" applies to boundary setting in this tradition. That is to say, where one enters a study puts in motion the process through which a study then unfolds. For example, suppose you are interested in understanding the experiences of students with mobility impairments on college campuses. If you begin your study in a cold climate, the experiences differ greatly from those in a warm climate, and each study would therefore yield different knowledge.

If you bound your study by the construct "post-traumatic stress disorder in adults who were spanked as children," you have already delimited your study conceptually as well as through the informants you seek.

The implications of boundary setting in mixed method studies are dependent on how the investigator designs a study. Limitations inherent in both experimental-type and naturalistic traditions may be replicated in mixed method studies, or the researcher proceeding from this tradition may seek to address the limitations of each single tradition through purposive design. Suppose, for example, that the findings from the study of mobility impairment in cold-climate campuses were then used to develop a survey to be administered broadly to a range of geographic areas. The narrow parameters of the initial study would therefore be tested, perhaps affirming no difference among climate zones or yielding new knowledge that then would require more expansive theory building regarding mobility access on campuses.

Specifying the Scope of Participation

One of the most important ways a researcher sets limits in a study is determining who or what will make up the scope of a study. In experimental-type design, this process is referred to as developing inclusion and exclusion criteria. The inclusion and exclusion criteria define the population (or group) to whom the study results are directly applicable, reflect the underlying purpose of the research endeavor, and reflect the research question. Although the specific criteria are not contained in the research question, the population is specified and thus, as discussed, forms the basis for determining external validity.

Within the naturalistic tradition, boundaries are fluid and purposive, and who or what is included at the beginning may vary as the study proceeds.

Assume you are planning a study that reflects a Level 2 question (see Chapter 8). You intend to investigate the level of functional ability in a population of adults with chronic health conditions and then to study the relationship of their functional ability to their earned income over two points in time: 1 month and 12 months after hospitalization for acute illness. First, the purpose of the study limits the inquiry to examining two concepts, "physical function" and "earned income." Second, the purpose also limits the study to investigating these concepts in one particular population—specifically, "adults who have experienced an acute health episode." You choose to specify age range between 21 and 70, all genders, a full range of levels of physical function, cognitive status within normal limits, and chronic conditions that impair mobility and manipulation as inclusion criteria for the participants you seek to involve. Your criteria for excluding people involve certain health conditions such as multiple sclerosis, which has periods of remission, and geographic locations that do not provide the option of public transportation. Both types of criteria, those that include and those that exclude, establish the boundaries for sampling and recruiting individuals into your study. (Chapter 14 describes

sampling plans in greater detail.) For the purposes of this example, however, you use a "sample of convenience." Doing so involves identifying and recruiting any individual who fits your criteria and who has been discharged from one of three area hospitals.

Your next effort is to determine a way to identify appropriate study subjects and a mechanism to involve them in your study. You want to ensure that your sampling and recruitment procedures are systematically followed so that bias is not introduced into your study; that is, you want to ensure that every person who is truly eligible for your study has an opportunity to be identified and is asked to participate. One recruitment strategy may involve asking discharge coordinators and case managers at each participating hospital to use your study criteria to identify and screen individuals as they leave the hospital. You might develop a simple form that can be easily completed by the discharge coordinator. For each person identified by the coordinator, you seek permission to contact the individual and ask his or her willingness to participate in your study.

This set of steps may sound simple. However, suppose the coordinator is busy one week and is unable to screen patients who are being discharged; or assume the coordinator does not refer some patients who fit the study criteria because they are perceived as uncooperative by staff. Both cases may occur in experimental-type studies and introduce bias into the recruitment process. Selecting individuals for experimental-type study requires constant monitoring of the implementation of these recruitment procedures by the investigator. •

In experimental-type designs, there is a high level of specificity in bounding the study. In contrast, usually only broad inclusion and exclusion guidelines are established before engaging in naturalistic designs, if at all. However, the structure of boundaries and the extent to which they are established depend on the particular type of naturalistic design. For example, in a phenomenological study, the researcher may bound a study only by identifying the type of experience that is of interest to the researcher. The only criterion for participating in the study may be that an individual has experienced the phenomenon of interest. Other factors, such as age, gender, or ethnicity, may not be specified or used as criteria to include or exclude individuals from the study because they may not even be known. Likewise, in a large-scale ethnography, only the context or natural setting may be initially specified or bounded, whereas the participation of individuals in the natural context may not be restricted, at least initially. In a focused life history, however, individuals who meet specific criteria are selected purposively for study participation, and these criteria are articulated before data collection begins.

Mixed method studies may apply scope bounding techniques from one or both traditions depending on the purpose of the study and the questions/queries to be answered and addressed.

Involving humans in health and social service research and establishing participation criteria have important ethical considerations that must be fully understood and carefully thought out by the researcher. When developing a research study and writing a proposal to carry it out (see Chapter 23), whether of the experimental, naturalistic, or mixed method type, the researcher must address numerous ethical concerns of involving humans, as examined in Chapter 4.

General Guidelines for Bounding Studies

The extent to which a study is bounded depends on your preferred way of knowing, research purpose, question, and/ or query, and practical considerations such as monetary resources, context, and time constraints. It is important to recognize that there is nothing inherently superior about any one boundary-setting approach. The strengths and limitations of a boundary-setting technique depend on its *appropriateness* and *adequacy* in how well it fits the context of the particular research problem and aim of the study.

Appropriateness is defined as the extent to which the method of boundary setting fits the overall purpose of the study, as determined by the research problem, purpose, and the structure of the research design. For example, it would be inappropriate to use a random sampling technique when your purpose is to understand how individuals interpret their experience of illness. In this case, the purposeful selection of informants who can articulate their feelings may

provide greater insight than the inclusion of a sample with predetermined characteristics. Purposive selection to bound the study facilitates understanding, which is the underlying goal of the study.

Adequacy is defined as the extent to which the boundary setting yields sufficient data to answer the research problem. In experimental-type designs, adequacy is determined by sample size and composition. In naturalistic designs, adequacy is determined by the quality and completeness of the information and the understanding that is obtained in the selected domain. "Saturation," reaching a point in the inquiry in which no new information is obtained, is one important cue that the boundary has been fully met and the investigator has achieved a complete understanding of the identified context.

Subjects, Respondents, Informants, Participants, Locations, Conceptual Boundaries, Virtual Boundaries

Are individuals who are involved in a study the *subjects, respondents, informants,* or *participants*?[4] Are you focusing on *locations*, concepts expressed in text or image, or the virtual world?[5] Subjects, respondents, informants, and participants refer to humans or the individuals who agree to become part of a research study. Each term reflects a different way that an individual participates in a research study and a different type of relationship that is formed between the individual and the investigator. Locations, *conceptual boundaries*, and *virtual boundaries* are viable boundaries as well, used to delimit studies in experimental-type, naturalistic, and mixed method approaches.

First, we discuss the distinction among the four terms that describe humans' roles in research. In experimental-type research, individuals are usually referred to as subjects, a term that denotes their passive role and the attempt of the investigator to maintain a removed and objective relationship. In survey research, individuals are often referred to as respondents because they are asked to respond to very specific questions. In naturalistic inquiry, individuals are usually referred to as informants, a term that reflects the active role of informing the investigator as to the context and its cultural rules. Participants can refer to those individuals who enter a collaborative relationship with the investigator, who contribute to decision making about the research process, and who inform the investigator about themselves.[4] This term is often used in endogenous and participatory action research.

Locations, conceptual boundaries, and virtual boundaries all are terms that are used to denote non-human delimiters of a study. Similar to descriptors of humans in a study, these terms overlap as well. For example, suppose you are interested in looking at stigmatizing spatial designs. You would use built environment spaces and the imagery and objects contained within them as place-based and conceptual boundaries, respectively, to how visual design and place might impart and communicate stigma.

Although there are no specific rules to guide the use of these terms, you should select the one that reflects your preferred way of knowing and the role that individuals play in your study design.

Some Words About Setting Boundaries in Mixed Methods

As we introduced earlier, the next two chapters detail boundary setting in the experimental-type and naturalistic traditions. Integrating strategies from both chapters creates the tools for setting boundaries in mixed method designs. There are many combinations and permutations of strategies that can be used to set boundaries in mixed methods. However, the boundary-setting criterion for mixed methods is singular. That is to say, purpose is always held as the guide for choosing boundary-setting techniques. Therefore, when you read the next two chapters, think of how and why you might use the strategies presented in both to enter and set boundaries in a mixed method project. We will return to illustrate mixed methods in Chapter 16.

Summary

Boundary setting refers to the action process of determining and enacting selection criteria for study participants, study concepts, or study phenomena. Setting boundaries is one of the first action processes that occurs in experimental-type research. In naturalistic inquiry, boundary setting occurs throughout the data collection and analytical action phases and is an ongoing process. Boundary setting in mixed methods is variable depending on the purpose of the study

design. Boundary setting may occur at the beginning and/or throughout the full study.

One crucial way in which experimental-type studies are bounded is developing inclusion and exclusion criteria for the involvement of human participants. Each tradition handles human involvement differently, with inductive designs initiating boundary setting with individuals by selecting a point of entry and then letting the limitations unfold and mixed methods delimiting a study by its purpose.

Given the ethical considerations of working with human subjects in an inquiry, protection from risk is a critical consideration (see Chapter 3). Ethical decision making is also critical in how the knowledge from the study will be interpreted and used in professional practice.

EXERCISES

1. Identify a research article that tests an experimental intervention. Describe how the authors bound their study with regard to the inclusion and exclusion criteria and recruitment procedures. Identify specific limitations to generalizability of their study given how it was bounded.
2. Identify a research article that reports findings from an ethnographical study. Describe how the authors bound their study. Identify specific boundary scope, strengths, and limitations.
3. Identify a research article that reports findings from a mixed method study. Describe how the authors bound their study. Identify specific boundary scope, strengths, and limitations.

References

1. Agar MH: *An ethnography by any other name*, 2006. http://www.qualitative-research.net/index.php/fqs/article/view/177/395.
2. Rubin HJ, Rubin IS: *Qualitative interviewing: the art of hearing*, Thousand Oaks, Calif, 2012, Sage.
3. DePoy E, Gilmer D: Adolescents with disabilities and chronic illness in transition: a community action needs assessment. *Disabil Stud Q* (Spring), 2000.
4. Hall A: *What's in a name,* 2014. Prim&r's Ampersand, http://primr.blogspot.com/2014/01/whats-in-name-research-participant.html.
5. Bennett J: *Vibrant matter*, Durham, NC, 2010, Duke University Press.

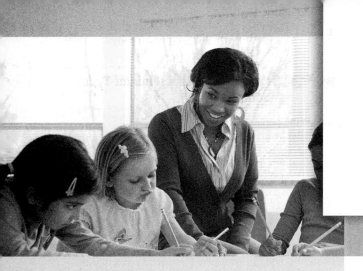

Chapter 14
Boundary Setting in Experimental-Type Designs

KEY TERMS

Cluster sampling
Convenience sampling
Effect size
External validity
Nonprobability sampling
Population
Probability sampling
Purposive sampling
Quota sampling
Sample

Sampling
Sampling error
Sampling frame
Simple random sampling
Snowball sampling
Statistical power
Stratified random sampling
Systematic sampling
Target population

CHAPTER OUTLINE

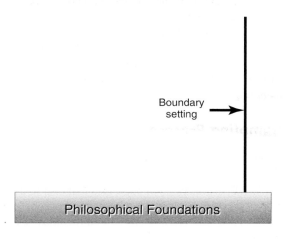

Boundary setting

Philosophical Foundations

As discussed in Chapter 1, setting boundaries is one of the first action processes that occurs in experimental-type designs. Think about what you have learned thus far about experimental-type designs. What do you think are the characteristics of the process of setting boundaries in this research tradition? If you said the process is primarily deductive, prescribed, and determined before entering the field, you are correct.

The aim of experimental-type boundary setting is to select a group of study participants, subjects, or objects who adequately represent the target population of the study. This purpose is a critical point on which all boundary-setting procedures are based in this tradition. Now we examine how researchers who use the range of experimental-type designs enact the action process of selecting people, groups, or other entities for study participation.

As previously introduced, in experimental-type design, the boundary-setting action process is basically deductive. Using this logic structure, the researcher begins with a clear idea of what or whom he or she wants to study. The study group of interest to the investigator is called a *population*, defined as a group of persons, elements, or both that share a set of common characteristics as specified by the investigator. The researcher clearly delimits the characteristics of the population, including individuals or units to be studied and those to be excluded. Then, a set of procedures is specified by which to select a subset or sample of the population who will participate in the study. Unless the entire population is studied, the individuals or units from the population who are directly involved in the study are called a *sample*, which is a subset of the population. The process of selecting a subgroup or sample is called *sampling*.

Sampling Process

The main purpose of sampling is to select a subgroup that can accurately represent the population as defined and delimited by the investigator. The intent of sampling is to be able to draw accurate conclusions about the population by studying a smaller group of elements (sample). The problem for the experimental-type researcher is how best to select a sample that is most accurate in representing an entire population. Precise representation is critical if an aim of a study is to apply or generalize findings from the study sample to the larger group (population) from which the sample is drawn.[1,2]

For the most part, sampling designs or procedures in the experimental-type tradition are structured to increase the chances of selecting individuals or elements most representative of the larger population from which they are drawn. The more representative the sample, the more assured the researcher will be that the findings from the sample apply, within a degree of certainty, to the population. The extent to which findings from a sample apply to the population is called *external validity*, as discussed in Chapter 13. When the intent of a study is to generalize from

---

> **BOX 14-1** *Five Steps in Experimental-Type Sampling*
>
> 1. Define population by specifying criteria
>   a. Inclusion criteria
>   b. Exclusion criteria
> 2. Develop sampling plan
>   a. Probability
>   b. Nonprobability
> 3. Determine sample size
> 4. Implement sampling procedures
> 5. Compare critical values of sample to population

a sample to a population, most researchers conducting experimental-type designs attempt to maximize external validity by using one of the sampling procedures discussed in this chapter.

Investigators follow many action processes to draw a sample from a population. In this chapter, we discuss five basic steps common to the various experimental-type sampling processes (Box 14-1). The first step in sampling involves the careful specification of a population. As presented earlier, in the experimental-type tradition, a population is defined as the complete set of elements that share common characteristics and do not possess any attributes identified by the researcher as "not to be included." Examples of elements are persons, households, communities, hospitals, outpatient settings, websites, and, in meta-analysis, research studies on a common topic. The "element" is the unit of analysis included in the population, regardless of its type. For example, in meta-analysis, an investigator would specify the essential elements for each study that would be included, as well as characteristics of studies that would be excluded.

> In a study of the management practices of hospitals, the investigator is interested in the hospital as a whole, rather than the people in it. In this case, the hospital is the unit of analysis, and the sample is the specified number of hospitals participating in the study. However, in a study of the characteristics of older persons admitted to hospitals in the summer months, each patient, not the hospital as a whole, is the unit of analysis, and the sample is composed of the set of individuals selected for the study. •

New investigators often ask how populations are identified and delimited. In experimental-type design, two issues are important to consider: (1) the purpose of the study and (2) the literature support for selecting or excluding population parameters. Thus, it is the investigator who uses previous work and a purposive lens to define or choose the characteristics or parameters of the population that are important to study. Consider the following two examples.

> You are interested in studying the needs of parents of children with chronic illness. The first step in selecting your study sample would be to identify the specific characteristics of the population you are interested in examining. To identify population characteristics, you identify the purpose of your inquiry and then consult the literature to see how other investigators have conceptualized the important population characteristics that need to be included and excluded. •

> Now consider this example. You are conducting a needs assessment study as the basis for implementing a hospital-based transition intervention to assist parents of children with cystic fibrosis in their parenting. Because of the hospital policy regarding the age range of children in their cystic fibrosis unit, you decide to include parents of children between ages 3 and 8 years who have been diagnosed within the past 6 months. On the basis of the literature, you may also decide to exclude cases in which both parents do not reside together, both are unemployed, or more than one other sibling is in the home. By establishing these inclusion and exclusion criteria, you will have defined a target population from the universe of parents with a child who has been recently diagnosed with chronic illness. •

By some definitions, the target population is an "ideal" only because the investigator cannot access such a population.[3] However, in this chapter we define the *target population* as a useful entity, referring to the group of individuals or elements from which the investigator is able to select a sample. Each element of the target population may possess characteristics other than those specified by the

> ## BOX 14-2 *Three Criteria for Elements of a Target Population*
>
> - Must possess all the characteristics that the investigator has identified as "inclusion criteria"
> - Must not possess any of the characteristics that the investigator has defined as "exclusion criteria"
> - Must be available, at least in theory, for selection into the sample

investigator. However, each element must fit three criteria (Box 14-2).

How do investigators using experimental-type designs identify a population? First, the research question guides the investigator. Remember in Chapter 10, we stated that all properly articulated experimental-type questions include the population in which the variables and their relationships are being studied. Thus, the research question contains the basic lexical identification of the population. Second, the researcher uses the literature to clarify and provide support for establishing population parameters.

> If an investigator is interested in studying persons with chronic mental illness, a vast body of literature provides clear descriptions and definitions of this broad category of individuals. An astute investigator may choose a well-accepted source, such as the *Diagnostic and Statistical Manual of Mental Disorders* (DSM-V),[4] for a definition of chronic mental illness to structure parameters based on this knowledge. •

The literature also helps to identify those characteristics that the investigator may want to exclude from the targeted population.

> To isolate and not confound the major population parameter of interest, "chronic mental illness," individuals may be excluded from the target population if they possess a primary physical diagnosis along with a psychiatric diagnosis, or if the mental illness is a secondary consequence of a traumatic head injury. •

BOX 14-3 *Guiding Questions in Identifying a Population in a Study of Individuals with Quadriplegia*

- Should I include both men and women in the study?
- Should all persons with quadriplegia be included, regardless of functional level?
- In what type of setting should the persons included in the study reside (e.g., community, independent living center, institutional setting)?
- In which geographic location should they live? What ages, ethnic groups, and occupational groups should be included?
- Should persons with additional diagnoses be excluded?

Consider another example. You are interested in understanding the daily routines of persons with quadriplegia. What would be the steps you would follow to obtain a sample of this population? First, you would define the specific population characteristics (parameters) of the group you want to study. Some guiding questions you would ask are listed in Box 14-3. •

Reading how other researchers bound their studies is helpful in answering these questions. Your responses will lead to the development of specific criteria by which to include and exclude individuals. In addition, as indicated earlier, to answer these questions, consider your purpose in conducting the study. Finally, refer to the practice and research literature for definitions of terms such as "quadriplegia" and "functional level."

Defining a population is a critical step in sampling and is done carefully and thoughtfully. How an investigator identifies a population shapes the nature and findings of a study.

Suppose you are interested in examining the health literacy of veterans who were wounded in Afghanistan. In your study, you define your population broadly as all soldiers who have returned home from Afghanistan within the past 2 years and are admitted to Veterans Administration hospitals for treatment of physical injuries sustained in battle. You are surprised when you find an extremely low literacy level. In a similar study, your colleagues study the same population of wounded veterans but exclude those who have visual impairments and who speak English as a second language. The level of health literacy revealed in this study is very high, and thus the findings appear to contradict those from your study. •

As illustrated, including or excluding different population characteristics can change the outcomes of a study. In the example just given, including English-language competency and excluding potential confounding parameters, such as the inability to see print material, had a major impact on study findings. You should clearly articulate the criteria used for bounding your study. Also, when comparing findings from studies on a similar topic and target population, whether used in literature review or formal meta-analysis, you should carefully evaluate the differences in boundary setting among studies.

The second major step in boundary setting in experimental-type design involves drawing a sample from your specified population through the use of a sampling plan. There are two basic categories of sampling plans, probability sampling and nonprobability sampling. Table 14-1 provides an overview of the commonly used sampling plans discussed in this chapter.

Probability Sampling

Probability sampling refers to those plans that are based on probability theory. This type of sampling is used when the investigator wants to maximize external validity (the degree to which the sample represents the population from which it was selected). The two basic principles of probability theory as applied to sampling are as follows: (1) the parameters of the population are known and (2) every member or element has an equal probability or chance of being selected for the sample.[3] A third rationale, related to probability reasoning, but not specific to guiding action processes in this essential, is the theoretical assumption that equal probability of being selected

TABLE 14-1 Summary of Common Sampling Plans Used in Experimental-Type Research

Probability Sampling	Nonprobability Sampling
Parameters of a population are known	Parameters of a population are not known
Sampling frame is used	No sampling frame is available
Every member/element has the same probability of being selected for sample	Probability of selection is not known
Methods	
Simple Random Sampling	**Convenience Sampling**
Table of random numbers is used to randomly select sample	Available individuals enter the study
Systematic Sampling	**Purposive Sampling**
Sampling interval width is determined and individuals are selected	Individuals are deliberately selected for study
Stratified Random Sampling	**Snowball (Network) Sampling**
Subjects are randomly selected from predetermined strata that correlate with variables in study	Informants provide names of others who meet study criteria
Cluster Sampling	**Quota Sampling**
Successive random sampling of units is used to obtain sample	Individuals who are unlikely to be represented are included

To determine sampling error, we can derive a calculation called the "standard error of the mean," which reflects the standard deviation of the sampling distribution and is designated SE_m (see Chapter 20). Many statistical analytical tools used in experimental-type research are based on an assumption of probability: the assumption that a variable will be distributed in a population along a normal or bell-shaped curve. The bell-shaped curve is a graphic depiction of what is expected to occur in a typical group. In other words, it is most probable that the majority of observations will be similar and will cluster around the average. More extreme observations, or those that are further from the mean, are expected to be less frequent. The distance of a single score from the mean score is called "deviation."

 Assume you want to draw a sample of 50 older adults from a larger population of older persons with a diagnosis of cancer and evaluate their quality of life using a "life satisfaction" measure. Then you want to draw another sample of 50 older adults, then a third sample, and so forth. If you compute the mean score on life satisfaction for each sample, you will derive what is called a "sampling distribution of means." •

is accompanied by equal probability of being exposed to all influences that could otherwise provide potential confounding factors in your study.

The important point to remember about probability as it applies to sampling is that the probability of each element included in the study is known and greater than zero. By knowing the population parameters and the degree of chance that each element may be selected, an investigator can calculate the sampling error. *Sampling error* refers to the difference between the values obtained from the sample and the values that actually exist in the population. This error reflects the degree to which the sample is actually representative of the population. The larger the sampling error, the less representative the sample is of the population and the more limited is the external validity of the study. The purpose of probability sampling is to reduce sampling error and to increase external validity of a study.

Theoretically, the distribution of these means should be in a normal shape (bell-shaped curve). However, the means will most likely vary among the samples, simply as a result of chance error. You then calculate the standard deviation of each mean. In actuality, however, you will not draw several samples from the population to derive the standard error of the mean; a formula can be used with one sample to estimate SE_m. Also, the larger the sample, the smaller the SE_m. Likewise, the less the variability in a population, the smaller the SE_m.

Sampling error may be caused by either random error or systematic bias. "Random error" refers to those errors that occur by chance. Not much can be done about random error at the sampling stage of the research process except to calculate the standard error of the mean. "Systematic error" or "systematic bias," within the philosophical framework of experimental-type design, reflects a basic flaw in the sampling process and is characterized by scores of subjects that systematically differ from the population. Sampling plans based on probability theory are desirable because they are designed to minimize systematic error and thus are the standard when asserting external validity.

To use probability sampling, the investigator must be able to develop a sampling frame from which individuals or elements are then selected. A *sampling frame* is a listing of every element in the target population. Examples of sampling frames include name listings in online contact directories, a complete list of hospitals in a specific region, listing of studies to be included in a meta-analysis, or a complete roster of identified virtual phenomena. A sampling frame can range from simple to complex. A simple approach might involve defining the sampling frame as those population members the investigator can easily access. A more complex approach might be the development of a sampling frame to ensure that the investigator can access the total population. This approach can involve substantial time and money.

> Suppose you want to study the needs for adaptive sports equipment in a rural community. There are several ways to proceed with sample selection. The most expansive approach would be to obtain a list of all people who live in the community and then randomly select the appropriate number of people. This approach would allow you to generalize your findings to the total population in the community. However, suppose you decided to use the online contact directory as your sampling frame. Your sample will represent only the universe of those who are listed. •

Now let us turn to the four basic sampling procedures that can be used to select individuals or elements from a sampling frame (Box 14-4).

Simple Random Sampling

Simple random sampling (SRS) is the most basic method used to enhance the "representativeness" of a sample. In this case, the term "random" does not mean "haphazard." Rather, in concert with probability theory, random means that theoretically, every element in the population has an equal chance of

---

BOX 14-4 *Probability Sampling Methods*

- Simple random sampling
- Systematic sampling
- Stratified random sampling
- Cluster sampling

BOX 14-5 *Subset From a Table of Random Numbers*

345	687	798	143	203	107	654	176
241	267	925	007	115	003	409	115
076	861	623	351	090	065	190	325

---

being included in the sample. As we noted earlier, theoretically, if elements are chosen by chance, they also have an equal chance to be exposed to all conditions to which all other members in the population are exposed. This random nature of selection therefore precludes the possibility of the sample being selected because of a special trait that is uncommon in the target population, or because of exposure to an influence that does not theoretically affect the total population.

> Returning to sample selection from the rural community, both sampling approaches involve random selection, one from the roster of residents and one from the online contact directory, ensuring that each individual who meets the criteria for inclusion has an equal chance of being selected for the study. •

Most researchers who want to attain a large sample size use a table of random numbers to determine which elements should be included in the sample (Box 14-5). The table, only a small portion of which is displayed in Box 14-5, is carefully constructed through computer-generated programs such as Research Randomizer[5] to ensure a random listing of digits that appear with the same frequency. So how does an investigator use this table to select a sample?

You plan to survey all full-time, nonsupervisory professional providers in a selected rural hospital (target population). You obtain a complete listing of professional providers (the sampling frame) who fit the study criteria. You then assign a unique number to each provider on the list. If there are 150 providers, the list will run from 001 to 150. Because the numbers contain three digits, you select the random numbers in sets of three. Although you would most likely use an automated computer application, in order to understand the process, consider how you would proceed if randomizing manually. You would begin by selecting any starting point and then establishing a plan on how to move through a table of random numbers. Assume that you decide to start from the third column from the left and one row down (925) and proceed to read down each row. Numbers outside the range of the digits assigned to the providers on the list (e.g., numbers greater than 150) are ignored. Therefore, the first two numbers, 925 and 623, are outside the range and do not yield a selection. Moving to the top of the fourth row, numbers 143 and 007 reflect number assignments of providers in the sampling frame. You proceed through the table in this way until the total number of providers needed for the study have been selected. •

As we discussed earlier, there are numerous online programs that not only generate tables of random numbers and automate assignment, but also instruct you in how to use them.

Random sampling can be done with or without replacement. By "replacement," we mean that the selection of a unit will always occur from the total sampling frame. Thus, elements selected for the sample will be put back manually or digitally into the sampling frame before the next selection. Using a table of random numbers typically involves replacement because it is possible to select a number more than once. Random sampling without replacement can be as simple as drawing sample member names from a hat that contains all the names listed on a sampling frame.

Let us consider what may happen with smaller numbers in the sampling frame when random sampling without replacement is used. Suppose we have 10 persons in our sampling frame, and we want to select three persons for our sample. Before any

subject is selected, the chances are 1 in 10 that an individual will be chosen. However, once the first name is chosen and not replaced in the pool, the next individual has a 1 in 9 chance of being selected. As you can see, the rule of equal chance for selection is violated. However, if we replace the name of the subject who was selected for the subsequent two selections, the chance for sample selection remains 1 in 10. Replacement ensures the same probability of chance of selection for each element throughout the selection process.

Systematic Sampling

SRS can often be time-consuming and difficult to complete when drawing a large sample. However, it is indicated when feasible and purposive because *systematic sampling* offers a more efficient method by which to select elements randomly. After the identification and specification of your population parameters and sampling frame, this sampling approach involves determining a sampling interval width based on the needed sample size, then selecting every Kth element from a sampling frame.

Suppose, as a way to improve employment opportunity for people with mobility and sensory impairments, you are interested in developing a program to improve accessibility in small businesses. In surveying a sample of 60 small business owners from a total population of 300, a sampling fraction (the interval width), 60:300, or 1 in 5, is derived. Second, a random number between 1 and 5 is selected to determine the first participant in the sampling frame. Every fifth element from this starting point will be selected for inclusion in the sample (i.e., 8th, 13th, 18th, and so on). A number generated from a table of random numbers can also be used to determine the starting point. If the sampling fraction is not a whole number, the decimal is usually rounded upward to the next largest whole number.[6] •

When this sampling approach is used, it is critical that the sampling frame itself represent a random listing of names or elements. Also, there must be no hidden biases, purposes, or cyclical arrangements of the elements.

Now suppose by chance every 10th business owner on your list has just started his/her enterprise. If you used a sampling interval of five and started with the fifth person, you would select only novices, introducing systematic bias in your sample and increasing the sampling error. •

Stratified Random Sampling

Systematic sampling and SRS treat the target population as a whole. At this point, however, you might be asking how you can ensure that diverse subgroups in your population are represented in the correct proportion in your sample. *Stratified random sampling* is one way that investigators address the issues of diversity. In stratified random sampling, the population is divided into the smaller subgroups, or strata, that the researcher determines to be of importance on the basis of literature support. Once again, in order to avoid spurious or inaccurate conclusions, we emphasize the importance of selecting these considerations about population parameters on the basis of previous support for their relevance in the research literature. Elements are then chosen from each stratum.

Stratified random sampling is a more complex approach than either simple or systematic sampling. Stratified approaches enhance sample representation and decrease sampling error on a number of predetermined characteristics by increasing the homogeneity and by decreasing the variability in each subgroup. The more homogeneous a population, the fewer elements needed to enhance representation, and the lower the error in generalizing from part to whole. This principle makes common sense; imagine how complicated a sampling plan would be for the population of residents in New York City.

The Nielsen polls are an example of complex sampling frames and samples. The researchers clearly specify a multiplicity of characteristics that typify the television-watching population in the United States. Because this population is diverse, it is separated into strata based on characteristics such as geographic location, socioeconomic status, age, and gender. The

proportion of each subgroup or stratum in the total population is then determined. Sample subjects are drawn from each stratum in the same proportions represented in the population. For example, if the gender distribution in the population is 59% female and 41% male, then 59% of the subjects will be obtained from the female stratum and 41% from the male stratum. Proportionate stratified sampling is frequently used when it is known that a given characteristic appears disproportionately or unevenly in the population. •

If we only used SRS or systematic sampling for a diverse population, we might miss the influence on our study question of important characteristics as they exist in the population.

Consider how a researcher in health and human services may use this technique. Suppose in your population of persons with quadriplegia, only 20% are women. As just noted, the researcher will split the sampling frame into two strata representing male and female genders. As a result, 20% of the sample from the female group and 80% from the male group will be selected. This selection process will ensure that gender (defined as male and female in this study) is proportionately represented in the chosen sample. Without stratification, it is likely that the gender balance of the sample would not match the population. Characteristics are chosen for stratification on the basis of the assumptions supported by literature that they will have some effect on the variables under study. In persons with quadriplegia, investigators have posited that gender may be associated with the nature of daily routines. Thus, it would be important to ensure that a comparison between men and women could be made with regard to daily activity. •

Suppose in your study of veterans returning from Afghanistan, you wanted to test the outcome of an Internet support group on veterans' health and emotional well-being. If you did not stratify along literacy levels, you might miss the effect of reading capacity on participation, comprehension, and outcome of your text-based intervention. •

We keep emphasizing the importance of selecting strata on the basis of literature support. Consider how many extraneous variables could be used to stratify a sample—shoe size, eye color, and so forth. Without literature support, stratification can be perfunctory at best and prejudicial, essentialist, or harmful at worst.

As an example, suppose hair color and gender were used to stratify small business owners without support from the literature. A spurious finding in which blonde women held the most negative attitudes toward hiring disabled workers would only serve to perpetuate stereotypes.

Cluster Sampling

Also referred to as "multistage sampling" or "area sampling," *cluster sampling* is another subject selection plan that involves a successive series of random sampling of units. With cluster sampling, the investigator begins with large units, or clusters, in which smaller sampling units are contained. This technique allows the investigator to draw a random sample without a complete listing of each individual or unit.[3]

In testing a rehabilitation intervention for persons with cerebrovascular accident at inpatient rehabilitation settings, the researcher will first list the geographic regions of the United States. Using simple random selection procedures, regions will be selected from this list. Then, in each randomly selected region, the investigator will obtain a complete listing of the freestanding rehabilitation facilities and make a second random selection among these units, yielding a random sampling of hospitals within a random sample of regions. To obtain the individuals who will participate, the investigator will randomly select participants from a list of individual clients. •

Can you see how this approach is efficient in creating a random sample with a broad scope of external validity? Because each step of the sampling process was random, the sample of individuals at one hospital center theoretically represents the national population of inpatients who sustained a cerebrovascular accident.

Nonprobability Methods

In experimental-type design, probability sampling plans are preferred to other methods of obtaining a sample, when the research goal is to generalize from sample to population or, in other words, to increase the external validity of the study. Probability sampling plans provide a degree of assurance that the members selected for the sample will, within a reasonable degree of confidence, represent those who are not selected. These probability methods are often used in health and human service research for needs assessments, survey designs, and large-scale funded research projects. Moreover, these methods are held as important standards for evidence-based practice, given that this body of knowledge is meant to predict best outcomes from interventions in broad populations.

However, random methods are often impractical because, in order to use them, the researcher must have considerable knowledge about the characteristics and size of the population, access to a sampling frame, access to a large number of elements, and the ability to omit elements from the study for ethical reasons. Therefore, in health and human service research, various forms of nonprobability sampling techniques are frequently and efficaciously used in experimental-type designs.

In *nonprobability sampling*, nonrandom methods are used to obtain a sample. By "nonrandom," we mean that sample members are not chosen on the basis of equal chance to be selected from a larger sampling frame. Nonrandom or nonprobability methods are used when the parameters of the population are not known or when it is not feasible or ethical to develop a sampling frame. If you are unable to use probability sampling in your research, does that mean that your project is flawed? Not at all; the key to using nonprobability sampling is to attain your purpose, be it achieving the greatest degree of representation possible or investigating a phenomenon in a single group. The caution in using nonrandom sampling is to avoid claims that exceed what you can support with the sampling plan and to identify limitations in your discussion.

Suppose you want to study the attitudes of potential students in health professional programs toward working with persons with severe intellectual impairments. There are many ways to proceed to obtain a sample, but because you have access to students at your own university who have declared a major or have shown interest in a health professional program, you decide to use this group as your sample. This approach to sampling is a nonrandom process. In your study and report, you would clearly depict your sampling process, identify the applications and limits of your work, and indicate that generalization beyond the scope of your sample should not be attempted. Although you might suggest that your findings have applicability to similar populations and contexts, you would clearly state that further research should be done to verify the findings on other populations. However, your work would provide important information for the curriculum of your health professional program as well as contribute to theory to be further tested by others interested in the same phenomenon. •

There are four basic nonprobability sampling methods (Box 14-6).

Convenience Sampling

Also referred to as "accidental sampling," "volunteer sampling," and "opportunistic sampling," *convenience sampling* involves the enrollment of available subjects or elements as they enter the study until the desired sample size is reached. The investigator establishes inclusion and exclusion criteria and selects those individuals who fit these factors and volunteer to participate in the study in the case of human subjects, or that meet the criteria in the case of nonhuman elements. Sampling health professional students is an example of convenience

---

BOX 14-6 *Nonprobability Sampling Methods*

- Convenience sampling
- Purposive sampling
- Snowball sampling
- Quota sampling

---

sampling of human subjects. Other examples are interviewing individuals in a physician's office and enrolling subjects as they enter an outpatient setting to determine their health service needs.

Suppose you are interested in testing the literacy of health information websites. Nonhuman convenience sampling might involve selecting the first 20 websites that are listed in an Internet search using the keywords "health information."

Purposive Sampling

done (intentional or consciously)

Also called "judgmental sampling," *purposive sampling* involves the deliberate selection of individuals or elements by the researcher on the basis of predefined criteria. In your study of persons with quadriplegia, you may decide to choose purposely only those who can clearly audio record and wirelessly transmit their daily experiences to you. In this way, you purposely select individuals to represent insight into the daily routines of a larger group in a manner that is most parsimonious for your work.

Snowball Sampling

trust between participation

Also called "networking," *snowball sampling* involves asking subjects to provide access to others who may meet study criteria. This type of sampling is often used when researchers do not have direct access to a population. In our example of nonhuman sampling of literacy testing for health information websites, using links on existing health information websites would be an example of snowball sampling.

You are interested in studying the health and human service needs of drug-addicted women with young children. It is not likely that you would advertise for this sample and expect that people would readily come forward. Rather, you might ask counselors, members of the community where you know the women live, or agency personnel who work with this population to "nominate" informants, who in turn would be also asked to identify additional informants. In this way, you would be able to recruit a sample with techniques in which the women would not feel unsafe or publicly exposed. •

Quota Sampling

This technique is often used in market research. The goal of quota sampling is to obtain different proportions of subject types who may be underrepresented by using convenience or purposive sampling methods. In *quota sampling*, parameters of a population and their distribution in the population are known. The researcher then purposively selects a sample that is representative of the population, in that elements are selected to display parameters in the same proportions exhibited in the population. This type of sampling is the nonprobability analogue of stratified random sampling in that the investigator identifies the critical population parameters a priori and then attempts to obtain elements proportionally with these characteristics.

> You are interested in testing the effects of an innovative community program on the functional level of persons with schizophrenia living in the community. Because schizophrenia represents different types of syndromes, you first determine the proportions of varying types of schizophrenia in your population. On the basis of literature support, you then find that gender and age are distributed differently in each type. To ensure that your nonrandom sample is as representative of your population as possible, you set up a matrix of diagnoses, ages, and genders and select your sample by filling each cell in the same proportions that are exhibited in your population. •

Sampling Without Human Subjects

Throughout this chapter, we have referred to sampling elements that are not human. Examples involve selection of representative studies for meta-analysis, locations, virtual spaces, objects, images, and so forth.

> Consider this scenario. Suppose you wanted to conduct a self-esteem intervention in which adolescents used avatars to depict how they see themselves. To begin to describe avatar appearance and use, you decide to "lurk" on a website and rate avatars on their appearance using a theoretically supported scale that links self-esteem to avatar creation. In this example, you are not sampling human subjects but are studying anonymous virtual images that the adolescents have created. •

The investigator would follow procedures for defining population parameters, select a sampling strategy, and then identify the elements that would be included in the sample. The techniques for sampling would depend on the choice to use probability or nonprobability sampling, and conclusions would include the strengths and limitations of the approach. Because this study uses a public domain for investigation, consent is not indicated. Similarly, sampling studies for meta-analysis does not require consent if studies are published in professional journals or on the Internet.

We previously introduced an example of studying the meaning of mobility aids in the Gilded Age of America as the basis for informing redesign of stigmatizing assistive devices. In this study, the objects themselves are the elements in the sample.

Studies that involve nonhuman primates are regulated by research ethics but are beyond the scope of this text. There are many resources and texts available to guide you through processes in which living nonhuman subjects and elements are sampled. In all cases, sound sampling thinking and action are indicated, regardless of the nature of your sample. Although the techniques for selection of nonhuman sample errors are based on the same principles as sampling involving humans, the protection of human subjects and informed consent move into the background. Nevertheless, research ethics still require the investigator to consider how the sampling process will affect knowledge development, ethical application, and thus humans, whether directly or indirectly.

Sampling in the Virtual Environment

The Internet and virtual environments bring multiple options to investigators who have the potential to expand boundary-setting options while improving efficiency and decreasing cost. As in any boundary-setting action, the basic thinking and action principles for experimental-type traditions guide the process. However, unlike the physical world, the Internet is both far-reaching and limited. By far-reaching, we refer to the potential to obtain a global sample. Yet the limitations are significant, beginning with access to and competency with computers as critical concerns and then moving into how to manage sample elements so that the investigator obtains an accurate picture of the population.

For example, suppose you decide to conduct an Internet survey of adolescents to determine their attitudes toward substance abuse prevention in their local area. You first would need to consider penetration of the technology. Who has access and who does not? Second, how do you control for more than one person responding to a survey when you are not present? Even with password protection, you cannot see who is responding. Third, how do you account for varying degrees of comfort with and skill in using the computer?

Of particular concern is the identification, in the virtual context, of a sampling frame. In the physical world, sampling frames are often located through contact information such as cell phone numbers or addresses, many of which can be linked to an actual location. However, Internet sampling uses virtual addresses, networks, and content areas (websites) to delimit a population of interest. So identifying respondent characteristics is often dependent on respondent self-report. On the Internet, alternative identities can be created, and thus its accuracy for individuals reporting information is not known. Like any sampling technique, Internet sampling has limitations that can be noted by the investigator and integrated into the interpretation of the data. The key to efficacious use of the Internet for boundary setting is to select this strategy purposively. You would not use virtual boundary setting to study how individuals who live in remote areas without electricity or smartphones maintain their hygiene.

Drawing probability samples on the Internet would follow the principles for random selection.

Suppose you were interested in surveying health professionals about their views on the recent national health insurance strategies. To obtain a sampling frame, you contact professional organizations to obtain email addresses. You can then randomly select every Kth address using a table of random numbers. It would also be possible to include all addresses in your sample, at which point you would be accessing the whole population. As we have already noted and discussed in detail in Chapter 20, testing a population rather than a sample has implications for statistical testing.

The Internet provides many opportunities for nonprobability sampling. You can post a request for participation on a content-specific site; send an email, text, or message to a listserv; or use social networking sites such as Facebook and Twitter to recruit respondents.

For example, suppose you were interested in investigating the relationship between social networking use and self-esteem for persons who are unable to navigate outside their homes. There are many ways that you could approach this project. You might use nonhuman sampling methods to count postings on a selected Facebook site along with instrumentation to rate the emotive tone of posting, or you could directly recruit users of a particular Facebook or networking site to recruit users as participants in a direct, online survey.

The boundary-setting options for the Internet are only limited by one's imagination, purpose, budget, and, of course, literature support for selecting a sampling method. Remember, however, that although the techniques may use different technologies, the basic principles for boundary setting in experimental-type design must be followed to enhance external validity, transparency, and rigor.

Comparing Sample to Population

As we initially stated, major reasons for sampling are to ensure representativeness and the ability to generalize from sample findings to the target population. At this point, you might be asking why probability sampling is even used in light of the numerous nonprobability techniques. The power of probability sampling lies in its capacity to use and generate estimated population parameters from the sample based on statistical theory.

Five basic steps are involved in determining whether findings from the sample are representative of the population, as follows (Box 14-7):

BOX 14-7 *Steps to Compare Sample to Population*

1. State hypothesis.
2. Select level of significance.
3. Compute statistical value.
4. Obtain a critical value.
5. Accept or fail to accept null hypothesis.

1. State the hypothesis of no difference (null hypothesis) between the population and the sample being compared. This null hypothesis implies that the values obtained in the sample, such as on a depression scale, are the sample values that would have been obtained if depression had been measured in other samples drawn from the same population.
2. Select a level of significance, or the probability that defines how rare or unlikely the sample data must be before the researcher can "fail to accept" the null hypothesis. If the significance level equals 0.05, the researcher is 95% confident that the null hypothesis should not be accepted. Failure to accept the null hypothesis means that, with a degree of certainty, there is a difference between the sample and the population.
3. Compute a statistical value using a formula (see Chapter 30).
4. Compare the computed statistical value with a critical value. Although mostly calculated on computers with automated readouts on of the level of confidence at which a critical value is reached, you can also refer to most statistical texts to understand the conceptual process. Statistical texts still contain tables of critical values to which the researcher can refer and that make the process clear. The critical value indicates how high the computed sample statistic must be at a given level of significance to fail to accept the null hypothesis.
5. Accept or fail to accept the null hypothesis. If the computed sample value is greater than the critical value, the null hypothesis can fail to be accepted, and the researcher will conclude that a significant difference exists between sample and population. In many cases, the researcher wants to accept the

null hypothesis, as in situations when he or she wants to demonstrate that sample values mirror or represent the population from which the sample was selected. In other cases, the researcher prefers to "fail to accept" a null hypothesis, such as when he or she wants to demonstrate that a particular intervention changed the sample significantly from the values represented in the population.

Determining Sample Size

Determining the number of participants in the study or the size of the sample is a critical issue that often causes difficulty for new investigators. A common suggestion is to "obtain as many subjects as you can afford." However, a large sample size is not always the best policy and is often unnecessary. The size of your sample can influence the type of data collection techniques, procedures for recruitment, and the costs involved in conducting the study. Also, sample size needs to be carefully thought out so that you maximize external validity. Think of the articles that you have read in which claims are made on the basis of testing one group, albeit large.

> If you were a health or human service professional in a school setting, how likely is it that you would inform your intervention by a study that reported success in reducing problem drinking behaviors in only one urban high school sample?

Although many published research articles do not discuss the rationale for the size of the sample for a study, you should have a reason for the number you choose. A defense of your sample size is particularly important when you submit a proposal requesting funds to conduct an investigation. In the proposal you will need to provide justification for the number of subjects that will be included in your study.

Researchers determine the number of elements in a sample after the population and sampling frame have been identified. The determination of sample size may be based on the proportion of units from the population necessary to conduct statistical testing. The number of subjects needed to test a

---

BOX 14-8 *Considerations in Determining Sample Size*

1. Data analytical procedures that will be used
2. Statistical level of significance (usually chosen at 0.05 or 0.01 level)
3. Statistical power (.80 acceptable)
4. Effect size

---

hypothesis is directly related to *statistical power*, which is the probability of identifying a relationship that exists, or the probability of failing to accept the null hypothesis when it is false.

Assume you are testing the outcome of a new intervention. Without sufficient power to detect a difference between experimental and control group outcomes, there will be no use in conducting the study. You want to ensure an adequate number of subjects in the study to have the power to determine whether the intervention made a difference in the study outcomes. •

There are four considerations in determining the size of your sample (Box 14-8).

As noted, statistical power is the probability that a statistical test will detect a significant difference if one exists. An 80% statistical power level is considered the minimum level of acceptability. If a power analysis is calculated and statistical power is lower than 80%, the researcher runs the risk of a Type II error (described in Chapter 20) or the inability to detect significance if one exists. If statistical power is too low, it is not wise to conduct the study as planned.

In the 1970s, Cohen[7] advanced the technique of "power analysis." This step is still central to and followed in contemporary experimental-type research. Four factors must be considered in a power analysis: significance level, sample size, effect size, and power. If three of the four factors are known, the fourth can be calculated. Significance level and sample size are straightforward. The investigator sets both these parameters before data collection. Cohen has developed tables indicating power levels for

different sample sizes, significance levels, and effect sizes. *Effect size* refers to the strength of differences in the sample values that the investigator expects to find. These values are now available for automated calculation and application on Internet sites.

Consider a study that tests the benefits of a low-impact aerobic exercise program for elders. On the basis of empirical evidence from literature reviews and data from small-scale or pilot studies, the investigator hypothesizes that there will be a large effect of the program on muscle strength and a minimal-to-moderate effect on cardiovascular fitness. If the difference between values in experimental and control group subjects is large, only a few subjects will be needed in each group to detect such differences. If the effect size is small, a large sample size will be necessary to detect differences. •

The number in the sample is also determined by the number of units in the sampling frame. Practical considerations, such as time and financial support for conducting the research, may also provide guidelines on the number of units to be included in the sample.[8]

Summary

The purpose of boundary setting in experimental-type designs is (1) to complete the study in a timely, cost-effective, and manageable manner and (2) to use the findings about the subset (sample) to inform us about the larger group (population) from whom the sample was selected. A number of probability and nonprobability methods can be used to select a sample from a population. Probability sampling procedures are used to ensure that a sample reflects or is representative of the larger population from which it was extracted. Nonprobability methods are used when it is not possible to identify a sampling frame or when random selection is not feasible or desirable. Although boundary setting may sound simple, many decisions must be made along the way. Multiple print and virtual resources are available that provide in-depth discussions of each procedural step in experimental-type research, as well as the statistical theory guiding the various sampling plans. Furthermore, you should be aware that an investigator may use variations and combinations of these sampling plans, depending on the nature of the research question and the resources available to the investigator. When probability sampling is used, it is often wise to consult a statistical expert to ensure that the sampling plan maximizes representation.

Experimental-type designs increase external validity by achieving "representativeness" of the sample through probability sampling. However, in health and human service research, it is frequently not practical or ethical to use probability sampling techniques. Health and human service contexts may mediate against probability sampling, in which case researchers use nonprobability methods. Even with limited external validity, however, well-planned studies with conclusions consistent with the level of knowledge that the sampling can yield are extremely valuable.

EXERCISES

1. Find a research article that uses probability sampling. Describe the sampling plan.
2. Find a research article that uses nonprobability sampling. Describe the sampling plan, and then compare its usefulness for practice with the article in Exercise 1 that uses probability sampling.

What conclusions and guidance can you obtain from each, and for which groups? What are the ethical and methodological limitations and concerns of each?
3. Develop a sampling plan for a study on lifestyles of adults with chronic heart disease who live in their own homes. First, identify population parameters, then suggest how best to obtain a representative sample of that population.
4. Discuss how you might obtain a random sample of children, given the regulation that a child's legal guardian must consent to the child's participation in research.

References

1. Babbie E: *Practice of social research*, ed 13, Belmont, Calif, 2013, Wadsworth.
2. Monette DR, Sullivan TJ, DeJong CR, et al: *Applied social research*, ed 9, Belmont, Calif, 2014, Wadsworth.
3. Daniel J: *Sampling essentials: practical guidelines for making sampling choices*, Los Angeles, 2012, Sage.
4. American Psychiatric Association: *Diagnostic and statistical manual of mental disorders*, ed 5, Washington, DC, 2013, American Psychiatric Press (DSM-V).
5. Urbaniak GC, Plous S: *Research randomizer*, 1997-2008. http://www.randomizer.org/form.htm.
6. Thompson SK: *Sampling*, Hoboken, NJ, 2012, Wiley.
7. Cohen J: *Statistical power analysis for the behavioral sciences*, ed 2, New York, 1990, Academic Press.
8. Liu XS: *Statistical power analysis for the social and behavioral sciences*, New York, 2014, Routledge.

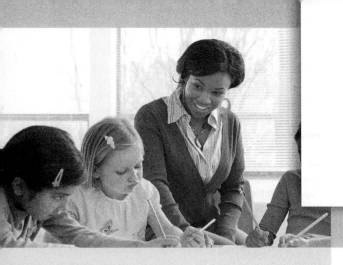

Chapter 15
Boundary Setting in Naturalistic Designs

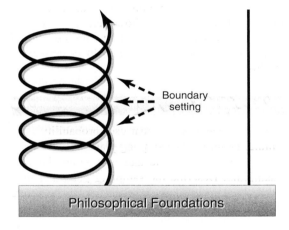

Boundary setting

Philosophical Foundations

Let us now look at the way in which a researcher engages in the action process of setting boundaries when conducting a study using naturalistic designs. In this tradition, setting boundaries is dynamic and inductive. The action process is flexible and fluid and may take from a short to a very prolonged period of time.

Because the purposes of naturalistic research are detailed, contextual exploration, understanding, description, and explanation, the researcher does not often know the specific boundaries of the inquiry or the particular conceptual domains before undertaking the study. Indeed, the very point of the study may be to uncover and establish the specific characteristics that bound or define a group of persons or explicate a particular concept or human experience. Thus, for most naturalistic designs, boundary setting is embedded in context; boundaries emerge and are set and reset as data collection and analysis occur. Remember, in naturalistic inquiry, these three processes often co-occur. The final determination of boundaries for a particular concept, or set of constructs, may not actually be known until the formal analysis and reporting phases of the study. Nevertheless, a researcher starts setting boundaries at the beginning of the process and makes decisions about what to observe, with whom to talk, and how to proceed in the context. Thus, depending on what knowledge emerges, boundary setting in naturalistic inquiry could change dramatically throughout the research process.

Ways of Setting Boundaries

Researchers working in the traditions of naturalistic inquiry consider bounding their study along a number of dimensions. These include the location or physical or virtual setting, groups and experiences of interest, the particular concepts that will be explored, the artifacts and images that will be examined, and the ways in which individuals are involved.

The Setting

Naturalistic studies can investigate a wide range of locations, from virtual settings (e.g., Second Life, Internet chat rooms, blogs, websites, Twitter feeds) to geographic locations and physical settings. Regardless of the setting, there are basic principles for creating boundaries. Choosing the initial boundary or location is a conscious decision on the part of the researcher. It is often followed by an expansion or change of setting as the inquiry unfolds.

Consider the following example of bounding a naturalistic study by setting. Let's say you want to examine how middle school students interact with peers. The initial boundaries of the research might be set broadly to include the social spaces of a particular school setting. You decide on the lunchroom and playground as your two points of initial observation. But as you observe and interact with the youth, you find that much of the interaction takes place in the hallways as students move from class to class and after school in other locations. You then notice that even when youth are in the same physical location, they are often not engaged in direct communication with one another. Rather, many are texting on their cell phones. In this case, an initial geographic location is identified to enter the study, but the knowledge that you acquire as the study proceeds leads you to realize that peer interaction does not necessarily rely on students being in the same physical space. As the study proceeds, your data collection takes you beyond the initial physical boundaries into other locations and electronic venues for interaction. Observations and collecting information also change as the contexts for interaction expand. This process is characteristic of boundary setting in naturalistic inquiry. •

The geographic location of schools in this case is an appropriate initial boundary, as that is where middle school–aged youth spend much of their time interacting with their peers. The identification of a specific locale, geographic region, or area is a customary way of initially bounding a study in the naturalistic traditions. It allows the investigator to enter the study, but as you see in this example, a physical location is only an entry point and may be expanded to other physical spaces and beyond as well.

Choosing the initial boundary or location is a conscious methodological decision, and the investigator, depending on purpose, resources, and the query, may choose to then expand or not expand the boundary. Consider the following example, in which the location remained very bounded throughout the study.

In her investigation of dying at a nursing home, Kayser-Jones[1] explains her boundary-setting decisions in this way (three facilities formed the initial boundaries of the study):

> Data were gathered in three facilities, two proprietary nursing homes (one with 174 beds and the other with 138 beds), and one government-owned facility. Facilities were chosen to provide variation in resident, provider, and setting characteristics.

The initial physical boundary of the nursing home was purposive in that the investigator was particularly interested in examining the experience of dying within the institution of a residential care facility.

By delimiting the study to this setting and focusing on the world within the nursing home, she achieved a rich or "thick" description of the multiple social realities of residents, their families, and nursing staff in that one locale. Also, by staying within that one setting, she was able to observe multiple interactions and uncover factors that made the dying experience difficult. For example, the heavy workload of nursing staff often resulted in communication between residents and staff that was terse and appeared disrespectful. She also found that pain was not well managed and thus there was significant need for attention to this critical part of palliative and end-of-life care. Regardless of the institutional requirements for providing meaningful activities, the staff neglected these quality-of-life issues as they struggled to provide physical care. Finally, the burden of family caregiving, often thought of as an in-home experience, was described as family often relinquished community and family time to take care of a dying loved one.

Thus, in the study conducted by Kayser-Jones, staying within the initial boundaries set at the beginning of the study was a purposive decision in that studying the experience of dying within the residential setting was her aim. You might notice, however, that the nature of informants changed from focus on the dying resident to move expansively, interviewing family and staff. This change led to important findings about caregiver burden.

Now let's apply the principles from these examples to a virtual location.

Suppose you are interested in identifying the experiences of students with mobility impairments on college campuses in the northeastern United States. Rather than spend time on multiple campuses, you choose to enter an online site that students with mobility impairments have created on a social networking site to discuss their experiences. Or suppose you wanted to theorize about how the construct of diversity is reflected in the virtual environment. You might enter a site such as Second Life and observe or interact to understand how avatars and interactions inform diversity differently than embodied, racial, or ethnic views of the physical world. •

You therefore choose your initial point of entry into the study as the interactive chat room on the website, setting this virtual location as your initial boundary.

Groups

Delimiting a study by groups is another way in which researchers in the naturalistic tradition may form their study's initial boundary and point of entry. In classic ethnography, cultural groups were the focus of interest. However, in the 21st century, groups are diverse. They may be considered cultures or may be defined through other shared characteristics such as age, interest, diagnostic category, market segment, or Facebook group.[2]

First, let us consider culture, as this definition of a group remains relevant today. A "culture" may be loosely defined as the customs and tacit knowledge held by individuals who belong to a group. Although it is often typical to think of culture as ethnic, racial, or even disability identity, any shared experience (e.g., parents of children with chronic illness, substance abusers) could constitute a cultural group. Culture may also be identified by the location in which it exists or as the rules, beliefs, and values that guide a person or group of people through a particular experience, such as the "culture of home care therapists," "culture of disability,"[3] or "culture of caregiving."[4]

Assume you want to study family interactions and the impact of caregiving among Cuban Americans, an ethic cultural group highly concentrated in Florida and in the southern United States. You begin your study in one region of Florida but are uncertain of the impact of "southern" values and culture on interaction patterns. You may want to expand or redefine the boundary of your study to include other geographic locations with Cuban American communities to tease out the potential influence of the Southern culture of the United States. •

Or consider the large literature developing on disability culture. There are numerous scholarly websites that display productions of this culture. For example, look at the first goal of the Disability Cultural Center at Syracuse University:

> *Establish and celebrate a community that fosters pride in one's identity and creates a culture of inclusion.*[3]

If you wanted to identify who was considered a member and then study the essence, rituals, and meanings of this cultural grouping, you might set your boundaries specific to the group and then, rather than going to a geographic location where these individuals reside, you might begin to enter the culture on websites such as the Disability Cultural Center site.[3]

As a researcher collects information about a group, he or she may refine the boundaries of the study to obtain a fuller understanding of the membership. In the previous example, you could decide to travel to Cuba to understand the cultural underpinnings and historical forces that have shaped your Cuban-American study group. Or as in the example of disability culture, a researcher also might use virtual sites to expand cultural boundaries, such as websites devoted to a particular cultural group.

Suppose you were interested in an age grouping that was not portrayed as a culture. Think back to the examples of mobility equipment that we discussed. Regardless of the ethical, racial, geographic, or common interest characteristics that create a group, you are interested in promoting fitness engagement. So you define your group by age boundaries and mobility equipment need.

Experiences of Interest

In studies that focus on the exploration of a particular experience, the phenomenon immediately sets the boundaries for what will be examined; that is, the boundaries of the inquiry lie within the realm of the particular experiences described by the individuals. Experiences such as suffering, healing, aging, poverty, a rite of passage, and terminal illness are examples of potential areas of exploration from a phenomenological perspective. In phenomenological studies, the goal is to understand the experiences of a small set of individuals from their own perspectives or "lived" experience.[5] For example, a

phenomenologist who wants to describe the experience of a parent who has a child with a terminal illness may choose to interview and observe that parent. There are many experiences related to health, illness, adaptation, coping, mental health, and so forth that are important to understand from the "inside" or emic perspective—that is, how people with specific conditions experience those phenomena and how lived experience can inform health and human service practices. For example, Eleck[6] conducted her study to examine the experiences of mothers who had a terminally ill child as the basis for improving nursing care for this group.

Suppose you are interested in the following experience.

 To explore the different meanings of the experience of trauma resulting from exposure to war, you might identify soldiers (and/or civilians) from one or more wars with varying levels of exposure to traumatic experiences. Many possible directions are available for you to take. If your purpose is to understand the variability in the experiences of trauma, you would want to maximize the variability of persons and experiences examined. If, however, your intent is to explore a more select or targeted aspect of traumatic experiences (e.g., prisoners of war), you would select individuals accordingly. You might even choose to lurk or be active on a Second Life virtual world site that was developed for this experience, as a boundary-setting technique.[7] •

Concepts

As in the previous example, some forms of inquiry explore a particular concept. Thus, it is the particular concept that initially bounds the scope of the study in these types of inquiries. Eleck's study was bounded by the concept of impending loss of a child.[6]

In other types of naturalistic inquiries, the investigator "casts a wide net" and is interested in understanding underlying values or beliefs that guide behaviors.[8] In these forms of inquiry, the concepts of interest may not be immediately identified and may emerge only in the course of the study as a consequence of the analytical process.

As an example, consider the concept of mobility aid. One example of this broad approach is a study by Gitlin and colleagues, who were interested in discovering the meanings attributed to the use of mobility aids and other special assistive devices for persons after their first stroke.[9] The concepts that explicated particular meanings were uncovered from an analysis of interviews with 102 individuals receiving rehabilitation services. Concepts such as social "stigma," "biographic management," and "continuity of self" emerged as important analytical domains that explained the dimensions of meanings associated with device use. Each concept had been defined and developed by other researchers involved in disability studies. Gitlin and associates did not initially bound the study to these conceptual domains; rather, these concepts emerged as important focal points in the analytical phase of the study.[9] Based on this and other literature, DePoy and Gilson bounded their study of mobility equipment to stigmatizing appearance and user preferences as the foundation for equipment redesign.[10] Some studies, however, begin by setting conceptual boundaries. They then expanded their conceptual boundaries to the design and branding of disability not only through adaptive equipment design but also through many other methods such as place branding, imagery, and policy branding.[10]

The following example illustrates the process of setting conceptual boundaries in naturalistic research. In his classic but still relevant study of the culture of a nursing home, Savishinsky[11] was originally interested in describing the behavioral responses of nursing home residents to pet therapy. He stated:

> *The approach that I took began with two concepts at the very heart of pet therapy-companionship and domesticity. In the broadest terms, I came to realize that the study had to be a cultural and not just a behavioral one. ... It had to look at meanings and not simply actions.*[11]

As you can see, the initial boundaries of the study—observing actions during pet therapy—became modified and expanded as the study proceeded to the nursing home culture as a whole, including not only behavioral patterns but also meanings embedded within that culture.

Objects

As we have introduced previously, studies may be bounded by the meaning of objects.[12] According to Berger,[12] objects take on life and meaning in the increasingly visual culture of the 21st century. Objects can involve pictures/photos, materials, environmental contents, clothing, equipment, and so forth. Consider the work of Sobchack[13] and Smith and Mora.[14] They bounded their work by the object of prosthesis, looking at its diverse meanings of devices as functional assistive devices, body sculpture, bodily augmentation, and contributions to rethinking the contemporary body as cyborg (part human, part machine).

Using objects as your boundaries, let's suppose you are interested in learning about how older adults use their living space to accommodate limitations that are experienced as a result of aging bodies. Objects and their placement in homes, cars, and so forth can provide important knowledge about functionality and how elders adapt to differences in health status as they age in place. You might look at bathrooms, for example, to see what objects are used for bathing and what other additions have been made to prevent falling. Examining where medications are placed and stored offers insights as to their salience in the person's daily routines. Artifacts such as eyeglasses and reading lamps provide information about vision. Even looking at the presence of devices such as computers and tablets might be important data to enter a study about how function is augmented in one's home.

Narrative Boundaries

Naturalistic researchers may define boundaries by narratives.[15] Naturalistic meta-analysis is one example. In this design, the researcher enters the study by identifying specific narrative reports that have common content, such as reports of the narratives or life histories of cancer patients or newly injured veterans.

Print materials such as written documents set the initial boundaries of an inquiry. They may include but are not limited to historical documents, journals, or diaries, Take, for example, Theophano's[16] exploration of women's lives through the cookbooks they used and wrote in from the 17th century to the present. Cookbooks and the letters and notes stuck in their pages were the sole source of data, from which Theophano was able to uncover rich stories about families and friendships and how food and cooking were linked to everyday life in different countries and time periods.

Images

Images are visual representations that hold meaning. Initiating and bounding a study with image is increasingly used by researchers who seek to understand meaning and how it is communicated in diverse venues, including but not limited to art, film, screen-mediated visual, logo, and photograph.[17,18] As an example, Blynn[19] identified visual archives of freak shows to set the initial boundaries to study how cultural and artistic meaning depicted in "extraordinary bodies" shaped the meaning of avant-garde in America.

> Suppose you are interested in finding out about the attitudes towards disabled students at a university. You could distribute an attitude survey, but you are concerned that your study will be confounded by socially desirable responses. So you decide to examine photos of students, faculty, and spaces to see if any contain visual images of students with impairments. •

As you can see, there are numerous ways to bound naturalistic studies. So now, let us begin to look not just at what researchers use but at how they go about choosing people, objects, images, and spaces to begin their inquiries.

The Process of Setting Boundaries

Involving research participants, selecting artifacts, narratives, and images are critical in shaping how a naturalistic study will unfold.[15] It is often believed that researchers who engage in naturalistic inquiry simply select any individual or object on the basis of convenience. This belief is a misconception and an inaccurate understanding of the actions undertaken by researchers to involve participants and delimit

other forms of data. There is nothing haphazard about the process of boundary setting in naturalistic inquiry. The use of a convenience selection strategy is only one of many important approaches used by researchers working from these multiple traditions. Selecting individuals and objects is a purposeful action process, and the investigator must be acutely aware of the implications of his or her selection decisions. Boundaries stem from either the investigator's theoretical perspective or the study's purpose and the research query, or selection is informed by judgments or interpretations that emerge in the course of fieldwork.

There are important differences between experimental-type research and naturalistic inquiry with regard to setting boundaries in research. Knowing these differences provides a basis for a better understanding of the decision-making process used by naturalistic researchers. The concern in identifying subjects in experimental-type research is "representativeness," as discussed in Chapter 14. Basically, the principle of representativeness suggests that the larger the sample size or the more elements involved in a study, the better the chances of achieving representation of the target population and detecting group differences or patterns.

In naturalistic inquiry, however, usually the concern is with the selection of humans or nonhuman elements with the potential to illuminate a particular concept, experience, or context. The number of participants, objects, narratives, or images in a study is not as important to the naturalistic investigator as the amount of exposure to participants and opportunities to explore phenomena in depth. The investigator therefore develops selection strategies that ensure richness of information and complexity of understanding. The concern is not with selecting a sample that represents a known population; rather, naturalistic inquiry is characterized by entering a study through the most productive venues and then being open to revision as the data unfold and reveal new findings.

Although some researchers label the approaches used in naturalistic inquiry as sampling techniques, we see this word as a misnomer. Sampling in experimental-type designs is based on the premise of representation of and/or randomization from a population whose parameters are already known and determined. In many naturalistic designs, the aim is to discover who and what make up a group. Because the logic of boundary setting in naturalistic inquiry is inductive, population parameters are not known or even relevant to methodology. Therefore, using the term "sampling" in naturalistic inquiry is misleading and does not capture the intent of the decision-making process within these traditions. We prefer the term "strategies of engagement" over "sampling."

The way in which individuals and other forms of information are selected for study participation in naturalistic designs depends on the study's purpose and design. Individuals and artifacts may be involved differently at distinct points in the study process. This variability is especially the case for large ethnographical studies or forms of naturalistic inquiry that occur over a long period and that focus on a broad domain of concern. In any case, researchers working from the traditions of naturalistic inquiry use a wide range of strategies for involving participants, objects, images, and so forth, and these strategies emerge within the context of carrying out inquiry. Occasionally, probability or nonprobability sampling techniques may be integrated into naturalistic studies when these approaches are appropriate and fit the structure of the study's purpose and design. These types of strategies have typically been used in large ethnographical studies and after the investigator has identified particular patterns that warrant further explication through the use of these sampling approaches. The ethnographer can use these sampling techniques to determine the representativeness of the particular concept or domain of concern within the cultural group, community, or context. When sampling methods are used in naturalistic designs, we take the position that the design moves to the category of "mixed methods."

The specific processes of boundary setting in naturalistic research are diverse but for the most part follow five principles (Box 15-1). Boundary setting begins with the investigator determining an entry point into the inquiry. In classical ethnographies, the process of entering a study context has been referred to as *gaining access*.[20,21] When we use that term, we are referring not only to ethnographic research but to initiating a naturalistic study in a context that may

---

BOX 15-1 *Five Guiding Principles in Boundary Setting*

1. Inductive process is used.
2. Each selection decision informs the next decision.
3. Boundaries are adjusted throughout the study.
4. A range of strategies is used to select individuals, events, artifacts, and concepts throughout the study.
5. Boundary setting occurs throughout the research process until redundancy or saturation is achieved.

---

or may not involve direct contact with human participants. Remember that health and human service research is concerned with humans even when they are not directly involved. Examining objects, images, narrative, and other forms of data provides important information about human experience that can be applied to understand and improve health and human experience.

An investigator will frequently seek introduction to a context through a member of a group. This member acts as a facilitator, or a bridge between the life of the group and the investigator. From that entry point, which could be (but is not limited to) establishing rapport with other group members, examining a concept, or observing a location in which the group lives, communicates, and performs, the researcher collects information or data to describe the boundaries. Gaining virtual entry may involve identifying a particular website, Twitter feed, set of blogs, or other Internet-based group or collection of materials that becomes the initial focus of and entry into the proposed inquiry. Deciding on what artifacts to use as an entry point is a similarly purposive decision. Some researchers use formal collections of artifacts if they are bounding their study by object (as in the case of prosthetics), and others integrate strategies such as object reading and observation of images into studies involving humans in context.[18]

After a researcher has gained initial access to the context of the study, other boundary-setting issues emerge. For example, although the researcher may be initially accepted into a cultural group or community, it may take a prolonged period before participants will share intimate information or before the meanings of objects, rituals, narratives, and images become clear enough that the researcher knows how to focus.

Entering a study context is not an easy action process. Much literature has been written on this important research action. The approach to gaining entry will differ depending on the context and whether the investigator is a member (emic) or stranger (etic) in the context.

> You can think of gaining entry as going to a party or new school where you do not know anyone and you are unfamiliar with the rules of behavior and what is acceptable. How would you approach the "scene" or situation? How would you learn about the underlying rules that are governing the partygoers' or students' behaviors? You may choose to stand outside the group and make observations, or you may try to identify someone nearby to introduce yourself and strike up a conversation. How do you think you would feel? Most likely, you would feel unsure of yourself and ask, "What is going on in this 'context' that I am now a part of?" In many respects, this common experience (which we all have had) is similar to gaining access to a group, virtual site, or geographic location for research purposes. •

In the process of discovery and within the context of the field, the naturalistic researcher continually makes boundary decisions as to whom to interview, what to observe, and what to read. There may be an overwhelming number of observational points and potential individuals to interview. Selection decisions are based on the specific questions the researcher poses throughout the research process and the practicalities of the field, such as who is available or willing to be interviewed or observed. Decisions may also be influenced by a theoretical framework that is guiding the study or that is being elaborated on or refuted.

Boundary setting in naturalistic inquiry begins inductively, and as concepts emerge and theory development proceeds, the researcher assumes a more deductive way of selecting observations, individuals, or artifacts to observe and the types of

questions or probes to ask. For example, observational points may be chosen to ensure representation of what the researcher observes.

> Assume you want to examine the quality of life of residents with dementia on a separate unit in a nursing home. As part of your study, you might purposely select different times of the day and night to make your observations to ensure representation of time and behaviors. If you have limited resources or access to the context you want to observe, you may need to make less frequent and intense observations and then query participants about how well your observations reflect routine or daily occurrences. •

Throughout a study, the researcher is actively determining which sources will be most helpful to gain an understanding of the particular question and to derive a complete perspective of individuals or a group, practices and rules of behavior, and experiences. Thus, once in the context, the investigator uses other techniques and approaches to establish the boundaries of the study. For example, to understand certain practices, an ethnographer may seek a key actor or informant to represent the group. This individual is selected because of his or her strategic position in the group or because the person may be more expressive or able to articulate what the researcher is interested in knowing. A researcher may involve a key informant at critical junctures in a study to confirm both emerging insights and understandings.

One could ask what the impact of any one or more key informants have on the interpretive framework that emerges. If other individuals were selected, would the same understandings emerge? This is a question that the investigator must continually ask. Selecting one or more key informants is very purposeful, and one's reasons for selection should be carefully explicated. As noted earlier, one strategy in ethnographic design is to begin broadly. The investigator initially "samples" what is immediately accessible or in view. As fieldwork and interviewing proceed, questions and observational points become increasingly focused and narrowed. The investigator may use a "snowball" or "chain" approach to identify informants, search for extreme or deviant cases, or purposely sample diverse individuals or situations to increase variation.[20]

The process of selecting and adding pieces of information through interview, observation, and review of literature and artifacts, as well as analyzing the data for discovery and description of the boundaries of the phenomenon being examined, helps the researcher understand, in depth, specific occurrences within the domain of the study.[15] The domain or focus of a study must be clearly understood to ensure that findings or interpretations are meaningful. For example, a domain may be a culture, a context, a group, a concept, or a set of experiences specified by the researcher as the major concern in a study.[15] Although no claim is made about the "representativeness" of a domain in naturalistic inquiry, principles are explicated that may be relevant to other settings. We now turn to the specifics of involving humans and nonhuman sources in studies.

What or Whom to Choose and on What Basis

Patton[22] and others[15,18] have suggested many distinct strategies that can be used separately or in combination for involving individuals and sources in naturalistic inquiry. The following six strategies are commonly used to identify informants. (Some of these strategies are discussed in Chapter 14 and involve nonprobability methods, such as convenience, purposive, and snowball sampling.) A researcher may begin with one strategy, such as identifying the source that best maximizes variation, and then switching to another strategy, such as identifying a disconfirming case to challenge emerging interpretations.

Maximum Variation

Maximum variation is a strategy that involves seeking individuals or sources for a study who are extremely different along dimensions that are the focus of the study. That is, in using this strategy, the researcher attempts to maximize variation among the broadest range of experiences, information, and/or perspectives. Maximizing differences and variability challenges the researcher and attempts to involve a universe of experiences and meanings.

From the differences that are unveiled, the researcher attempts to identify common patterns that cut across variations, as well as to determine the study's boundaries. The challenge for researchers using this approach is uncovering the universe of variations.

Assume you are interested in understanding and developing a theory of adaptation to life-altering disabling conditions. A grand theory needs to be based on adaptation to many types of conditions and must involve an examination of individuals from vastly different life circumstances. You will want to maximize variation of disabling conditions and experiences to ensure that a theory of adaptation is comprehensive and captures the broadest possible swath of human experience. In this case, you may attempt to vary context as well. •

Homogeneous Selection

In contrast to maximum variation, *homogeneous selection* involves choosing sources that are similar, such as humans with similar experiences. This approach reduces variation and thereby simplifies the number of experiences, characteristics, and conceptual domains that are represented among study participants and sources. Focus groups are often conducted with homogeneous groups of informants in order to achieve consensus on a domain of study.[23]

It is important to note that the selection of a homogeneous focus group does not mean that everyone in that group will express and interpret the experience similarly. The researcher usually discovers wide variation and diversity in expression and interpretation of an identified experience, even among a group initially selected for similarities. DePoy and Gilson[2] referred to this phenomenon as "diversity patina." That is, grouping people by characteristics that are obvious, such as race, class, gender, disability status, and age, may reveal some differences among groups but barely scratch the surface of the diversity within these groups. Thus, homogeneous selection provides an approach by which to uncover diversity within a particular group of individuals initially selected for their similar characteristic(s), or to uncover what DePoy and Gilson refer to as "diversity depth."

Theory-Based Selection

Theory-based selection involves choosing sources that exemplify a particular theoretical construct for the purposes of expanding an understanding of the theory. Theophano's study exemplified this approach.[16] Through examining "food narrative," the investigator was able to elucidate the properties of women's lived experiences. DePoy and Gilson[10] used a theory-based selection approach to examine disability as an artifact of design and branding. Their study sought to illustrate theory as it appeared in multiple domains that had been named "disability context."

Confirming and Disconfirming Cases

Confirming cases and *disconfirming cases* are strategies in which the investigator purposively searches for sources that will either support or challenge an emerging interpretation or theory posited by the investigator. Using disconfirming cases allows the investigator to expand or revise an initial understanding of the phenomena under study by identifying exceptions or deviations. Using data from sources that may provide alternative views and experiences engages the investigator in a process of elaborating and expanding on an understanding that accounts for a fuller range of diverse phenomena than would have been revealed without this purposive strategy. On the basis of this expanded understanding, concepts, theories, or interpretations are rethought and developed. Sobchack's work[13] provides an example of this point. She contrasted her interpretation of prosthesis with that of Mullins.

 Assume you are interested in developing a theory of parental caregiving of children with disabilities. You may begin your inquiry with in-depth interviews of parents with a child who is severely disabled. As you develop guiding concepts, you may choose to verify and contrast them by interviewing a few parents who have never had a child with a disability. These interviews will offer important contrasts that will help further bound the emerging concepts relevant to parenting children with disabilities. They will confirm or highlight the uniqueness of the experience of families of children with disabilities, or they will reveal similarities to the experience of families without disabled children. If the latter occurred, you would need to rethink your theoretical design because your data would not support a theory that families with a disabled child have experiences that differ from those of families without a disabled child. •

Extreme or Deviant Case

In the extreme case, or *deviant case*, the researcher selects a case that represents an extreme example of the phenomenon of interest.

 Suppose you were interested in understanding how body image emerges and develops in girls with congenital amputations. To explore body image, you might select an individual who had a severe congenital amputation resulting in the absence of both arms. By selecting this informant, you would be expecting that every aspect of life for this person is different from that for a girl with a typical body structure. The extreme case would provide a basis for understanding the development of body image in a girl who does not experience what is typical for most girls. •

Typical Case

In contrast to the deviant case, an investigator may choose to select a *typical case*. A typical case is one that typifies a phenomenon or represents the average.

In your body image study, you might choose to identify girls who typify girls' experiences in a particular cultural group. On the basis of the information you gather, your next selection strategy may be to choose an atypical or deviant case within that group. •

How Many Study Participants and/or Sources?

There are no specific rules in naturalistic inquiry to assist the researcher in selecting the number of persons or nonhuman sources needed for interviewing or observation in a study. No procedure for naturalistic inquiry is comparable to a "power analysis" for experimental-type research. Can you guess the reasons for this based on your knowledge thus far of the naturalistic tradition?

Remember that the concern in naturalistic inquiry is *not* with numbers in a study but rather with the types of opportunities and extent of exposure for in-depth observation and interviewing. Some guidelines, however, can be used to determine the number of sources to include in a naturalistic study. If the intent is to examine a shared experience, meaning, or concept, a homogeneous strategy should be used to obtain study participants. Given that the naturalistic researcher is minimizing variation, only a small number of individuals or objects (e.g., 5 to 10) may be necessary to include in the study. The small number provides a "representative picture" of the phenomenon or focus of the study. In contrast, if the intent is to examine approaches to a heterogeneous phenomenon such as family caregiving of patients with dementia and to develop a theoretical understanding of caregiver management techniques, the naturalistic researcher may want to maximize variation in experiences and approaches to derive the broadest understanding of this activity. Thus, a larger number of caregivers (e.g., 50 to 100 individuals) from diverse backgrounds may be required, each representing different life circumstances and stages of caregiving. In the historical study of the meaning of walking sticks in the Gilded Age currently being conducted, the researchers are planning to engage a large number of artifacts, narratives, and images, given that these objects theoretically have such different meanings to those who design and use them. This knowledge is intended for application in current times, and thus a detailed understanding of the historical domain is necessary to provide useful knowledge for contemporary mobility device design and use.[10]

Note that in naturalistic inquiry the term "representation" does not refer to or imply external validity as used by experimental researchers to mean the generalizability of knowledge or its application to others. Rather, it refers to developing a comprehensive understanding of what may be typical of or common to a group, shared experience, artifacts, images, or virtual or geographic location.

Ethical Considerations

There are numerous ethical considerations in making boundary decisions for naturalistic inquiry. Consider the following examples.

> You are observing interactions between therapists and families on an inpatient unit of a hospital; the therapists and family members have granted permission for you to make such observations. Suppose a disoriented and cognitively impaired individual interrupts a therapeutic session you are observing. This interruption is of great interest to you because you want to see how both the therapist and family member handle it and then reconnect. However, the person who interrupted the scene has not been approached about your study, and he has not given you permission to make systematic observations of his behavior. What do you do? •

> You are observing a community-based program for persons with cognitive disabilities, and you have selected several key informants who attend the program. The inclusion and exclusion of select individuals within the program may be offensive to other participants and may create jealousy or distrust of those selected. Thus, your decision making may have a direct impact on the context you want to observe and may have both positive and negative consequences for those you engage. How should you handle this naturalistic design issue? •

> You are studying a group of substance-addicted individuals to learn how their interactions contribute to prolonged addiction. Part of your study is an examination of the meaning of drug-related artifacts such as needles and other paraphernalia. What if possession of some of these objects is illegal and unsafe? What do you do? •

Other ethical issues in naturalistic inquiry involve how to enter and exit the context and how to draw appropriate boundaries between the researcher and the individuals who are being studied. This point is particularly important as global research expands and investigators enter nations, geographies, and cultures with customs, expectations, beliefs, and values that differ from those of the investigator's country of origin. Thus, the researcher must carefully frame the purpose and scope of the study and be clear and transparent in the relationships that are forged. Engagement in naturalistic inquiry is intense, personal, and often prolonged, and researchers, once involved in a study, may have difficulty extricating themselves from the relationships forged. Also, individuals may come to expect certain favors or ways of behaving that are outside of the boundary of being an investigator.

Suppose you are conducting a longitudinal study that involves observations of mothers and their children with disabilities and how parenting decisions are made. Over time, you will naturally become involved in numerous family occasions and will learn about and share personal and intimate aspects of their daily life. Consider some of the ethical dilemmas you may confront. •

The boundaries of relationships and even nonparticipant observations in naturalistic research can easily become tenuous, especially in times of personal and political duress over the course of the research process.[15,20]

Summary

Boundary setting in naturalistic research is an ongoing and active process. It is part of the process of doing this type of study and emerges inductively from data collection and analysis. Research is undertaken not only to address a research problem but also to promote further understanding and descriptions of the boundaries of the research. The naturalistic researcher is constantly making decisions and judgments about who should be interviewed and when and what to observe. The investigator uses a range of selection strategies in a study. The selection strategy used to choose an individual to interview, event to observe, or artifact to review is based on the specific focus of the investigator, and this focus usually emerges in the course of the study. These strategies may include probability and nonprobability techniques, as well as others developed specifically for naturalistic inquiry (e.g., typical case, deviant case). Although initially a boundary may be defined globally, the investigator delimits the nature of the group, phenomenon, artifacts, or concepts under investigation through ongoing data collection and analysis.

EXERCISES

1. To understand boundary setting in naturalistic inquiry, select a public place, such as a shopping mall, virtual chat room, or restaurant. Spend at least 1 hour observing, and then determine patterns of human behavior in the location. Look at the artifacts and how they are used. Record the images. As you observe, record how and why you choose to focus on specific elements of the location. Reflect on the range of strategies you use. What did each strategy provide in terms of understanding the setting? Reflect on what information and observations you might have missed by your boundary decision making.

2. After leaving the location in Exercise 1, write a list of events, images, objects, and behaviors that you believe will be important to observe on another occasion to confirm your emerging understanding.

3. Develop a research plan to examine the experience of being a health professional working at a managed care facility. Identify three strategies for involving study participants, and provide a rationale for using each approach.

4. Select a theory to investigate through naturalistic inquiry. Identify the initial entrée into the study. Whom and what will you choose to study?

References

1. Kayser-Jones J: The experience of dying. *Gerontologist* 42:11–19, 2002.
2. DePoy E, Gilson SF: *Human behavior theory and applications: a critical thinking approach*, Thousand Oaks, Calif, 2012, Sage.
3. Syracuse University: *Disability Cultural Center*, 2012. http://sudcc.syr.edu.

4. Thissen J, Zwijneberg R, Zijlmans K: *Contemporary culture*, Amsterdam, 2012, Amsterdam University Press.
5. Detmer D: *Phenomenology explained: from experience to insight*, Chicago, 2013, Carus.
6. Eleck L: *The lived experience of parents surrounding the death of a child with hospice services*, 2013, Dissertation, St Joseph College.
7. Institute for Creative Technology: *Coming home*, 2012. http://projects.ict.usc.edu/force/cominghome.
8. Neuman L: *Social research methods: qualitative and quantitative methods*, ed 7, Boston, 2009, Allyn & Bacon.
9. Gitlin L, Luborsky M, Schemm RL: Emerging concerns of older stroke patients about assistive device use. *Gerontologist* 3:169–180, 1998.
10. DePoy E, Gilson SF: *Branding and designing disability*, London, 2014, Routledge.
11. Savishinsky JS: *The ends of time*, New York, 1991, Bergen & Garvey.
12. Berger A: *What objects mean*, Walnut Creek, Calif, 2009, Left Coast Press.
13. Sobchack V: A leg to stand on. In Candlin F, Guins R, editors: *The object reader*, London, 2009, Routledge.
14. Smith M, Mora J: *The prosthetic impulse*, Cambridge, Mass, 2006, MIT Press.
15. Denzin N, Lincoln Y: *2011, Sage handbook of qualitative research methods*, Thousand Oaks, Calif, 2011, Sage.
16. Theophano J: *Eat by words: reading women's lives through the cookbooks they wrote*, New York, 2002, Palgrave.
17. Harper D: *Visual sociology*, New York, 2012, Routledge.
18. Rose G: *Visual methodologies*, Los Angeles, 2012, Sage.
19. Blyn R: *The Freak-garde: Extraordinary Bodies and Revolutionary Art in America*, 2013, University of Minnesota Press.
20. Spradley J: *Participant observation*, New York, 1980, Holt, Rinehart & Winston.
21. Geertz C: *The interpretation of cultures: selected essays*, New York, 1973, Basic Books.
22. Patton MQ: *Qualitative evaluation and research methods*, ed 3, Thousand Oaks, Calif, 2001, Sage.
23. Liamputtong P: *Focus group methodology*, Los Angeles, 2011, Sage.

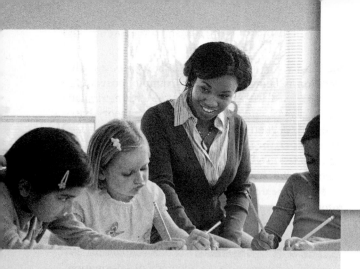

Chapter 16
Collecting Information

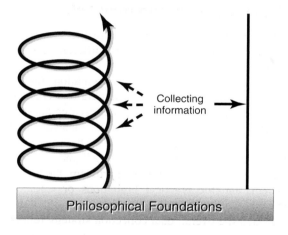

Collecting information

Philosophical Foundations

You now have a better understanding of the methods for involving individuals, events, observations, and artifacts in your study. Now let us explore the various strategies you can use to collect information or data. This chapter provides an overview of the action process of gathering evidence to answer research questions or queries. A number of strategies are discussed, some of which are used primarily in either experimental-type research or in naturalistic inquiry and all of which can be used in mixed methods, of course depending on purpose. Subsequent chapters examine the specific approaches used in each research tradition and then examine how they can be integrated in mixed methods.

In experimental-type research, data collection is a distinct action phase that represents the crossroads between the thinking processes involved in question formation and development and implementation of design, and the action process of analysis. Strategies for data collection involve specific activities that are pertinent to the research problem and consistent with the design. In turn, the types of data collected and the methodological approach used to obtain information shape both the type and nature of the analytical process and the understandings and knowledge that can emerge.

In naturalistic inquiry, gathering information is shaped by the initial query. However, it is embedded in an iterative, abductive approach (depending on the design) that involves ongoing analysis, reformulation, and refinement of the initial query. The configurations used in mixed methods are purposive and diverse, as both experimental-type and naturalistic methods of obtaining information complement one another.

Principles of Information Collection

Three basic principles characterize the process of collecting information within the different research traditions (Box 16-1).

First, the aim of collecting information, regardless of the tradition, is to obtain data that are both relevant and sufficient to answer a research question and/or query. Second, the choice of a data collection or information-gathering strategy is based on four major factors: the researcher's paradigmatic framework, the nature of the research problem, the type of design, and the practical limitations or resources available to the investigator (Table 16-1). Third, although the overall data collection strategy reflects the researcher's basic philosophical perspective and logic structure, a specific procedure, such as observation or interview, may be used by researchers conducting a naturalistic, an experimental-type, and/or a mixed method study. Thus, the logic structure, not

the format of information itself, determines what tradition is being used.[1,2] For example, observation may be used in experimental-type and naturalistic inquiry, but if rated with a preexisting, theory-based scale, it is deductive and thus fits within experimental-type data collection. If treated inductively, observation is often used as the basis for developing or fitting theory within naturalistic inquiry.

Many researchers find it useful to collect data and information with more than one procedure or technique to be able to answer a question or query more fully. The use of multiple collection techniques is referred to as "triangulation" or "crystallization" and is useful for increasing the accuracy of information.[3] We discuss this technique in subsequent chapters.

In general, the action process of data and information collection uses one or more of the following strategies: (1) looking, watching, listening, reading, and recording; (2) asking; and (3) obtaining and examining materials. Each of these strategies can be structured, semistructured, or open-ended, depending on the nature of the inquiry (Table 16-2). Also, each strategy can be used in combination with another.

Looking, Watching, Listening, Reading, and Recording

One important data-collection and information-gathering strategy involves systematic observation. The process of *observation* includes five primary activities, which may be interrelated: looking,

---

BOX 16-1	Basic Principles for Collecting Information

1. Information needs to be relevant and sufficient to answer the question or query.
2. Selection of collection strategies needs to be purposeful.
3. Use of a single strategy or combination of strategies must enhance validity or trustworthiness.

TABLE 16-1	Factors Influencing Choice of Strategy for Collecting Information

Factor	Specific Issue
Paradigmatic framework	Relationship of investigator to what is being investigated
Research problem	Question or query
Design type	Naturalistic inquiry, experimental-type, mixed methods research
Practical limitations	Time Money Access to research population

TABLE 16-2   *Summary of Strategies for Collecting Information*

Method	Structured	Unstructured
Watching and listening	Checklists Rating scales	Participatory Nonparticipatory
Asking	Closed-ended questions	Open-ended questions
Examining materials	Coding schemes	Open-ended observation

watching, listening, reading, and recording. The record produced by the investigator forms the data set. The way in which the researcher looks, watches, reads, and listens may range from being structured to unstructured, participatory to nonparticipatory, narrowly to broadly focused, and time limited to ongoing and fully immersed.[4]

In the experimental-type tradition, observation is usually time limited and structured. Criteria to look, watch, listen, read, and record are determined a priori to gathering data, and the data are recorded as a structured measurement system. For example, checklists may be used that indicate the frequency (or only the presence or absence) of a particular behavior or object under study. Or a text may be read, and the occurrences of a particular phrase to denote "power language" might be counted and recorded. Phenomena other than those specified before entering the context are omitted from or remain outside the investigator's record. Rating scales may also be used to record observations; the investigator rates the observed phenomenon on a scale with a predetermined point system (see Chapter 17).

Looking, watching, listening, reading, and recording take on an inductive quality in naturalistic designs, with varying degrees of participation and interaction between the investigator and the phenomena of interest. The investigator broadly defines the boundaries of observation (e.g., a community health center), then moves to a more focused observational approach (e.g., particular locations, navigation patterns, staff-client interactions, language, signs, images) as the process of collecting and analyzing information from previous observations unfolds.

🔍 Let us examine the concept of "intelligence" to illustrate different observational approaches. In experimental-type studies, intelligence testing relies largely on the use of a structured instrument that involves paper-and-pencil or computer-based tests and a tester observing a subject's performance in a "laboratory setting." Measurements are obtained on dimensions that have been predefined in the literature as composing the construct of intelligence. Typically, a score or set of scores will denote the magnitude of an individual's intelligence. In a naturalistic approach, however, rather than using predefined criteria, the investigator may watch and listen to persons in their natural environments to reveal the meaning of intelligence and the ways it is recognized and responded to in a particular culture. Each approach has its value in addressing specific types of research questions or queries. Structured observation of intelligence is appropriate for the investigator who wants to compare populations or individuals, measure individual or group progress and development, or describe population parameters on a standard indicator of intelligence. In contrast, naturalistic observation of intelligence is useful to the researcher attempting to develop new understandings of the construct. Mixed methods might be used to ascertain the relevance of predefined constructs of intelligence in a particular domain in which intelligence is defined differently than how it is approached through measurement. •

Asking

Health and human service providers routinely ask a wide range of questions to obtain information for professional purposes. Similarly, in research, "asking" is a systematic and purposeful aspect of a data collection plan. As in observation, questions can vary in structure and content, from unstructured and *open-ended questions* to structured and *closed-ended questions* or fixed-response queries that use a predetermined response set.

🔍 An example of an open-ended question is, "How have you have been feeling this past week?" or "How is it now for you compared with before your stroke?" In contrast, examples of structured or closed-ended questions are, "In this past week, how would you rate your health: excellent, good, adequate, fair, or poor?" Or, "Compared to how you generally felt before your stroke, how do you now feel on average (select one that best describes you)? sadder than I did before my stroke, happier than I did before my stroke." •

BOX 16-2 *Response Alternatives for Closed-Ended Questions*

- Dichotomous ("yes" or "no") questions
- Multiple-choice answers
- Rank-order questions (Guttman scale)
- Four or more graded responses (Likert-type scale)

Naturalistic research relies more heavily on open-ended types of asking techniques, whereas experimental-type designs tend to use structured, fixed-response questions. Focused, structured asking is used to obtain data on a specified phenomenon, whereas open-ended asking is used when the research purpose is discovery and exploration. However, as we mentioned earlier, the method of obtaining data does not determine the tradition in which the data fit. Rather, the logical analytical approach, deductive for experimental-type and inductive or abductive in naturalistic inquiry, are tradition specific. In mixed methods, one source of data can be analyzed from both inductive and deductive perspectives.

Asking typically occurs through two methods, *interviews* or *questionnaires*. We look at both now.

Interviews

Interviews are conducted through verbal communication; they may occur face-to-face, by telephone, or through virtual communication, and may be either structured or unstructured. Interviews can be conducted with individuals or groups. Group interviews may include a range of persons, such as those conducted with couples, families, and work groups to focus groups with five or more people. Deciding on which way to proceed depends on the research question or query. Individual interviews are used when interaction and groupthink are not desirable, whereas family interviews may be warranted to observe communication methods. In focus group methodology, the interaction of individuals is key to the information the investigator wants to obtain. This technique is particularly useful in attitudinal and participatory research in which groupthink is desirable.[5,6] An audio recording of the group interview is transcribed, and the narrative (along with investigator notes) forms the information base, which is then analyzed. (See Chapter 18 for more detail.)

Structured interviews rely on a written questioning protocol (sometimes referred to as an interview schedule) in which maximum researcher control is imposed on the content and sequencing of questions. Each question and its response alternatives are developed and placed in sequential order before an interview is conducted. Interviewers are instructed to ask each question precisely as it is written in the protocol. Most questions are closed-ended or fixed; that is, subjects select one response from a predetermined set of answers. Closed-ended questions vary with regard to the type of response alternatives (Box 16-2). Each response set forms a different type of scale, as discussed later in this chapter.[6]

In a structured interview, the investigator may use a few open-ended questions. However, responses are then examined to derive categories, which are coded and, in effect, changed into a closed-ended response set on a post hoc analytical basis; that is, the investigator develops a numerical coding scheme based on the range of responses obtained and assigns a code to each subject. The numerical response is then analyzed.

You are interested in examining the social support of a group of veterans with posttraumatic stress disorder. To minimize respondent burden, you choose to use a semistructured interviewing approach by asking the veterans who volunteer to participate in your study to talk about the important people in their lives and the roles that each plays. However, to obtain a score of the level and nature of support for each respondent, you analyze the recorded interview by scoring it according to a preexisting scale of social support. This example illustrates how open-ended questioning, typically thought of as naturalistic, can be used in deductive designs. •

Unstructured interviews are primarily used in naturalistic research and in exploratory studies with experimental-type designs. The researcher initially presents the topic area of the interview to a respondent, then uses probing questions to obtain the desired level of detailed information. The interview may begin with an explanation of the study purpose and a broad statement or question such as, "Could you please describe your experience using this mobility device?" Other probing questions emerge as a consequence of the information provided from this initial query. *Probes* are statements that are intended to be neutral, to the extent possible, and thus attempt to avoid influencing the respondent to answer in any particular way. Probes are used to encourage the respondent to provide more information or to elaborate. A probe (e.g., "Tell me more about it," or simply repeating a question) encourages a respondent to discuss an issue or elaborate on an initial response.[6]

Quantitative researchers sometimes use unstructured interviews in pilot studies to uncover domains and response codes for future inclusion in a more structured interview-and-question format.

In mixed method studies, various combinations and formats can be integrated to answer questions and queries.

Questionnaires

Questionnaires are text-based instruments and may be administered face to face, by proxy, through the mail, or over the Internet. Similar to interviews, questionnaires vary as to whether questions are structured or unstructured. (The process of developing questionnaires is examined in Chapter 17 as part of the discussion on measurement in experimental-type research.)

Each way of asking—structured or unstructured—has strengths and limitations that the researcher must understand and weigh to determine the most appropriate approach. There is no "best way" of collecting information. The strengths and limitations of structured (closed-ended) questions must be evaluated in terms of the researcher's purpose (Boxes 16-3 and 16-4). Consider the following example.

As the basis for promoting healthy behaviors among elders residing in a rural community, you are

---

BOX 16-3 Strengths of Structured (Closed-Ended) Questioning

1. Honest responses can be obtained.
2. A large cohort can answer questions in a short period.
3. Responses can be compared across groups.
4. Statistical analysis can be conducted to describe and compare responses.

BOX 16-4 Limitations of Structured (Closed-Ended) Questioning

1. The researcher is uncertain how respondents interpret or understand the questions.
2. Issues relevant to respondents may not be captured.
3. Respondent answers may reflect socially desirable responses.

BOX 16-5 Strengths of Open-Ended (Unstructured) Questions

1. Highly sensitive issues can be explored.
2. Nonverbal behaviors can be captured and analyzed.
3. Issues salient to respondent can be identified.
4. Meaning of questions to respondent can be identified.

---

planning to study their activity patterns. You decide to use a structured interview approach in which you provide an activity monitor to each respondent for automated activity tracking and wireless transmission to your computer. As you suspect, this inquiry documents a low level of activity. In planning your intervention, however, you realize that more information is necessary to determine how to structure the intervention. To obtain the answers to explain why the activity level was low and how to address it, you therefore decide to conduct an unstructured (open-ended) group interview of all community residents meeting your inclusion criteria.

Using this example, now consider the advantages of open-ended (unstructured) questions (Box 16-5). Then, identify the limitations of an open-ended

---

BOX 16-6 *Limitations of Open-Ended (Unstructured) Questions*

···

1. Respondents may not want to address sensitive issues directly.
2. Extensive time is required to conduct interviews and analyze information.
3. Responses across groups cannot be readily compared.

---

approach and see whether you can apply these to the example (Box 16-6).

As you can see, both structured asking and unstructured asking have merits and limitations, depending on the research purpose, phenomena to be studied, and study population.

Obtaining and Examining Materials

Materials are defined as objects, information, imagery, phenomena, or data that already exist. There are numerous reasons to seek out and use existing materials. First, direct observation and interview may not be possible, and thus an investigator may try to answer the research question by seeking a data set that has already been generated in the topic area of interest. Consider the investigator who is conducting inquiries of a sensitive nature, where informants may not want or be able to share their experiences. Seeking information that has already been obtained and organized not only makes sense for the researcher but also saves further discomfort on the part of respondents. Second, the use of existing materials eliminates the attention factor, or the *Hawthorne effect*[7] (change in respondent's answer as a consequence of participating in the research process). Third, using existing materials allows the researcher to view phenomena in the past and over time, which may not be possible with a primary data collection strategy that occurs at one point. Finally, as articulated by Rose,[8] archaeologists and now material culture investigators can derive great knowledge from the visual and material worlds.

As with asking and observing, securing and examining materials in experimental-type design are structured by criteria before the research is activated.

In naturalistic inquiry, the selection of materials to observe or examine emerges as a consequence of the investigative process. Although there are many ways to use existing materials, we organize them here into three distinct approaches: (1) unobtrusive methodology, (2) secondary data analysis, and (3) artifact review.

Unobtrusive Methodology

Unobtrusive methodology involves the observation and examination of documents, objects, and environments that bear on the phenomenon of interest.[9] This methodology is nonreactive; that is, there is minimal or no discernible investigator effect in the research setting. More recently, visual sociology and material culture methods such as object reading have become increasingly integrated into health and human service research.[8]

Consider these examples. To estimate the danger of ambulation in rural community geographies as the basis for informing policy and practice for advancing community safety, an investigator might observe wear spots on stairs, carpets, pathways, roadside walkways, and so forth. This approach can be used to confirm information obtained from another source. The researcher may have used unobtrusive observation to confirm information obtained from the emergency-room records of patients who have been injured by falling.

Consider also the investigator who examines text and interactions on social networking websites to ascertain the answer to a research question. Investigators may use many sources for text-based materials in their analysis (Box 16-7). Or consider the investigator who examines the degree of abandonment of protective helmets on the basis of their visual appearance. Look at Box 16-8 for sources of material data.

Secondary Data Analysis

In *secondary data analysis*, the researcher reanalyzes one or more existing data sets.[10] By "data set," we mean information that has been obtained and organized for the purpose of research.

- Diaries or personal journals
- Text on diverse information technology such as podcasts, blogs
- Medical records
- Clinical notes
- Historical documents
- Minutes from meetings
- Letters
- Newspapers, magazines, and professional journals

BOX 16-8 *Examples of Material Sources*

- Objects
- Images
- Geographies
- Architectures
- Clothing

A health care researcher may examine client medical records to obtain data or may combine the data of two studies for subsequent analysis. Also, a social work researcher may examine clinical process recordings as a basis for understanding therapeutic interaction in family therapy. •

The purpose of a secondary analysis is to ask different questions of the data from the data set analyzed in the original work. Researchers use several large, national health and social service data sets for secondary data analysis. For example, the census tracts, Kids Count, National Health Interview Surveys, National Health Care Data Set, Medicare and Medicaid data, Annual Housing Survey, Disability Statistics, and court report recordings are important sources for secondary analysis in health and human service research.

Geographic Data

Geographic data are increasingly being used to answer research questions of interest to health and human service providers. With the expansion and advancing sophistication of computer applications that can map and depict levels of spaces and geographies, questions regarding the public health and service needs of regions, as well as place-related epidemiology, risks and strengths, health disparities, and resources, can be systematically informed. Because health and human service problems, needs, and efforts are most frequently geographically situated, contemporary statistical modeling methods and geospatial inquiry delimited to local communities provide the tools through which to develop models relevant to health and human service questions. Moreover, these models can be statistically manipulated to predict the relationships among social and health problem prevalence and the availability, proximity, and nature of prevention resources in a geographic area.[11]

There is a wide range of applications and complexity in geographic analysis, from static, slice-in-time snapshots to temporally changing dynamic modeling.[11] What all geographic data have in common are the use of visual spatial locations as delimiters of information and analysis. The Geographic Information System (GIS) relies on two overarching spatial paradigms, raster and vector. Raster GIS carves geography into mutually exclusive spaces and then examines the attributes of these. Thus, the attributes of one space can be represented and compared with the attributes of another.

Vector GIS relies on location points. This approach locates points and identifies spaces and the attributes delimited inside of them by the lines that connect the points. Each approach has its strengths and limitations, but both have valuable applications.

For example, suppose you are interested in the causes of underage drinking, and you ascertain that geographic areas differ. To look at the different attributes from the raster approach, you would obtain a frequency count of the number of establishments that sell alcoholic beverages in delimited areas and then depict by color the number of establishments in that area. However, from the vector approach, you would identify the addresses or geographic coordinates of each alcohol sales establishment and plot it on your map.[12] Each of these approaches answers the relational question in a different way, and depending on the purpose, research questions, and application, you would choose one or even both methods for analysis. •

Information in the Virtual and Information Technology Environment

As we have discussed throughout this chapter and the book, the Internet, among other digital formats such as podcasts, cloud computing, text messaging, and other wireless interactivity, is becoming a major source of information and thus provides a rich environment for obtaining information in all research traditions. Experimental-type, naturalistic, and thus mixed methods on the Internet can parallel the structure and content of data in the physical world. Therefore, survey data can be generated, secondary data can be obtained, and data for naturalistic observation and analysis can be developed and/or unobtrusively accessed, as we have discussed. However, some information can only be created or accessed virtually, as exemplified by geospatial data that are rendered in multidimensional layers. Two major advantages of conducting research in the virtual environment are reach and multiplicity of formats.

Reach refers to the global scope of the Internet. Information can be obtained instantaneously from across the continent, the ocean, or even beyond. We can now connect to the Internet and cellular towers while traveling in airplanes, allowing information to be obtained and considered from locations that are not even situated on terra firma.

Consider this example.

> Suppose you were interested in comparing attitudes toward accessibility standards in the United States, Canada, the United Kingdom, and Japan. You might create a survey to measure favorability. Although you could post the survey on the Internet in English to the English-speaking countries, you would be able, through programs such as Google Translate and BabelFish, to use automated free software to translate your survey into Japanese even if you do not read or speak the language. Similarly, responses could be translated back into English, and you would never need to have a bilingual person at your disposal. With the omnipotence of mobile devices and their connectivity, investigators can now reach respondents and participants in their shirt pockets, purses, eyeglasses, and watches where these devices are carried. •

Multiplicity of formats refers to the capacity of the virtual environment to present information in text, orally, and in images. Because the virtual environment is a digital medium, the survey in the previous example could be obtained in text, oral, or image format on multiple devices. Of course, you would test differences related to format in your research, because device preference and use could be confounding variables or influences in shaping knowledge.

Artifact Review

Artifact review, most recently referred to as material culture methods,[8] comprises a set of techniques primarily used to ascertain the meaning of objects in research contexts. For example, archaeologists examine ruins to learn about ancient cultures. Material culture theorists examine objects for emotive meanings, to identify conferral and response. Artifact review in health and human service research may include the examination of personal objects in a patient's hospital room or client's home to determine interests and preferred ways of arranging the environment as a basis for intervention planning.

Sobchack[13] contrasted the meaning of lower extremity prostheses in an object reading methodology. In contrast to Mullins, a model and athlete known for running on bilateral "cheetah legs" who sees prosthetics as wearable sculpture, Sobchack's prostheses meant rejoining typical functioning and ambulation.

Summary

Three basic principles guide the action process of obtaining information: (1) collecting relevant and sufficient information for the research question or query; (2) choosing an information-gathering or data-collecting strategy that is consistent with the research question, epistemological foundation, design, and practical constraints of the research effort; and (3) recognizing that methods can be shared across traditions. The categories of collecting information in all designs are looking, watching, reading, listening, and recording; asking questions; and examining materials.

We are now ready to examine specific data collection strategies in experimental-type design (Chapter 17) and gathering information in naturalistic design (Chapter 18).

EXERCISES

1. You want to study the level of function in individuals with spinal cord injuries immediately after hospitalization. Identify and describe two data collection strategies you may use. Evaluate the strengths and limitations of each.
2. Conduct a brief interview with an older adult. Ask the person to rate his or her health on a 5-point scale (excellent, very good, good, fair, poor) and then to explain the rating in narrative. Compare and contrast the type of information you obtained by asking a structured question and an unstructured question.
3. Select a website for analysis. Ask a question that can be answered by examining the frequency of a particular word or phrase. Then ask a question that can be answered through inductive analysis. What are the strengths and limitations of each approach when analyzing the same virtual data set?

References

1. Agamben G: *The signature of all things: on method*, New York, 2009, Zone Books.
2. Audi R: *Epistemology*, New York, 2011, Routledge.
3. Denzin NK, Lincoln YS: *Sage handbook of qualitative research*, ed 2, Los Angeles, 2011, Sage.
4. Patton M: *Essentials of utilization-focused evaluation*, Los Angeles, 2012, Sage.
5. Liamputtong P: *Focus group methodology*, Los Angeles, 2011, Sage.
6. Gubrium JF, Holstein JA, Marvasti AB, et al: *The SAGE handbook of interview research: the complexity of the craft*, Los Angeles, 2012, Sage.
7. Babbie E: *Practice of social research*, ed 13, Belmont, Calif, 2012, Wadsworth.
8. Rose G: *Visual methodologies: an introduction to researching with visual materials*, Los Angeles, 2012, Sage.
9. Lee RM: *Unobtrusive measures in the social sciences*, Boston, 2000, Open University Press.
10. Vartanian MT: *Secondary data analysis*, Oxford, UK, 2011, Oxford University Press.
11. Gilson S, DePoy E: Geographic analysis for the social sciences. *Int J Interdisc Social Sci* 1, 2007.
12. Harder JC, Ormsby T, Balstrom T: *Understanding GIS*, New York, 2013, ESRI Press.
13. Candlin F, Guins R: *The object reader*, London, 2009, Routledge.

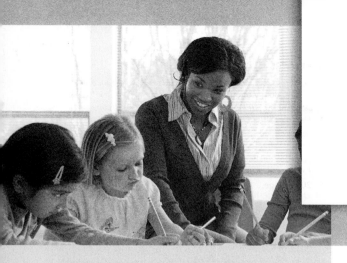

Chapter 17
Collecting Data Through Measurement in Experimental-Type Research

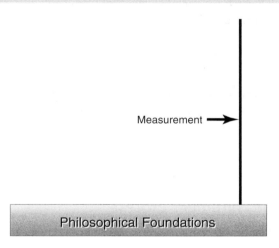

Think about the nature and scope of experimental-type designs. What would you say is the purpose of data collection using these research designs? This chapter addresses that question.

In experimental-type designs, the purpose of data collection is to learn about an "objective reality." (Revisit Chapter 4 for a discussion of objectivity.) In this tradition, the investigator is viewed as a separate entity from that which is being studied, and an attempt is made to ensure that the researcher's own perspective and biases are not interjected in the conduct of the research. As in all essentials in the experimental-type tradition, there must be strict adherence to a data collection protocol as well. In this research tradition, "protocol" has a specific definition. It refers to a series of procedures and techniques designed to remove the influence of the investigator from the data collection process and ensure a "nonbiased" and uniform approach to obtaining information. In order to accomplish objectivity, numbers are assigned to denote a "measured reality." To generate numbers, the investigator develops or selects instruments that are reliable and valid or which have a degree of correspondence to an objective world or truth. Therefore the process of measurement is central to experimental-type thinking and action. Measurement is intended to promote objectivity by standardizing data as quantitative indicators. Consider weight, for example. The "subjective" observer might judge body size on the basis of appearance and preference. However, standardizing weight in numeric units—pounds or kilograms—allows assessment and thus comparison of body sizes without opinion. Once generated, numeric data can then be submitted to statistical procedures to test relationships, hypotheses, and population descriptors. This knowledge is viewed as representing objective reality.

In this chapter, we examine the measurement process and concepts, such as reliability and validity, that are critical to the experimental-type research tradition.

Measurement Process

What is measurement? In research, measurement has a precise meaning. Broadly speaking, *measurement* can be defined as the translation of observations into numerical values or numbers. It is a vital action process in experimental-type research that links the researcher's abstractions or theoretical concepts to concrete variables that can be empirically or objectively examined and quantified. In experimental-type research, concepts must be made operational; in other words, they must be put into a format such as a questionnaire or interview schedule that permits structured, controlled observation and measurement. The measurement process involves a number of steps that include both conceptual and operational considerations (Fig. 17-1).

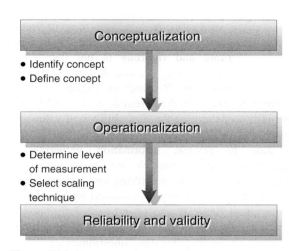

Figure 17-1 Measurement process.

The first step in measurement involves conceptual work by the researcher.[1] The researcher must identify and define what is to be measured. Although this may seem obvious, it is often a difficult initial first step that involves asking, "How will I conceptualize the phenomenon I want to study?" or "How will I define these concepts in words?" Consider such basic concepts in health and human service research as adherence, self-management, attitude, depression, anxiety, mastery, function, disability, wellness, quality of life, or adaptation. Each has been defined in many ways in the research literature. After the researcher identifies a concept, such as "anxiety," "depression," or "well-being," the literature must be thoroughly reviewed to decide on an appropriate definition that fits within the theory selection of the researcher.

The second step in measurement involves developing an operational definition of the lexically defined concept. This operational step involves asking, "What kind of an indicator will I use as a gauge of this concept?" or "How will I classify and quantify what I observe?" A "measure" is an empirical representation of an underlying concept. Because, by definition, a "concept" is never directly observable, the strength of the relationship between an "indicator" and an underlying concept is critical. This relationship is referred to as "validity." In other words, does the measurement assess what it claims to measure? Also, it is important for the indicator to measure the underlying concept consistently. The consistency of a measure is referred to as its "reliability." The greater the reliability and validity, the more desirable and rigorous is the instrument. Reliability and validity are two fundamental properties of indicators. Researchers engage in major efforts to evaluate the strength of reliability and validity to determine the desirability and value of a measure,[2] as discussed later.

Just to review, information gathering in experimental-type research, an important action process, begins with identifying key concepts from the literature. This step is followed by developing conceptual (lexical) and operational definitions of these concepts. On the basis of these definitions, specific indicators (scales, questionnaires, rating forms) are chosen or newly developed. These indicators represent the source of information or data that will be collected.

Levels of Measurement

The first step in developing an indicator involves specifying how a variable will be operationalized. This action process involves determining the numerical level at which the variable will be measured. *Level of measurement* refers to the properties and meaning of the number assigned to an observation.

There are four levels of measurement: nominal, ordinal, interval, and ratio. Each leads to different types of manipulations. That is, the way in which a variable is measured will have a direct bearing on the type of statistical analysis that can be performed. The decision regarding the level of measurement of a variable is thus a critical component of the measurement process. It is important to understand that the way in which you measure a particular concept dictates the type of analytical approach you will be able to pursue.

> 🔍 You need to collect information on a person's age. What are some of the ways you could ask about age? You could categorize people as being either young, middle-aged, or old; you could develop categories that reflect specific ranges of ages (17-35, 36-55, 56-65, 66-75, 76+); or you could record actual ages reported or dates of birth and then calculate age in years. •

The level of measurement, whether you use age categories or the full range of possible ages measured in years, will determine the types of analytical approaches you can use, as you will learn here and in Chapter 20.

Several principles are used to determine the level of measurement of a "variable." The first is that every variable must have two qualities: (1) a variable must be exhaustive of every possible observation—that is, the variable should be able to classify every observation in terms of one or more of its attributes; and (2) the attributes or categories must be mutually exclusive.

Exhaustive

"Exhaustive" refers to the complete measurement of the construct and no more. That is to say, there must be enough categories that all the observations will fall into one. A simple example is the concept of gender. If the classic lexical definition of "male" or "female" is used, those two categories must be included in the measurement scheme. But what if McDermott's[3] definition of gender is used, defined as six categories (feminine, masculine, androgynous, transsexual, cross-dresser, and culturally specific genders)? The two categories that have previously represented the full range of attributes for the concept of gender must be expanded to include all six or the exhaustive criterion will not be met.

Mutually Exclusive

The second quality of a variable is that the attributes must be mutually exclusive.

Returning to the previous example, there can be only a male attribute or a female attribute in the classic definition and six attributes with no overlap in the McDermott definition.[3]

The second principle in determining a variable's level of measurement is that variables can be characterized as being either discrete or continuous. A *discrete variable* is one with a finite number of distinct values. Again, gender is a good example of a discrete variable. Gender, as classically defined, has either a male or a female value. There is considered to be no "in-between" category. Using McDermott's definition, there are six discrete categories with nothing in between.[3]

A *continuous variable,* in contrast, has an infinite number of values.[1,4] Age (measured in years) and height (measured metrically or in feet and inches) are two examples of possible continuous variables in that they can be measured along a numerical continuum. It is also possible to translate a continuous variable into discrete categories, such as the classification of the age variable as young, middle-aged, or old or the height variable as tall, medium, or short.

Discrete and continuous structures represent the natural characteristics of a variable, although sometimes these can be differently interpreted and assigned by researchers as just illustrated for age and height. However, the characteristics of a variable do have a direct bearing on the level of measurement that can be applied. We now examine each level in greater detail.

Nominal

Nominal measurement, exemplified by assigning numbers to gender as female or male or as one of six categories, represents the most basic, simplest, or lowest level of measurement. This level involves classifying observations into mutually exclusive categories. Nominal means "name"; therefore, at this level of measurement, numbers are used, in essence, to name attributes of a variable. This level merely labels attributes, and these attributes are not ordered in any particular way.

 Your cell phone number, the number on your sports jersey, and your Social Security number are used to identify you as the attribute of the variables "person with a cell phone," "athlete," or "taxpayer." All are examples of nominal numbers. •

Variables at the nominal level are discrete. For example, we may classify individuals according to their political or religious affiliation, gender, or ethnicity. In each of these examples, membership in one category excludes membership in another, but there is no order to the categories. One category is not higher or lower than another. Box 17-1 provides examples of mutually exclusive categories.

For data analysis, the researcher assigns a numerical value to each nominal category. For example,

BOX 17-1 *Examples of Nominal-Type Variables*

Yes or no
Male or female
Democrat, Republican, or Independent
White, African American, Hispanic, or Asian

"male" may be assigned a value of 1, whereas "female" may be assigned a value of 2. The assignment of numbers is purely arbitrary, and no mathematical functions or assumptions of magnitude or ranking are implied or can be performed. Many survey analyses, conducted by phone, mail, on the Internet, or face to face, use nominal-level questions. The intent of these surveys is to describe the distribution of responses along these discrete categories. This level of measurement therefore is also referred to as "categorical," because the assignment of a nominal number denotes category membership.

A survey may provide answers to questions such as how many men versus women have low back pain and how many unemployed versus employed people have health care insurance. In these examples, the nominally or categorically measured variables are "gender" and "employment," respectively. A respondent must (and can) only belong to one gender category and one employment condition. •

Ordinal

The next level of measurement is *ordinal.* As designated in its name, ordinal means "order" and thus can be remembered as the numerical value that assigns an order to a set of observations. Ordinal numbers allow the ranking of phenomena. Variables that are discrete and conceptualized as having an inherent order at the theoretical level can be operationalized in a rank-order format. Variables operationalized at the ordinal level have the same properties as nominal categories in that each category is mutually exclusive of the other. However, in addition, ordinal measures have a fixed order so that the researcher can rank one category higher or lower than another.

Income may be ranked into categories, such as 1 = poor, 2 = lower income, 3 = middle income, and 4 = upper income. Using this ordinal variable, we can say that middle income is ranked higher than lower income, but we cannot say anything about the extent to which the rankings differ. •

The assignment of a numerical value is symbolic and arbitrary, as in the case of nominal variables, because the distance or spacing between each category is not numerically equivalent. However, the numbers do imply magnitude—that is, one is greater than the other. Because there are no equal intervals between ordinal numbers, mathematical functions such as adding, subtracting, dividing, and multiplying cannot be performed. The researcher can merely state that one category is higher or lower, stronger or weaker, or greater or lesser than others.

Many scales useful to health and human service researchers are composed of variables measured at the ordinal level. For example, the concept of self-rated health may be ranked from 1 = very poor to 5 = excellent. Although the numbers imply a state of being in which 5 is greater than 1, it is not possible to say how much greater the distance is between responses. Also, the difference in magnitude between 5 (excellent) and 4 (very good) may be perceived differently from person to person. Thus, you must be careful not to make any assumptions about the degree of difference between numerical values.

Consider the Cantril Scales. To quantify and compare the well-being of citizens around the globe, Gallup developed a measure of well-being. The lexical definition of well-being measured by this scale is as follows: judgments of life or life evaluation.[3] Originally, an 11-point self-rating was developed, but for ease and clarity of reporting, the scores from 0 to 10 were translated into three ordinal responses: thriving, struggling, and suffering. The three are ranked from least to most desirable, are mutually exclusive, and are exhaustive.

We want to raise a caution here to remind you that ordinal data must denote mutually exclusive phenomena. A common mistake in creating categories from higher order numbers such as interval measurement (we discuss this level next) is the inclusion of the extreme points of an interval in more than one category. For example, let's say a questionnaire asks us about our age using categories of years, such as 1-10, 10-20, and 20-30. What category do you check if you are 10, 20, or 30 years old? These numbers incorrectly appear in two categories. The investigator should have specified mutually exclusive intervals, such as 1-10, 11-20, and 21-30.

Note that both well-being and age have been illustrated as both interval and ordinal. This point illustrates the point made earlier. Although some variables may fall into natural levels of measurement, it is the researcher's prerogative to assign what best measures the variable to fit the purpose and theory of the study.

Interval

The next level of measurement shares the characteristics of ordinal and nominal measures but also has the characteristic of equal spacing between categories. This level of measurement indicates how much categories differ. *Interval* measures are continuous variables in which the 0 point is arbitrary. Although interval measures are a higher order than ordinal and nominal measures, the absence of a true 0 point (the score at which none of the construct exists) does not allow statements to be made concerning ratios. However, the equidistance between points allows the researcher to say that the difference between scores of 50 and 70 is equivalent to the difference between scores of 20 and 40.

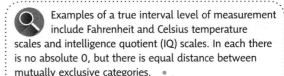

Examples of a true interval level of measurement include Fahrenheit and Celsius temperature scales and intelligence quotient (IQ) scales. In each there is no absolute 0, but there is equal distance between mutually exclusive categories. •

Once again illustrating investigator control of the level of measurement is the example of behavioral or attitudinal scales in the social and behavioral sciences. There is considerable debate as to whether these scales represent interval levels of measurement. Typically, such scales have a Likert-type response format in which a study participant responds to one of four to seven categories, such as strongly agree, agree, uncertain, disagree, or strongly disagree. Researchers who accept this type of scaling as an interval measure argue that the distance between "strongly agree" and "agree" is equivalent to the distance between "disagree" and "strongly disagree." Others argue that there is no empirical justification for making this assumption and that the data generated should be considered ordinal. In the actual practice of research, many investigators assume such scales are at the interval level to use more sophisticated and powerful statistical procedures that are only possible with interval and ratio data. You should be aware that this issue continues to be controversial among experimental-type researchers. If you choose this type of scaling, think about the most purposive assignment of numeric levels to your response set.

Ratio

Ratio measures represent the highest level of measurement. Such measures have all the characteristics of the previous levels and, in addition, have an absolute 0 point. Income is an example of a ratio measure. Instead of classifying income into ordinal categories, as in the previous example, it can be described in terms of dollars. Income is a ratio measurement because someone can have an income of 0, and we can say that an income of $40,000 is twice as high as an income of $20,000. Similarly, age can be measured as ratio because an individual cannot "unlive" or be less than 0 years old.

Determining Appropriate Level

Table 17-1 summarizes the characteristics of each level of measurement.

Experimental-type researchers usually strive to measure a variable at its highest possible level. However, the level of measurement should also best reflect the researcher's concepts when obvious. If political affiliation, gender, and ethnicity are the concepts of interest, for example, nominal measurement may be the most appropriate level because magnitude does not typically apply to these concepts.

Measurement Scales

Now that we have discussed the properties of numbers, let us examine the different methods by

TABLE 17-1   Characteristics of Experimental-Type Levels of Measurement

	Level of Measurement			
	Nominal	Ordinal	Interval	Ratio
Mutually exclusive categories	X	X	X	X
Fixed ordering	X	X	X	
Equal spacing	X	X		
Absolute 0	X			

BOX 17-2   Examples of Useful Scales

Dyadic Adjustment Scale (measure of marital adjustment)[5]
Self-Rating Anxiety Scale (measure of clinical anxiety)[6]
Family Adaptability Cohesion Scale[7]
State-Trait Anxiety Scale[8]
Session Evaluation Questionnaire[9]
CES Depression Scale[10]
SF-36 (measure of health status)[11]

CES, Center for Epistemological Studies; SF, Short Form.

which data are collected and transformed into numbers in experimental-type research.

Scales are tools for the quantitative measurement of the degree to which individuals possess a specific attribute or trait. Box 17-2[5-11] lists examples of scales frequently used by health and human service professionals in research.

Scaling techniques measure the extent to which respondents possess an attribute or personal characteristic. Experimental-type researchers use three primary scaling formats: the Likert approach to scales, Guttman scales, and semantic differential scales.[2] Each has its merits and disadvantages. The researcher who is developing a scale needs to make basic formatting decisions about response-set structure, whereas the researcher selecting an existing scale must evaluate the format of the measure for his or her project.

Likert-Type Scale

In the *Likert-type scale,* the researcher develops a series of items (usually between 10 and 20) worded favorably and unfavorably regarding the underlying construct that is to be assessed. Respondents indicate a level of agreement or disagreement with each statement by selecting one of several response alternatives (usually five to seven). Researchers may combine responses to the questions to obtain a summated score, examine each item separately, or sum scores on specific groups of items to create subindices. In developing a Likert-type format, the researcher decides how many response categories to allow and whether the categories should be even or odd in number. Even choices force a positive or negative response, whereas odd numbers allow the respondent to select a neutral or middle response.

> The Dyadic Adjustment Scale-R3 is an example of a Likert-type scale with several even-numbered response formats. The first set (six separate items) has six response categories: always agree, agree a lot, agree a little, disagree a little, disagree a lot, and always agree. The instructions read: "Most persons have disagreements in their relationships. Please indicate the approximate extent of agreement or disagreement between you and your partner for each item on the following list."[5] •

> In contrast, the Family Adaptability and Cohesion Scale IV, which measures family function, is an example of a scale that allows a neutral response by structuring responses into five ordinal categories: almost never, once in a while, sometimes, frequently, and almost always. The "sometimes" category is the middle response and receives a score of 3.[7] •

Social science researchers frequently use Likert-type scaling techniques because they provide a closed-ended set of responses while still giving the respondent a reasonable range of latitude. As mentioned, Likert-type scales may be considered ordinal or interval, depending on what is being measured and which analytical procedures are selected. A disadvantage of Likert-type scaling is that there is no way to ensure that respondents have the same understanding of the magnitude of each response.

Guttman Scale

used to measure attitudes
& public opinion

The *Guttman scale* is referred to as "unidimensional" or "cumulative."[1,2] The researcher develops a small number of items that relate to one concept. The items form a homogeneous or unitary set and are cumulative or graduated in intensity of expression. In other words, the items are hierarchically arranged so that endorsement of one item means an endorsement of those items below it, which are expressed at less intensity. Knowledge of the total score is predictive of the individual's responses to each item.

> Consider a series of items in a classic but still relevant measure level of political tolerance.[12] If a person answers "no" to each of the three items in Box 17-3, he or she is most tolerant. On the other hand, a person who answers "yes" to all three questions is the least tolerant. Another person who answers "no" to item 2 will probably answer "no" to item 1. •

Thus, in the Guttman approach to scaling, items are arranged according to the degree of agreement or intensity in ascending order, such that each subsequent response along the scale assumes the previous one.

BOX 17-3 *Examples of a Guttman Scale*

1. Assume this admitted communist wants to make a speech in your community. Should he be banned from speaking?
2. If some people in your community suggest that a book he wrote favoring government ownership should be taken out of your public library, would you favor removing the book?
3. Suppose he is a clerk in a store. Should he be fired?

Modified from Stouffer SA: Communism, conformity and civil liberties, New York, 1955, Doubleday.

Semantic Differential Scale

The *semantic differential scale* is usually used for psychological measures to assess attitudes and beliefs.[13] The researcher develops a series of rating scales in which the respondent is asked to give a judgment about something along an ordered dimension, usually of seven points. Ratings are "bipolar" in that they specify two opposite ends of a continuum (e.g., good-bad, happy-sad). The researcher sums the points across the items.

The Session Evaluation Questionnaire used in a study of Internet-based psychotherapy is an example of a semantic differential scale.[9] The scale measures two constructs, "depth" and "smoothness," related to clients' perceptions of clinical counseling sessions in which they have participated. The scale also measures two postsession mood constructs, "positivity" and "arousal." The scale includes 24 items, 12 each for the two sections. One item related to the session reads:

> *The session was:*
>   *Bad-Good*

> One post-session item reads:

> *Right now, I feel:*
>   *Happy-Sad*

> The respondent is instructed to place an X in the space that most accurately depicts his or her feelings. •

Semantic differential scaling is most useful when natural phenomena can be categorized in opposite or contrary positions. However, it limits the range of responses to a linear format.

Confidence in Instruments

In selecting a scale or other type of measurement, the researcher is concerned about two issues: (1) whether the instrument consistently or reliably measures a variable and (2) whether the instrument represents an adequate or valid measure of the underlying concept of interest.

Reliability

Reliability refers to the extent to which the results obtained from an instrument are stable. You will want to be assured that if you were to measure the same variable in the same person in the same situation over and over again, your results would be similar. More formally, reliability refers to the degree of consistency with which an instrument measures an attribute.[1,2] Reliability is an indicator of the ability of an instrument to produce similar scores on repeated testing occasions that occur under similar conditions. To ensure that changes in the variable under study represent observable variations and not those resulting from the measurement process itself, reliability of an instrument is important to consider. If an instrument yields different scores each time the same person is tested, the scale will not be able to detect what is referred to as the "objective" value or truth of the phenomenon being examined.

It is easy to understand the concept of reliability when you consider a physiological measure such as a scale for weight. If you weigh an individual on a scale, you can expect to derive the same weight on repeated measures if the subject steps on and off the scale several times without doing anything to alter weight between measurements. Instruments such as a weight scale or blood pressure cuff must be consistent to assess an accurate value that approximates a "true" physiological value for an individual. Consider an example involving human behavior to see how this principle applies.

Suppose you are interested in measuring the level of depression in a group of inpatients who are in an experimental intervention program. You want to determine whether depression scores decline after participation in the program. You need to administer a depression scale before beginning the program and after its conclusion. Thus, it is important that the depression measure you select be reliable. If the measure is reliable, any change in depression scores that is observed after the intervention will indicate a "true" alteration in level of depression rather than a variation on a scale. •

However, there is always some error in measurement. A scale may not always be completely accurate. Suppose you measure a person's weight when he or she is wearing shoes; the next time you measure the person's weight without shoes. As another example, consider a tape measure that is not precisely held at the same place for each measure. This error is "random" in that it occurs by chance, and the nature of the error may vary with each measurement period.

Reliability represents an indication of the degree to which such random error exists in a measurement. A formal representation of *random error* in measurement is expressed by examining the relationship among three components: (1) the "true" score (T), which is unknown; (2) the observed score (O), which is derived from an instrument or other measurement process; and (3) an error score (E). An observed score is a function of the "true" score and some error. This tripartite relationship can be expressed as follows:

$$O = T + E$$

As you can see in this equation, the smaller the error term (E), the more closely O will approximate T. The standardization of study procedures and instruments serves to reduce this "random error" term. In a questionnaire, for example, a question that is clearly phrased and unambiguous will increase the questionnaire's reliability and decrease random error.

> You want to know whether your client is feeling depressed. You ask, "How do you feel today?" The client answers, "Fine," and then begins to weep. Obviously the client and you do not have the same question in mind, even though you both heard the same words. If you ask the client, "Do you feel depressed today?" you may be more likely to obtain the desired information. Although both questions refer to the same psychological state to you, the second question eliminates room for interpretation by the client. The client understands what you are asking and gives the answer that you seek. •

The point just illustrated holds true for measurement as well. Reduction of ambiguity decreases the likelihood of misinterpretation and thus error. Also, the longer the test or the more information collected to represent the underlying concept, the more reliable the instrument will become.

> If your client answers that he or she is not depressed but breaks down in your office and weeps, you may experience some cognitive dissonance. However, if you administer a scale to the client that asks multiple questions, all of which measure aspects of depressive behavior, you may be able to obtain a more accurate picture of your client's mood. •

Because all measurement techniques contain some random error (error that occurs by chance), reliability can exist only in degrees. The concept of reliability is thus expressed as a ratio between variation surrounding T (a "true" score) and variation of O (an observed score), as follows:

$$O = T + E$$

Because we can never know the "true" score, reliability represents an approximation to that "objective" reality. Reliability is expressed as a form of a "correlation coefficient" (we discuss these in detail in Chapter 17) that ranges from a low of 0 to a high of 1.00. The difference between the observed coefficient and 1.00 tells you what percentage of the score variance can be attributed to error. For example, if the coefficient is 0.65, then 0.35 reflects the degree of inconsistency of the instrument, and 65% of the observed variance is measuring an individual's "true" or actual score.

To assert reliability, experimental-type researchers frequently conduct statistical tests. These tests of reliability focus on three elements: stability, internal consistency, and equivalence (Table 17-2). The choice of a statistical test depends on the nature and intended purpose of the instrument.

Stability

Stability involves the consistency of repeated measures. "Test–retest" is a reliability test in which the same test is given twice to the same subject under the same circumstances.[4] It is assumed that the individual being tested should score the same on the test and retest. The degree to which the test and retest scores correlate (or are associated) is an indication of the stability of the instrument and its reliability.

TABLE 17-2	*Three Elements in Tests of Reliability*
Element	**Applicable Tests**
Stability	Test–retest
Internal consistency	Split-half technique Cronbach's alpha Kuder-Richardson formula
Equivalence	Interrater reliability
Alternate forms	

This measure of reliability is often used with physical measures and "paper-and-pencil" scales. (Note that we put quotation marks around the term "paper and pencil" to denote that it does not refer to the material of the instrument but rather to tests in which multiple items are completed by respondents. These may be delivered electronically as well.) The use of test–retest techniques is based on the assumptions that the phenomenon to be measured remains the same at two testing times and that any change is the result of random error.

Usually, physiological measures and equipment can be tested for stability in a short period, whereas text-based tests are retested in a 2-week to 1-month period. This approach to measuring reliability is not appropriate for instruments in which the phenomenon under study is expected to vary over time. For example, in the measurement of mood or any other transitory characteristic, we anticipate variations in the "true" score at each repeated testing occasion. Thus, a test–retest approach is not an appropriate way of indicating stability.[1,13]

Tests of Internal Consistency

Also referred to as "tests of homogeneity," tests of internal consistency are primarily used with "paper-and-pencil" instruments. In these tests, the issue of consistency is internally examined in relation to a composite score.

In the split-half technique, instrument items are split in half, and a correlational procedure is performed between the two halves. In other words, the scores on one half of the test are compared with the scores on the second half. The higher the correlation or relationship between the two scores, the greater

the reliability. Tests are typically split in half by comparing odd-numbered with even-numbered responses, by randomly selecting half of the items, or by splitting the instrument in half (e.g., questions 1 through 10 are compared with questions 11 through 20). This technique assumes that a person will consistently respond throughout a measure and therefore demonstrate consistent scores between the halves.[2]

Cronbach's alpha test and the Kuder-Richardson formula are two statistical procedures often used to examine the extent to which all the items in the instrument measure the same construct. The statistic generated is a correlation coefficient between the values of 0 and +1.00 in which a 0.80 correlation is interpreted as adequate reliability.[1] An "80% correlation" basically means that the test is consistent 80% of the time and that error may occur 20% of the time. A score close to +1.00 is most desirable because it indicates minimal error and maximal consistency.

Equivalence

Equivalence examines the extent to which the results of a test are consistent with measures that have been accurately used in the same population.[2] Two tests of equivalence are most often used by researchers: interrater reliability and alternate forms. The interrater reliability test involves the comparison of two observers measuring the same event. A test is given to one subject but scored by two or more raters, or the same rater observes and rescores an event on two occasions. The total number of agreements between raters or rating iterations is compared with the total number of possible agreements and multiplied by 100 to obtain the percentage of agreement. Eighty percent or above is considered to be an indication of a reliable instrument. As in the other tests of reliability, a higher score is more desirable than a lower score.

Consider the hypothetical data in Table 17-3. There are four potential chances for agreement, but only two occur among the raters. Agreement occurs in the ratio of 2 to 4 (2/4), or 1 to 2 (1/2), so interrater reliability is 50%. This would be an unacceptable finding, indicating that the researcher should not use this test under these circumstances. •

TABLE 17-3	*Example of Data for Interrater Reliability*
Rater 1	**Rater 2**
30	35
25	25
31	32
33	33

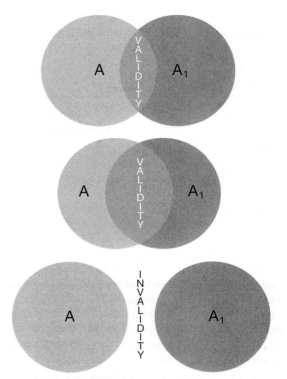

Figure 17-2 Three degrees of validity.

The alternate forms test, or "parallel forms" test, involves the comparison of two versions of the same "paper-and-pencil" instrument. In this case, two equivalent forms of one test are administered to one subject on the same testing occasion. The use of this technique depends on the availability of two equivalent versions of a form.

Equivalence may also be assessed by comparing the scores of two different instruments that measure the same construct, providing that the lexical definitions for each scale are the same as well.[14]

Validity

An indicator or measure must not only be reliable but valid as well. Referred to as instrument validity, this criterion addresses the critical issue of the relationship between a concept and its measurement. It asks whether what is being measured is a reflection of the underlying concept or to what extent are you measuring what you claim to be measuring. Figure 17-2 diagrams three degrees of validity and highlights how instrumentation (A1) only approximates the underlying concept (A). The closer an instrument comes to representing the "true" definition of the concept, the more valid the instrument.

Researchers argue whether the Wechsler Adult Intelligence Scale,[15] the traditional indicator of adult intelligence, actually measures what it purports to and whether it is valid for different cultures and populations. As with reliability, researchers can only approximate a perfectly valid instrument. Moreover, validity may vary with the intended purpose of the instrument and the specific population for whom it is developed or intended.[2] Thus, the Wechsler Adult Intelligence Scale may be a valid measure of intelligence as it has been traditionally defined for some groups and not for others.

Unlike reliability, the validation of an instrument occurs in many stages, over time, and with many populations. For example, a scale that assesses problem solving that is validated with college students may need further validation before being used with middle-aged and older persons. A scale that measures cognitive status in an older urban group may not be valid for rural Latino elders. Also, a scale that is valid is necessarily reliable, but the opposite may not be true. In other words, a scale may reliably or consistently measure the same phenomenon on repeated occasions, but it may not actually measure what it is intended to assess. Thus, validation of an instrument is extremely critical to ensure, to the extent possible, accuracy in measurement.

Whereas reliability is a measure of the random error of the measurement process itself, validity is a measure of systematic error, or "nonrandom error." *Systematic error* refers to a systematic bias or an error that consistently occurs. A weight scale that systematically and consistently weighs individuals 5 pounds heavier than an accurate scale is an example of systematic error and an invalid measurement. Note that, despite its invalidity, the scale is reliable as it is stable in its measurement.

A measure that systematically introduces error is a poor indicator of the underlying concept it intends to represent. Validity is therefore inversely related to the amount of systematic error present in an instrument: The smaller the degree of systematic error, the greater the validity of the instrument.

There are three basic types of validity that examine the degree to which an indicator represents its underlying concept: content, criterion, and construct.

Content Validity

Content validity is sometimes referred to as "face validity." It is considered the most basic form by which an instrument is validated. This type of validity addresses the degree to which the indicator reflects the basic content of the phenomenon or domain of interest. Ideally, the steps to obtain content validity include (1) specification of the full domain of a concept through a thorough literature search and (2) adequate representation of domains through the construction of specific items.

If all domains are known, the investigator can sample items that reflect each. The problem with content validity is twofold. First, for most concepts of interest to health and human service professionals, there is no agreed-on acceptance of the full range of content for any particular concept. Concepts such as wellness, poverty, health-related quality of life, depression, self-esteem, or physical function have been defined and conceptualized in many ways, but there is no unified understanding of the domains that constitute any of these concepts. Second, there is no agreed-on "objective" method for determining the extent to which a measure has attained an acceptable level of content validity. One way to obtain some degree of assuredness of content validity is to submit constructed items or drafts of a scale for review by a panel of experts. This review process can be repeated until agreement has been obtained as to the validity of each item. However, this process does not yield a coefficient or other statistical indicator to

discern the degree of agreement or the extent to which an instrument is content valid.

Criterion Validity

Criterion validity involves demonstrating a correlation or relationship between the measurement of interest and another instrument or standard that has been shown to be an accurate indicator of the same concept or construct being measured.[1] Central to the validation effort is that scores on a given construct should correlate with conceptually related constructs. Two types of criterion validity sought by researchers are concurrent and predictive.

Concurrent In concurrent criterion validity, there is a known standardized instrument or other criterion that measures/demonstrates the same underlying concept of interest (lexically defined in the same way). It is not unusual for researchers to develop instrumentation to measure concepts, even if prior instrumentation already exists.[1]

> Assume you are interested in developing your own measure of self-esteem. To establish concurrent validity, you will administer your instrument along with an accepted and validated instrument measuring the same concept to the same sample of individuals. The extent of agreement between the two measures, expressed as a correlation coefficient, will tell you whether your scale is accurately measuring the same construct operationalized in the validated scale. •

This form of validity can only be used if another criterion (existing validated instrument) exists. If so, the concurrent form is only as good as the validity of the selected criterion.

> You have developed a measure of physical functioning that you believe is more precise than existing measures. You are interested in examining the relationship between your measure and previously evaluated instruments, and you expect a strong relationship because they should be measuring the same underlying construct. •

Predictive Validity Predictive validity is used when the purpose of the instrument is to predict or estimate the occurrence of a behavior or event. For example, this type of validity can be used to evaluate whether an instrument designed to assess risk of falls can predict the incidence of falling. Agreement between the instrument and the criterion (a fall, or an established assessment of the risk of falling) is indicated by a correlation coefficient.

Discriminant

To establish validity, it is important to show not only that the instrument is associated with measures of the same concept but also that it is not associated with measures of concepts that are different. In establishing discriminant validity, you first need to hypothesize what measures you expect to be different from your instrument. Then you examine the level of agreement between the instrument and the criterion, as indicated by a correlation coefficient. In this case, you would want to see a correlation coefficient that is small and not statistically significant (see Chapter 20 for a discussion of statistical significance).

Construct Validity

Construct validity represents the most complex and comprehensive form of validation. Construct validity is used when an investigator has developed a theoretical rationale underlying the test instrument. The researcher moves through different steps to evolve supporting evidence of the relationship of the test instrument to related and distinct variables. Construct validity is based not only on the direct and full measurement of a concept, but also the theoretical principles related to the concept. Therefore, the investigator who attempts construct validity must consider how the measurement of the selected concept relates to other indicators of the same phenomenon.

> The researcher who is developing a measure of depression will base a set of expectations of the measurement outcome on sound theory about the nature of depression. If the instrument is a self-report of depression derived from cognitive-behavioral theory, the researcher will hypothesize that certain behaviors and thoughts, such as lethargy, agitation, appetite changes,

and melancholia, will frequently be found in subjects who score as "clinically depressed." Thus, the relationship of the scale score to other expected relationships will be measured as an indicator of construct validity. •

Validating a Scale

There are many complex approaches to establishing construct validity, including various types of factor analysis (see Chapter 20) and confirmatory structural equation modeling. This last procedure is very complex, so we refer you to advanced statistical resources for a detailed description of this technique.[16]

When validating a scale, it is good practice to consult with a psychometrician or statistician who is familiar with measurement development. The validation of a scale is ongoing; each form (content, criterion, and construct) builds on the other, occurs progressively or sequentially, and must be tested with different populations if the scale is to be widely used.

Considerations in Selecting a Measure

A basic action process in experimental-type research is selecting a measure to use in a study. A vast array of measures are available to health and human service researchers, and the selection of one measure over another should be based on a conscious recognition of the type of information that each measure will yield and its relative strengths and limitations.

Purpose of Assessment

In choosing a measure for your study, you first match the purpose of your investigation to the intent of a particular instrument. This step is the most elemental but critical action process for choosing a measure. You clearly articulate what you want to measure and why.

> Suppose you want to assess the physical function of older adults who enter your subacute rehabilitation facility after having a stroke. You decide on

the definition of physical function, which aspects of physical function you want to measure, and why. Assume you are introducing new clinical treatment guidelines for helping people who have experienced strokes with daily ambulation, and you anticipate being able to document significant improvements in mobility functioning at discharge. There are many measures of physical function,[17] but not every measure will match your specific purpose and the domain you need to target. You will need to select a measure that includes the ambulation items specific to your treatment focus and that rates physical performance using a response set that is sensitive enough to detect the types of changes in function that you are expecting will occur. For example, a measure that rates functional difficulty using a three-point scale (1 = no difficulty, 2 = some difficulty, 3 = cannot do at all) may not adequately detect small but clinically important changes from a treatment approach. However, a measure that scores level of dependence with more response options, such as a seven-point scale (7 = complete independence to 1 = complete dependence), may offer greater specification and opportunity to detect change before (pre) and after (post) rehabilitation. Similarly, a measure that involves observation of discrete movements could also be considered. •

The purpose of measuring a particular phenomenon is the initial driving force for selecting an instrument. If the purpose of measurement is not clear, then an inappropriate measure may be chosen, which in turn will significantly limit what you will be able to conclude from your study.

Psychometric Properties

After you have clearly articulated your study's purpose, you can focus on whether a particular instrument conforms to adequate standards of measurement. It is important to select measures that have stable characteristics and that have demonstrated reliability and validity, rather than using tools that lack adequate psychometric properties for the population you intend to study.[18] Given that the validation process occurs over time in multiple studies, it is important to examine what level of validation has been established for the measure you are selecting and for which populations. You can feel somewhat secure in using a new measure if it performs adequately compared with a well-tested measure, even if only convergent validation (the extent to which two measures of similar constructs are related) evidence is available. However, a tool for which only content validity has been established should be used with caution and the limitations identified in final reporting.

Population

The choice of a particular measure also largely depends on the study population you plan to recruit and enroll in your study. Diverse personal characteristics (e.g., age, cognitive status, background) may affect your decisions about the measure and the approach you choose to obtain information about the phenomenon of interest.[1]

You want to assess activities of daily living of individuals undergoing rehabilitation for stroke. In assessing mobility and navigation, you decide not to use self-report because individuals may not yield reliable ratings if they are unaware of changes in their own mobility. Also, the level of exposure of a particular person or group to the items included in a measurement protocol may be important to evaluate. Of this present cohort, a woman in her 90s may not have had prior experience with financial management (a typical question in measures assessing activities of daily living), so questioning her on level of performance in this area may not be particularly useful. The use of a standard measure that includes self-report and fiscal competency items would therefore provide an inconclusive understanding of actual performance and potential capabilities of the population you are testing. •

Also of concern is whether the measure has a "floor" or "ceiling" effect, such that it is not possible to obtain an adequate rating.

"Ceiling effect" is defined as "a measurement limitation that occurs when the highest possible score or close to the highest score on a test or measurement instrument is reached, thereby decreasing the likelihood that the testing instrument has accurately measured the intended domain"[4] (p 133). Thus changes in function for high scorers on pretest may not be observable, given that there is little room for improvement on the instrumentation.

A "floor effect" is similar to the ceiling effect but occurs at the lower end of the scoring range.[13] Most measures do not differentiate the types and levels of difficulty that may be present among healthy elder persons who do not experience difficulties or dependencies in traditional items of daily function that are assessed. Thus, for highly impaired persons who require total assistance in basic areas of daily activities, traditional measures may not sufficiently assess the components of a particular task that these persons can perform. Thus, there is a floor effect such that this population scores at the lowest level of the scale, with little differentiation possible within this group. •

Another population-related consideration is whether to select a measure that is useful for the population at large or a measure that is specific to a particular diversity issue.

Suppose you are interested in studying stress associated with providing care to persons with a severe impairment. You will need to decide between a general measure of stress or one that includes items specific to the experience of caregiving. A general measure may be preferred if your purpose is to compare caregiver and non-caregiver stress levels. However, if your purpose is to understand the specific aspects of caregiving that serve as stressors, a condition-specific stress measure would be more useful. •

Information Sources

Another consideration in selecting a measure is the source from which evaluative judgments will be obtained. Four basic sources of information are self-report, proxy, direct observation, and chart extraction (e.g., medical records, claims data). Each source has its own strengths and limitations. Your decision of source from which to obtain information will be influenced not only by your purpose but also by your resources (e.g., time, money, expertise).

Self-Report

Self-report involves asking persons to rate themselves using a standard metric. Self-report information can be obtained by a face-to-face or phone interview or through a "paper and pencil" survey. The use of a self-report approach usually does not require special expertise, although some interviewer training is helpful. This is a quick, relatively simple, and cost-effective approach for obtaining information.

Self-report has some limitations, however, and may not be useful for all study populations.[19]

If you are interested in obtaining functional status information, research has shown that community-living older people tend to overestimate their abilities, underestimate their level of dependence, and may be unaware of unsafe interactions in carrying out daily activities within their living environment.[17] Also, poor sense of personal mastery and feeling depressed may lead to underestimating performance capabilities. Persons with cognitive impairment also tend to be "unreliable" sources of information about their health and functioning, often reporting greater functional ability than that reported by their caregivers. •

Also, the test–retest reliability of self-report is unclear; certain domains of living may be more amenable to self-report than other domains, and the validity and reliability of obtaining self-report are unclear when using different modalities (e.g., phone interview vs. home visit).

Nevertheless, increasing evidence supports the important contribution of the self-report perspective to derive a comprehensive understanding of a person's health and well-being. Self-reports on health and function are highly predictive of actual performance, mortality, psychological well-being, and future expenditures for health care.[20]

Another benefit of self-report is that this method often allows for a type of causal attribution when a researcher cannot structure a true experiment. Let us look at how this might occur.

Suppose you are interested in determining the extent to which your new intervention was responsible for improving the symptoms of clinical depression. You select a sample of convenience from your client group who meet the inclusion criteria for that diagnosis and conduct a pretest, posttest only design using a standardized depression inventory that meets your lexical definition of depression (see Chapter 10). Because this design can only examine change in scores, you add the following closed-ended question to the posttesting protocol:

Please rate the extent to which your participation in this program improved your mood:
   Not at all; slightly; somewhat; a great deal

Although subject to the limitations of self-report and social desirability, this type of evaluative questioning provides some evidence for attribution that would not be possible with the constraints of the testing conditions. Cautious reporting and highlighting the limitations of this strategy would be warranted.

Proxy

The use of a *proxy*, or informant, is another important source of information, particularly in a clinical setting. This approach involves asking a family member, a health care professional, or an individual familiar with the targeted person to rate that person on the phenomenon of interest using a standard measure. As in self-report, ratings from a proxy may be obtained through a face-to-face encounter, phone interview, or "paper and pencil" survey. Proxies play a critical role in obtaining health information, particularly for individuals who may not be able to self-report or evaluate their performance accurately.

At issue, however, is the validity of informant responses and the specific factors that may inflate or otherwise influence proxy ratings. Proxy ratings may be affected by factors such as the relationship of the informant to the person, gender, or co-residence.[21] Although the specific role of gender, education, age, and relationship is unclear, evidence suggests that co-residency may enhance the accuracy of proxy responses.

Direct Observation

Measures that use direct observation of real-time performance tend to be task oriented, highly structured, and accurate. The performance of each step or component of an activity can be observed and numerically rated for its successful completion along a series of dimensions, including the time for activity completion and the need for verbal and tactile cueing. Performance-based measures tend to yield precise judgments of particular aspects of an activity and can be accomplished under supervision for safety. These measures also offer an exacting assessment tool to guide intervention and may be especially useful when self-report and proxy are not possible or not good choices.[22]

Nevertheless, direct observation does have several important limitations. First, performance-based measures need to be administered by highly trained raters and thus are often more costly to administer. Second, direct assessment of a specific area of activity may require special setup or stations in a clinic (e.g., use of the cafeteria) or home setting that may not be feasible to implement. Third, this approach can be time-consuming, even though only a few select skill areas may be observed. Fourth, observing an individual simulate an activity in one setting may still not provide an assessment of how an individual performs in another setting. There is little research to date from which to determine whether a simulated context is ecologically valid or whether ratings derived in the constructed settings reflect daily performance. Fifth, timed performance-based measures have a wide range of test–retest reliability, particularly for unfamiliar tasks or tasks that do not have discrete start and stop points.

Chart Extraction

Another common source of information, particularly in clinical research, is extraction of recordings from provider notes and charts, many of which are now electronic and easily accessible with permission. This method is an inexpensive, relatively simple approach from which to derive specific types of information, such as health status, numbers and types of medications, physical function, and psychological well-being. However, professionals may rate phenomena differently, and it is not clear whether ratings in health records reflect the outcome of a standard assessment or whether they are anecdotal and based on casual observations.

Online Surveys

With the ubiquitous use of the Internet on mobile devices and computers, online surveys are now a major source from which to obtain data. Many instruments that had been administered through the mail or in person through actual paper and pencil methods are now hosted on websites in electronic format. For example, the Wechsler Adult Intelligence Scale (WAIS IV) now is offered in digital format. Look at this description:

> To administer a test in Q interactive, the examiner and examinee use wireless tablets that are synched with each other so that the examiner can read administration instructions, time and capture response information (including audio recording), and control the examinee's tablet. The examinee tablet displays visual stimuli and captures touch responses.[23]

When developing and hosting your own survey, there are many easy-to-use apps and software to facilitate the development of items, dissemination of the survey, and subsequent analysis and summary of results. Online surveys are easy to create, but of course all of the principles discussed earlier about sound instrumentation apply.

In developing an online survey, you first need to have a clear purpose and understanding of what you want to measure. Items must be brief and clear. Testing items for their clarity before executing an online survey is important to ensure that questions can be easily understood. When developing digital surveys, items should be brief, taking anywhere from 10 to 20 minutes of a responder's time. Holding the interest of the responder is important. Promising that participation will be brief can be an important consideration for a potential responder. The researcher does not have any control over when a potential responder will see and then participate in an online survey, who actually is responding, and whether the items are answered completely and honestly. Keeping the survey brief and adding features that enable the responder to see how far he/she has advanced are simple techniques to increase the response rate for your Web survey.

Another consideration using an online approach is the targeted population. First, consider whether the persons from whom you seek data would participate in the format of an online survey. Second, consider who you will be missing by using this data collection technique; you may want to reach persons who for many reasons will not or cannot respond to digital formats.

Item Selection

Another important consideration in selecting a measure is determining whether the items you have included are adequate for the purpose of your study. We addressed this point earlier, in the discussion of validity. Remember that your items must be exhaustive as well as mutually exclusive.

Consider the study previously cited on the physical functioning of people who have had strokes, specifically their ability to ambulate after a therapeutic regimen. If you are interested in deriving ratings of "level of dependence" in ambulation and transferring, you will need to ensure that your selected functional measure includes the items that are important to your purpose. •

Consider another example. A number of health and fitness assessments, such as the YMCA Fitness assessment, measure physical endurance and cardiovascular health for standard bodies. Individuals who use mobility devices or do not have both lower extremities may be in excellent health, but the items will not only fail to capture their high level of fitness but will likely place them in an unhealthy category. Asking about mobility ability and endurance by restricting its operational definition to specific types of activities such as walking, cycling, performing sit-ups, and so forth is a source of instrument invalidity for specific populations. •

Response Sets

You not only have to consider which items are included in a measure but also whether the response set is suitable for your study purpose. A response set is defined as the tendency for respondent to answer questions in a preferred or similar fashion regardless of the content of the question.

It is likely that most if not all of us have been asked to rate our courses on a standardized measure. We might even have rated everything as highly desirable even if we did not like the class. This last point brings us to the structure and crafting of an instrument.

Constructing an Instrument

Health and human service professionals frequently find that measures must be newly constructed to fit the study or clinical research purpose. The development of a new measure in experimental-type research should always include a plan for testing its reliability and some level of validity (content, at the minimum) to ensure a level of accuracy and rigor to the study findings. These tasks can be complex and time-consuming, and investigators often develop different strategies to address measurement issues. Some investigators combine previously tested and well-established measures with a newly constructed measure to test their relationships and relative strengths in the study and provide evidence of reliability and validity.

The development of new instrumentation is, in itself, a specialty in the world of experimental-type research. We have introduced the basic components of the measurement process and have provided some principles for ensuring that your items are reliable. However, constructing an instrument and its components is a major research task (Boxes 17-4 and 17-5). Many sources of error interfere with the reliability and validity of an instrument.

Let us consider the process illustrated in Box 17-4. As we have discussed, literature review is the first step. A theory is identified that fits with your view of reality and meets the purpose of your study. Selecting and lexically defining the full range and scope of constructs to be measured are the next tasks. The format of the instrument is then decided (e.g., survey, interview schedule), and items are then developed with response structures that provide the desired data. Once developed, the instrument is tested for psychometric properties.

Of particular importance, as presented in Box 17-5, is the clarity of both the items and the response structures. We now introduce some basic rules for fixed-response questions.

First, avoid double-barreled questions. These types of questions are really two or more questions with only a single response. How would you answer the following question:

Do you like chocolate and vanilla ice cream? (select one response)
   Yes   No

In this example, what if the respondent only likes one of the flavors? How is he/she going to answer? And how will the investigator know what the answer means?

Second, don't ask questions that have an obvious or desired answer. How would you answer the following?

Don't you think that your health provider is competent?

Third, do not ask vague questions. How might you answer this question?

Did the exercise program work?
   Not at all   Somewhat   Totally

BOX 17-4   *Basic Steps in Constructing an Instrument*

1. Review the literature for relevant instrumentation.
2. Identify the theory from which to develop a new instrument.
3. Specify the concept or construct to be operationalized into an instrument.
4. Conceptually define the full range and content of the concept.
5. Select an instrument format.
6. Translate the concept into specific items or indicators with appropriate response categories.
7. Test the instrument.

BOX 17-5   *Considerations in Developing an Instrument*

1. Format or design of the instrument
2. Clarity of the instrument
3. Social desirability of the questions
4. Variation in administration
5. Situational contaminants
6. Response set biases (all "yes" or all "no" responses)

Here the investigator did not specify the desired outcome. Did the program work to do what?

Make your questions understandable. How might you answer the following?

Rate the extent to which you did not like the class.
  Not at all   Very much

These are only some basic examples of question construction errors. We refer you to the excellent resources on instrument construction in the references for more detailed information. For novices and even seasoned researchers, it is often a good decision to consider consultation.

Administering the Instrument

An instrument in experimental-type research can be administered by self-report using "paper-and-pencil" methods, direct observation of the phenomena of interest, face-to-face interview of the subject or a proxy, or phone. Even video chatting, social networking, and research in virtual worlds such as Second Life[24] are being used by researchers to conduct their studies. Regardless of the medium, it is important to standardize the administration of an instrument, particularly when more than one person is obtaining information for a study. The influence of the data collector or venue can potentially confound the findings. Consider the following example.

You and another investigator are studying perceived quality of life in a nursing home environment. You both have a set of questions with a closed-ended response set to be answered by the subjects. You begin your interview with a "thank you" statement and then ask the questions, whereas the other interviewer discusses the respondent's poor health status before beginning the interview schedule. In your data analysis, you find that the subjects you interviewed tend to be more satisfied with their lives than those interviewed by the other investigator. Is it possible that the second investigator influenced the respondents by discussing potentially depressing issues before administering the instrumentation?   •

This scenario highlights the importance of training for data collectors. Training is essential (1) to ensure that data collection procedures are the same for all data collection action processes and (2) to reduce bias that can be introduced by investigator differences. Establishing a strict protocol for administering an interview and training interviewers in that protocol will result in standardization of procedures to ensure "objective measurement."

A Few Words About Big Data

Before we leave this chapter, we bring your attention to one more emergent source of data: big data, the huge repositories of data often generated through the Internet or other computer-assisted methods.[25] These sources provide valuable information for analyzing health and human service trends, needs, and patterns across the globe. We do not discuss these methods further here as they are beyond the scope of the text. However, because big data collection and analysis are major contemporary methods that can be subjected to precise measurement, they may have much to contribute to knowledge in health and human services.

Summary

Data collection instruments for experimental-type designs vary in structure (open or closed), level of measurement, objectivity (reliability and validity), structure, and scope. The purpose of data collection is to ensure minimal researcher obtrusiveness through the systematic and consistent application of procedures. The researcher minimizes systematic and random errors through validation and reliability testing, respectively. Other procedures are developed to ensure consistency in obtaining data (Box 17-6).

BOX 17-6 *Enhancing Consistency in Obtaining Information*
Establish testing procedures and protocols
Establish when and how subjects are contacted
Establish a script by which to describe the study

Reliability and validity represent two critical considerations when a data collection instrument is selected or developed. When experimental-type research is conducted, the researcher's first preference is the selection of instruments that have demonstrated reliability and validity for the specific populations or phenomena the investigator wants to study. In health and human service research, however, as in other substantive or content areas (e.g., diversity, disability, caregiving, gerontology, children, family function), instruments to measure relevant researchable concepts may be limited, particularly as new theory and understandings of health and well-being are developed. Because reliable and valid instruments may not be available to fit the purpose and theoretical orientations of a study, some professional organizations and agencies, such as the Health Resources and Services Administration and National Institutes of Health, have placed a high priority on funding research directed at the development of data collection instruments. As we discussed and demonstrated in some basic questioning errors, instrument development is a precise set of knowledge and skills and often calls for consultation.

We concluded with a few words about big data to bring your attention to this huge and productive source of data.

EXERCISES

1. Develop at least five questions on a Likert-type scale to measure job satisfaction among your peers. Ask at least three of your peers to respond to the questions. Ask each to indicate the clarity of the questions. Do you need to revise the questions? Did the questions appear to measure what you intended?
2. Using job satisfaction as your construct, develop a Guttman scale and a semantic differential scale. What are the advantages and disadvantages of each? Ask your peers to respond to these questions, and compare the responses.
3. With a peer, observe a child in a playground and independently attempt to determine the child's age. Record the criteria used to make your judgment. Compare your impressions with those of your peer to determine the extent of interrater reliability.
4. Identify an online survey website and create a survey on it. Try it out with your peers to evaluate its adequacy in measuring the construct that you hope to measure. Compare this digital medium to other forms of administration for ease of access, ease of creating a survey, likelihood of obtaining a large response rate, and limitations of this approach.

References

1. Babbie E: *Practice of social research*, ed 13, Belmont, Calif, 2012, Wadsworth.
2. DeVellis RF: *Scale development: theory and applications*, Thousand Oaks, Calif, 2012, Sage.
3. McDermott L: *Human sexuality*, Saddle River, NJ, 2006, Pearson.
4. Salkind N: *Tests & measurement for people who (think they) hate tests & measurement*, Los Angeles, 2013, Sage.
5. Crane DR, Middleton KC, Bean RA: Establishing criterion scores for the Kansas Marital Satisfaction Scale and the Revised Dyadic Adjustment Scale. *Am J Fam Ther* 28:53–60, 2000.
6. Zung WK: A rating instrument for anxiety disorders. *Psychosomatics* 12:371–379, 1971.
7. Olson DH: FACES-IV. *J Marriage Fam Ther* 3:64–80, 2011.
8. Spielberger CD, et al: Assessment of anxiety: the State-Trait Anxiety Scale. *Adv Pers* 2005-2008. <http://www.mindgarden.com/products/staisad.htm#about>.
9. Reynolds DJ, Stiles WB, Grohol JM: An investigation of session impact and alliance in Internet based psychotherapy: preliminary results. *Couns Psychother Res* 6:164–168, 2006.
10. Radloff LS: The CES-D Scale: a self report depression scale for research in the general population. *Appl Psychol Meas* 1:385–401, 1977.
11. Stewart AL, Ware JE, editors: *Measuring functioning and well-being: the medical outcomes study approach*, Durham, NC, 1992, Duke University Press.
12. Stouffer SA: *Communism, conformity and civil liberties*, New York, 1955, Doubleday.
13. Dunn-Rankin P, Knezek GA, Wallace SR, et al: *Tasks. Scaling methods*, ed 2, Englewood, NJ, 2004, Erlbaum, pp 11–38.
14. Trustees of the University of Indiana: *Reliability*, 2014. <http://nsse.iub.edu/html/reliability.cfm>.
15. *Wechsler Adult Intelligence Scale—Fourth Edition*, 2014. <http://www.pearsonclinical.com/psychology/products/100000392/wechsler-adult-intelligence-scalefourth-edition-wais-iv.html?Pid=015-8980-808>.
16. Kline RB: *Principles and practice of structural equation modeling*, ed 3, New York, 2011, Guilford.
17. Gitlin LN: *Physical function in the elderly: a comprehensive guide to its meaning and measurement*, 2005, ProEd Press.

18. Furr RM, Bacharach VR: *Psychometrics: an introduction*, Los Angeles, 2014, Sage.

19. Salkind N: *Encyclopedia of research design*, Los Angeles, 2010, Sage.

20. Pacala JT, Boult C, Urdangarin C, et al: Using self-reported data to predict expenditures of the health care of older people. *J Am Geriatr Soc* 51:609–614, 2003.

21. Elliot M, Beckett M, Chong K, et al: How do proxy responses and proxy-assisted responses differ from what Medicare beneficiaries might have reported about their health care? *Health Serv Res* 43:833–848, 2007.

22. Mitchell M, Miller JS, Woodward MS, et al: 2011, Regression-based estimates of observed functional status in centenarians. *Gerontologist* 51:179–189, 2011.

23. Daniel MH: *Equivalence of Q-Interactive-administered cognitive tasks, WISC-IV*, 2012. <http://www.helloq.co.uk/content/dam/ped/ani/uk/helloq/downloads/wais-iv-tech-report.pdf>.

24. Dean E: *Survey research in virtual worlds*, N.D. <http://www.rti.org/brochures/srvyresvirtualworlds.pdf>.

25. Sicignano M: *Big data analysis and quality improvement in social services*, December 21, 2012. <http://www.socialjusticesolutions.org/2012/12/21/big-data-analysis-and-quality-improvement-in-social-services>.

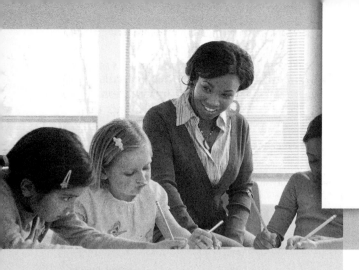

Chapter 18
Gathering Information in Naturalistic Inquiry

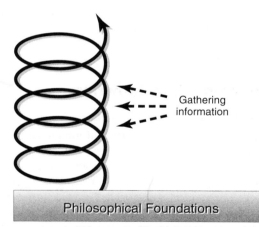

Gathering information

Philosophical Foundations

Gathering information in naturalistic forms of inquiry involves a set of investigative actions that are quite divergent in purpose, approach, and process from experimental-type research. In naturalistic inquiry, knowledge emerges from and is embedded in the unique and shared understandings of human phenomena in context.

The overall purpose of gathering information in naturalistic inquiry is to uncover multiple and diverse perspectives or underlying patterns that illuminate, describe, relate, and even predict the phenomena under study within the context in which phenomena occur. By "context," we mean the physical, virtual, intellectual, social, economic, cultural, spiritual, and other types of environments in which human experience unfolds. Thus, different from experimental-type approaches, which also aim to predict, the processes of collecting information in naturalistic inquiry serve as discovery and revelation in a contextual field, not verification or falsification of a theory through the specification, collection, and analysis of data in a carefully controlled environment. The investigator gathers sufficient information that leads to description, discovery, understanding, interpretation, meaning, and explanation of the rich mosaic of contextual human experiences.

As you now know, many distinct perspectives compose the rubric of naturalistic inquiry. Thus, there is wide variation in the information-gathering approaches used by researchers conducting studies in this tradition. For example, in semiotics the focus of data collection is on discourse, symbol, and context.[1] In classic ethnography, the focus of data collection may be broader than in semiotics and may include verbal exchanges, behavioral patterns, and physical objects.[2]

Four Information-Gathering Principles

Although the process of gathering information differs across the types of naturalistic inquiry, four basic principles provide guidance for action: (1) the nature of the investigator's involvement; (2) the inductive, abductive process of gathering information, analyzing the information, and gathering more information; (3) the time commitment in the actual or virtual field; and (4) the use of multiple data collection strategies.

Investigator Involvement

In experimental-type research, investigators implement a set of procedures designed to remove themselves from informal or nonstandardized interactions with study participants. Naturalistic inquiry, however, is based on *investigator involvement* and active participation (to a greater or lesser degree) with people

TABLE 18-1 *Investigator Involvement in Gathering Information From Study Participants in Naturalistic Designs*

Type of Naturalistic Inquiry	Investigator Involvement
Endogenous team decisions	Variable; flexible; depends on study
Participatory action team decisions	Variable; flexible; depends on study
Phenomenological	Active listener
Heuristic	Fully participatory
Life history	Active listener
Ethnographic	Fully participatory
Grounded theory	Fully participatory

and other sources of information, such as artifacts, written historical documents or virtual text and image, and pictorial representations. When working directly with humans, the quality of the data collected often depends on the investigator's ability to develop trust, rapport, and mutual respect with those participating in or being studied. The level and nature of the investigator's involvement with people and other sources of information, however, depend on the specific type of naturalistic study that is pursued (Table 18-1).

In most forms of naturalistic inquiry—but particularly in classic ethnography, life history,[3] grounded theory, and heuristic designs—the process of eliciting stories, personal experiences, and the telling of events is based on a relationship or bond that forms between the investigator and the informant. Some researchers characterize this bond as a "collaborative endeavor" or "partnership." In these approaches to inquiry, the primary instrument for gathering trustworthy information from study participants is the investigator.

The investigator as a data-gathering instrument is a logical extension of the primary contention of naturalistic inquiry. This position, shared by many forms of naturalistic inquiry, maintains that the only way to "know" about the "lived" experiences of individuals is to become intimately involved and familiar with the life situations or representations of those who experience them. The extreme of this position is found in heuristic inquiry, in which the investigator examines his or her personal lived experience.[4] In phenomenological research, the investigator develops rapport with study participants but engages in active listening to understand the experiences of others.[1] In ethnography, the researcher, as the primary data-gathering instrument, strives for intimate familiarity with the people and context in the study. By engaging in an active learning process through looking, watching, listening, participating, interviewing, and reviewing materials, the investigator enters the "life world" of others and uncovers what it means to live those experiences.[2]

In endogenous and participatory action research, the level of investigator involvement in data collection varies depending on the way in which the study team chooses to proceed. In these forms of naturalistic inquiry, the investigator tends to serve more as a facilitator of the research process and may or may not be directly involved in the various data collection strategies implemented by the team of participants.[1]

Naturalistic forms of inquiry may employ others in the data-gathering process in addition to the primary investigators. This strategy is particularly useful in studies involving multiple field sites or when the volume of interviews is high and requires assistance from others, who may be researchers, the subjects of the inquiry, or individuals trained in the rigorous procedures that characterize the study. In these cases, the investigator and data gatherers form a team and work together to develop consensus on methods and style to ensure similarity and consistency in the use of techniques for building rapport, as well as for probing and eliciting responses. To obtain a comprehensive understanding of the data, the team must also work together to share impressions, notes, and emerging analytical categories and themes.

For example, let's say you want to conduct a study to examine the attitudes of rural residents toward law enforcement's role in substance abuse prevention in a particular geographic region of the United States. Because the geographic area of interest is vast, more than one investigator is necessary to collaborate on the project and gather data. You form a team of investigators composed of parents, health and social service professionals, and students,

and you all meet every 2 weeks to discuss and agree on where to obtain interview data, how to conduct the interviews, and how to record and aggregate responses. Although each member of the team has a particular style and preferred methodologies, all agree on how best to identify and approach informants, type and level of probing questions, and initial analytic approach.

Information Collection and Analysis

In naturalistic inquiry, the act of gathering information is intimately entwined with analysis—that is, collecting data and conducting analysis reciprocally inform one another and are not sequences in a linear fashion.[1] Thus, once established in context, the investigator evaluates the information obtained through observation, examination of artifacts and images, recorded interviews, and participation in relevant activities. These initial analytical efforts detail the "who, what, when, and where" aspects of the context, which in turn are used to further define and refine subsequent data collection efforts and directions.

The dynamic process of ongoing data gathering, analysis, and more data gathering can be graphically represented by the "spiral" design used in this text. In the spiral, as analysis and data collection are refined, the investigator moves from a broad conception of the field to a more in-depth, richer, and "thick" understanding and, when indicated in the design, an interpretation of multiple field "realities."[5]

Time Commitment in the Context

The amount of time spent immersed in a physical or virtual context varies greatly across the types of naturalistic inquiry. In some studies, understanding a natural or virtual setting can be time-consuming because of the complexity of the initial query and the context that is being studied. In any type of naturalistic inquiry, however, the investigator must become totally immersed in the setting or involved with the phenomenon of study. "Immersion" means that the investigator must spend sufficient time in the context to ensure that a complete description is produced. In ethnographic research, spending time "hanging out"—interviewing, observing, and participating—has traditionally been called "prolonged engagement" in the field.[5] In classic and most forms of contemporary ethnography, prolonged engagement is essential to ensure that the investigator reaches an in-depth understanding of the particular cultural group of focus.[6] In other types of naturalistic design, engagement may be structured in diverse sequences, such as immersion on specific days and times or for specific events.

So how much time is necessary? The amount of time spent in the field may vary from specified hours each day or week to a few months to years, depending on the nature of the initial query and its scope, the availability of resources that support the investigator in the endeavor, the amount of time available to the investigator, and the specific design strategy that is followed.

Assume that you want to examine the initial meanings attributed to the diagnosis of breast cancer among women in their 20s. Using naturalistic inquiry even with such a focused query could require a few months of interviewing women in this age group who have recently learned of their diagnosis. Or you might even spend several hours in a group interview with this same group of informants, significantly reducing the time. Even if you plan to observe providers interacting with these women, your observations will be confined to this early treatment phase.

In contrast, assume you want to examine the experiences of women as they move through the stages of biopsy, diagnosis, surgery, chemotherapy, and the uncertainty of the future. Compared with the first study, this query is broader in scope and will require following a group of women over time. It may require up to 9 months or 1 year of the investigator's time to observe and interview women at each of these different stages, as well as to conduct interviews with their significant others and providers, to understand the full impact of the sequence of events. But what if you had limited resources and time, preventing you from engaging in face-to-face interviews with individuals or groups? You might enter the virtual field through an Internet site devoted to interaction among women newly diagnosed with breast cancer. Through the virtual field, you could access their interaction as a third-party observer or even participant. Your time commitment could therefore be reduced to specific hours of the day, text-based interactions, and so forth. •

Whether spending a short period or a long time in the study, the investigator must determine the point at which sufficient information has been obtained. At that point, the investigator leaves the context and engages in a final analytic or interpretive process that involves preparing one or more final reports. This point is sometimes referred to as *saturation*.[7] Indications of saturation include the investigator no longer being puzzled or surprised by observations, events, or by what people say; the investigator predicting behaviors or outcomes; and information becoming redundant compared with information already collected and learned by the investigator. When the researcher begins to hear the same story repeatedly, can predict what a respondent is going to say, or can anticipate image, text, and meaning, it is time to cease collection of data (see later discussion on saturation).

Multiple Information-Gathering Strategies

Some methodologists suggest that by its nature, all naturalistic inquiry is multimethod.[8] Because we define "multimethod" as the use of strategies from more than one research tradition, we disagree, because we do not see naturalistic inquiry as multimethod in itself. However, part of the naturalistic tradition is often characterized by the typical use of numerous data collection methods in a single study. Because different approaches are designed to derive information from numerous sources, the use of multiple methods to obtain information enhances the investigator's capacity to acquire a complex and rich understanding of the phenomenon under study. It is therefore common practice to use more than one data collection method even if a query is small in scope. Throughout and at the end of the data collection process, all sources of information are analyzed to ensure that they support a rich descriptive or interpretive scheme and set of conclusions.

Investigators can use varied data-gathering strategies, many of which are discussed later in the chapter. In most types of naturalistic inquiry, investigators may not know before entering the study exactly which strategies they will use. Although thought and planning occur in all phases of naturalistic inquiry, the final decision to use a particular approach to collecting information occurs as the research evolves. As noted, an important part of the naturalistic process of data collection occurs during inquiry, throughout which the investigator must decide which data collection techniques to use and at which point each should be introduced.

No standard approach is available to indicate which strategy should be used and when it should be introduced across the different forms of naturalistic inquiry. Data collection decisions are specific to the research query, the preferred way of knowing by the investigator, and the contextual opportunities that emerge. In a phenomenological study, for example, some investigators prefer to interview respondents first and then review written documents, virtual sources, journals, medical records, and other materials. In this type of study, it is considered critical initially to listen in an interview to the emotions and feelings naturally expressed by individuals asked to reflect on their experiences. Reading the literature or other textual sources before the interviewing process may introduce deductive thinking or preconceived analytical frames that may preclude attentive listening to the experiences of individuals. In contrast, some ethnographers prefer to begin by "hanging out" in the field and using the data collection strategy of observation before introducing interviewing or other collecting strategies. Still other investigators start with conducting open-ended interviews with key informants and then engage in observation. Other strategies, such as recordings, standardized questionnaires, or review of documents or images, may be introduced at subsequent stages of a study.[6]

Consider this example. Suppose you are interested in learning about the benefit of virtual-world interaction to individuals who interact on disability networks and blogs. There are numerous ways you could enter this field. You might join and virtually hang out as an avatar, or you might immediately start a conversation with another avatar in the virtual field. These methods would serve the purpose of gaining entry into the context of interest, but each would elicit a different scope of information and guide you in a different direction for further information gathering.

Overview of Principles

The hallmark of gathering information for the naturalistic researcher is that this action process is purposive and occurs in and is responsive to the context in which the study is taking place. Data-gathering actions are designed to examine context and all relevant phenomena that occur within it. No standardized data collection procedures structure studies. Rather, the critical components of information-gathering actions tend to be diverse, based on the particular form of inquiry and the investigator's ongoing judgments about what approaches can elicit the most relevant and illuminating data. Usually, the investigator is actively involved in the context over a prolonged time to ensure sufficient immersion. However, the level of investigator involvement varies depending on the form of inquiry. In all forms of naturalistic inquiry, best practice involves the use of multiple strategies to obtain information in an ongoing and integrated data collection and analytical process.

These basic components or guiding principles in data gathering yield descriptions, interpretations, and understandings of phenomena that are embedded in specific contexts and complex interrelationships. Complexity is preserved in all representations and reports by the nature of the data-gathering process. Let us examine how these principles are implemented and how obtaining in naturalistic inquiry actually proceeds.

Information-Gathering Process

What is the process of gathering information in the naturalistic tradition? Although the methods have been variably defined, we have built on the classic and enduring structure suggested by Shaffir and Stebbins[9] in the early 1990s because of its simplicity and comprehensiveness. Shaffir and Stebbins viewed the action process of data collection in naturalistic inquiry as four interrelated parts or considerations: context selection and "getting in the field," "learning the ropes" or obtaining meanings of the setting, "maintaining relations," and "leaving the field."[9] We have replaced the term "field" with "environment" and the term "learning the ropes" with "gaining familiarity" to depict the diversity of settings in which naturalistic inquiry is enacted and the topical areas that now extend naturalistic research beyond learning about remote cultures. Although these actions appear to represent distinct phases or research steps, the process is integrated; each component overlaps and shapes the other.

Selecting the Context

The first decision about data collection in naturalistic research is where or in what context information should be obtained. The researcher must "bound" the study by depicting a context that is conceptual, virtual, or locational (see Chapters 13 and 15). Because naturalistic research focuses on the natural research context, as well as what happens within it, selection of a context is an important factor in gathering data. The context may be the private lives of famous people, the interrelationships of a surgical team, the world of hospice specialists, the meaning of disability to avatars in a virtual disability world, or the meanings of caregiving to immigrant families.

Context selection may sound simple, but there are several important considerations. First, the specification of a context must be practical or realistic to study. For example, how realistic is it to propose an inquiry to study the private lives of famous people? Will you be able to gain access to such individuals? Will these people choose to participate in this type of study, given that agreement will jeopardize their privacy?

Second, in bounding a study to a particular context, the researcher must be careful not to limit the focus and thus the opportunity to obtain a full picture of the phenomenon under investigation. Consider the following examples.

> Assume you want to study how children with diagnoses of learning disabilities learn to adapt to their learning styles. Identifying the classroom as the main context of the investigation may be too narrow. It may enable you to identify and describe the strategies that children use in that context, but it may not enable you to understand the full range of adaptive mechanisms that are used in learning in other contexts and how these mechanisms are obtained. •

> Suppose you are interested in studying the interrelationships and behaviors of a surgical team. You initially plan to examine the interactions of the surgical team during surgery. However, observation of this context may be too limiting. It may not yield a complete understanding of the interprofessional relationships that inform interactions in the specific context of surgery. Examining professional behaviors in other environments, such as in the cafeteria, at staff meetings, or in social engagements, may provide important insights. •

> Consider a third example. You are interested in examining the functional capacities of persons with traumatic brain injuries. If the context for the study is the clinical rehabilitation setting, the informant may be maximally functional in this particular environment. The investigator who does not expand the scope to include other locations may not discover the functional incapacity that the person with traumatic brain injury often exhibits in less structured settings. •

It is important to recognize that identifying the context of a naturalistic study will depend, in part, on the nature of the query, the design strategy, and the characteristics of the persons being studied.

Gaining Access

After the context for the research endeavor is identified, the investigator must gain access to it. This is not as simple as it may sound. *Gaining access* to the context of the study may require strategizing, negotiating with key individuals who may serve as gatekeepers, registering for a virtual world and even creating an avatar, and perhaps renegotiating after initial entry has occurred. In some cases, the investigator may already be a part of the natural context (emic status).

Suppose you are a student and want to understand the process of becoming a health professional following graduation. As a student in health care, you are actually an "insider" (emic) of part of the particular context. Although access is not a problem in student professional socialization, access to other aspects of environments may be challenging.

However, even as an "insider student," you will have to work hard to understand how your new knowledge and previous experiences influence the information you gather and interpret.

> Consider a situation in which you are a regular reader of a listserv devoted to the discussion of disability rights and are examining the texts of postings to determine how rights are conceptualized and experienced. As a regular "lurker," you are knowledgeable about the lives and experiences of those who post. However, you must be careful to identify this information as different from analysis of the actual posted texts as you analyze the textual data for meanings. Moreover, as an insider, you will also analyze how your understandings, biases, values, and experiences influence your interpretation of Web-based text. ●

If the investigator is an "outsider" (etic), access must be obtained. Mechanisms for gaining access have been extensively discussed in the literature, particularly by ethnographers.[6,7,9] How the researcher gains access into a context can influence the entire course of the research process. Gaining access involves obtaining permission to enter and become part of a setting. Investigators may use different strategies, depending on the nature of the context and their initial relationship to the setting. Formal introduction to an informant by another, slowly building rapport through participation, joining a club or virtual context, liking a Facebook page, and gift giving are techniques used by investigators to enter an environment. Consider the following example.

> You want to conduct a study in a medical setting. To gain access, initially it will be important to discuss the nature of your study with the directors of the departments you want to include. This discussion will be followed by a more normal introduction to medical personnel in staff meetings. ●

Now consider the example of gaining access to a teen group where you are interested in studying the meaning of "hanging out" to the teens. Our students

> **BOX 18-1** *Considerations in Gaining Access*
>
> 1. Presenting study to participants
> 2. Ensuring confidentiality
> 3. Minimizing impact of investigator on natural context

conducted such a study, in which they asked teens what "hanging out" meant and what activities occurred in "hanging out." The information was less than compelling, and so they decided to text members of the group and ask, "What are you doing now?" The data that they obtained provided rich description of what this group meant by hanging out.

Gaining access may be simple but can also take time and hard work. You should clarify the ways you intend to be involved in the context and the implications of your study for the participants.

An important consideration in obtaining access is the degree to and the way in which the intent of your study is presented to participants (Box 18-1). The researcher decides on the extent to which the research activity is revealed to those being observed or interviewed. Although the purpose and scope of the research is most often disclosed to those informants who provide initial access, the specifics of the research activity may remain vague to others who are either observed or interviewed at different times in the course of the study. The extent of overt or covert research activities varies in any type of inquiry depending on the context, varies from study to study, and has important ethical concerns for researchers.

The other aspect of disclosure of research purpose is to assure your informants that the information they provide will remain confidential and will be useful. As Internet-based research becomes increasingly used, investigators consider confidentiality in different ways. As mentioned, websites can be easily accessed without the knowledge of those who post messages or interact online. Even if you gain access by registering to become part of a listserv and remain an anonymous participant, you still should take all measures to uphold the same ethic of confidentiality that you would exercise in other environments.[10]

Another consideration in gaining access is the impact of the investigator on the investigated.

Whether the researcher is initially an insider or out-sider, his or her presence may change the nature of the environment and how people present and live their experiences. The reactive effect of the investi-gator's presence on the phenomenon being observed is a major methodological dilemma for this type of research.

In his classic and well-known study of men who frequented urban street corners, Liebow described the effect of his presence:

> All in all, I felt I was making steady progress. There was still plenty of suspicion and mistrust, however. At least two men who hung around Carry Out—one of them the local numbers man—had seen me dozens of times in close quarters but kept their distance and I kept mine.[11]

Gaining Familiarity

After initial entry into the context has been made, the investigator obtains access to different infor-mants, personal stories and experiences, texts, images, and types of observations. Thus, gaining access remains an ongoing process that involves continued negotiation and renegotiation with members of the site or the individual or groups of individuals who are the focus of the study. This ongoing access process is part of the active work of conducting a study and has been referred to as "learning the ropes,"[9] "obtaining meanings," or obtaining an "intimate familiarity"[12] with the setting or study phenomena. We use the term "gaining familiarity" as a descriptor for this action process to be expansive and include contemporary forms and content of naturalistic inquiries.

In classic ethnography, the process of gaining familiarity may appear as if the investigator is simply "hanging out." However, a range of data-gathering strategies—including looking, watching, and listen-ing; asking questions; recording; and examining materials—is brought into play to describe or learn meanings within a setting. These strategies are pur-posely chosen, combined, and integrated, and are all part of the unfolding process of learning about the environment.

The choice of strategy depends on the ebb and flow of the contextual situation and the particular issue on which the investigator is focused. Any data-gathering strategy is designed to move the investiga-tor toward understanding and experiencing the meanings of symbols, language, and behavior within the environment. This process involves reflexivity.[13] That is to say, the investigator is constantly compar-ing and analyzing pieces of information and thinking about his or her role in the development of knowl-edge. Data collection strategies are designed to reveal the unknown and examine phenomena that the investigator does not understand or finds puzzling.

> Suppose you are studying families who are experiencing stress as a result of their efforts to meet the daily needs of a family member with dementia. As you interview a particular family, you surmise, on the basis of your own past experience with similar families, that the family will soon choose nursing home placement for the individual with dementia. You are surprised to learn, however, that institutionalization has never been considered by the family. •

This example represents what Agar referred to as a "rich point."[2] A *rich point* represents a problem in your understanding and the instance at which you learn that your assumptions or previous theory are not adequate to explain what you observe. Rich points reflect the active work of the investigator that bridges the distance between his or her professional and/or academic world and the focus of the study. Gaining familiarity involves using different data col-lection strategies that give rise to these rich points.

> Consider this example. With the recent passage of legislation legalizing gay marriage, an investigator has joined an online social network to learn about the experiences and meanings of divorce to individuals who are gay and lesbian. In anonymous reading of the postings, the investigator is confused by the diversity of opinions about divorce. To move further in the research process, the investigator must make a decision to identify herself, her purpose, and the acceptable actions that should ensue to be a more active participant in the network. •

Information-Gathering Strategies

Many information-gathering strategies are used in naturalistic inquiry. The main strategies introduced in Chapter 16—observing, asking, and examining materials—are used but are thought about through diverse logic structures when used in naturalistic inquiry.

Observing: Looking, Watching, and Listening

The process of looking, watching, and listening is often referred to as "observation." In naturalistic research, observation occurs within the natural context. In this data collection strategy, the investigator can be either a passive observer of people, places, objects, and images or a participant. Passive observation involves investigators situating themselves in the environment and simply observing what is present and what occurs. In contrast, active involvement or participation in combination with observation is immersion in an environment, and engagement with other humans if indicated, for the purpose of developing a depth of understanding.[12]

More recently, Tedlock (in Denzin and Lincoln[1]) suggested that the process of *participant observation* is a complex human action in which meaning and knowledge are generated by the interaction of the investigator, those investigated, and expansively to those who hear and read the research report. In participant observation, the investigator is not a passive observer but actively engages in the research context to come to know about it. The investigator begins with broad observations to describe what is seen and then narrows the focus to discover patterns and the meaning in what has been described. In descriptive observation, it is often helpful to think of the investigator as a digital still or video camera that records what it sees as it focuses or scans the boundaries of the research setting. This technique reminds the researcher that description, not interpretation, is the first step in participant observation.

Participant observation, which Tedlock renamed "observation of participation" to remind us of the need to observe ourselves in the process of the investigation, is based on the assumption that an important way of learning about a context and group of people is to participate in it or with others in their daily activities and personally experience and observe what occurs. Participant observation has many behaviors in common with what we do in newly encountered social situations. All of us participate and observe in social situations to a greater or lesser degree. As an investigator engaged in participant observation, however, the researcher seeks to become explicitly aware of the environment and what occurs within it. The researcher remains introspective or reflexive and examines the "self" in the situation and his or her experiences as both the insider participating in the event and the outsider observing the actions.[13]

As described by Rodwell in her classic book,[14] "It is in the doing of data collection that the understanding of the subject of interest is achieved." Gubrium and colleagues[15] elaborate further, suggesting that participant observation is a strategy used to reflect a context as it is seen through those who act within it.

In one of his early classic ethnographies on nursing homes, Gubrium described the multiple roles he assumed over several months as a participant observer:

> I took many roles, ranging from doing the rather menial work called "toileting" by people there to serving as gerontologist at staff meetings. I attempted to spend sufficient time in the setting to establish trust, to interact with as many people as possible, and to observe the varied facts of life at Murray Manor in their natural states.[16]

Some types of designs or situations warrant less participation in the observation process. Nonparticipatory observation can be used to obtain an understanding of a natural context without the influence of the observer. This approach is particularly relevant to inquiry in which text, image, object, and other nonhuman phenomena are the focus of the study.

Consider the previous example of the investigator examining the meaning of same-sex divorce. "Lurking," or reading Web postings without identifying oneself, would leave the interactive context of the social networking site intact. However, once the investigator actively enters the interaction, the virtual group and all subsequent interaction are expanded and changed.

Or consider a study in which the investigator is interested in exploring attitudes toward improving accessibility for mobility-impaired individuals in business environments with fewer than 10 employees. Asking the employer/owner might elicit a socially desirable response, so the investigator decides to examine the nonhuman environment to determine who can be included and who is excluded. Images, architecture, and built environment elements such as ramps and doorway sizes would be of interest and would lend themselves to nonparticipant observation. •

During the fieldwork process, looking, watching, and listening tend to move from broad, descriptive observations to a narrow focus in which the observer looks not only for more descriptive data but also for specific understanding of the meanings of what he or she has observed. The degree of participation in the context and the extent of immersion vary throughout fieldwork and are based on the nature of the inquiry, access to the setting, and practical limitations.

Asking

Asking in the form of interviewing is another essential strategy used in many types of naturalistic inquiry. Frequently, asking for information from key informants is the initial and primary data collection strategy in phenomenology, ethnography, and grounded-theory approaches. The investigator may use an asking strategy to obtain an example of a social interchange to clarify or verify the accuracy of observations or to obtain the informant's experience with and view of the phenomenon under study. Asking, unlike observation, involves direct or mediated contact with persons who are capable of providing information. Thus, to collect data by asking, the researcher establishes a relationship with the informant appropriate to the level of involvement.

Asking can take many forms in naturalistic research, from an informal, open-ended conversation to a focused or long in-depth interview. Asking can occur as a one-to-one interaction or in a group.[17] The timing of the interview in the research process, the purpose of the asking, and the nature of the relation-ship with the informant or informant group all influence the type of asking the investigator chooses.

The most common form of asking in naturalistic design is unstructured, open-ended interviewing. This type of interviewing is particularly important in the beginning stages of a study when the investigator is trying to become familiar with the phenomenon of interest.

In the investigation of the meaning of divorce to social network members, the investigator might post a broad question such as, "Tell me more about what the term 'divorce' means to each of you."

The open-ended interview may consist of informal conversation recorded by the investigator; face-to-face, telephone, or online "twosomes"; or small groups in which the investigator sets the context for the interview and the informants offer their knowledge.

Ethnographic interview is made up of strategies that frequently rely on face-to-face interviews. In ethnographic interview, the investigator seeks to understand a culture by talking with insiders (emic members) in the culture under study.[17] The investigator not only attends to the content of the interview but also examines the structural and symbolic elements of the social exchange between the investigator and the informant. Contemporary ethnographic interview acknowledges that meanings may be changed and may be made not only within the context of the interview itself, but also at any point from the initial communication through the consumption of the research report.[1]

Life history, or biography,[1,3] is a form of naturalistic interview that chronicles an individual's life within a social context. In the case of an investigator telling all or part of his or her own life story, the term "memoir" is used to name the data source. The investigator elicits information not only on the important events or "turnings" in an individual's life, but also on the meaning of those events within the contexts in which they occur. This form of interviewing can also serve as an independent design structure.

Common forms of group questioning include focus groups and group interviews with social units, such as families with more than one individual or a cohort of individuals who share a diagnostic condition.

Focus groups are a useful methodology to explore through group discussion a particular topic, experience, or phenomenon of interest. Focus groups can be composed in different ways depending on the researcher's purpose. In a *focus group*, the investigator sets the parameters for the conversation. The participants, usually a group of 6 to 12 individuals, then address the specified topic by responding to guiding probes or questions posed by the investigator. This approach is used when it is believed that the interactions and group discussions will yield more meaningful understanding than single, independent interviews.[14,18]

Suppose you were interested in learning about adolescent attitudes toward underage alcohol use. You decide to use a focus group because it seems most feasible to elicit participation from adolescents when they are not isolated, but rather in a social group, and interacting with one another as well as the researcher.

Group interviews with small social units are also useful in observing group dynamics and symbolic meanings exchanged among group members. In cultural descriptions, questioning social units can be most valuable in understanding the structural groups of a society. This form of interviewing can also be an independent design structure.[1]

Although the structured questionnaire is primarily used in experimental-type designs, it is occasionally incorporated into certain naturalistic inquiries. Investigators have found that structured or even semistructured questionnaires can provide important insights into specific questions that emerge in the course of conducting a study. The use of a standardized instrument or structured questionnaire also enables the investigator to determine the distribution of a particular phenomenon. Consider the following example.

You are conducting a study of the meaning of breast cancer among young women. In open-ended interviewing, you detect that many of the women may be exhibiting symptoms of clinical depression because their recurring statements suggest evidence of the disorder. To test your "hunch," or emerging hypothesis, you decide to administer a standardized depression scale. The scores that result provide an additional source of data that may or may not support your initial impressions. Also, the use of the scale will enable you to determine the distribution of depression among the study group. •

Although some methodologists maintain that standardized instrument use can be naturalistic, we would suggest that because of its deductive nature and theory testing purpose, the introduction of structured asking techniques that can be subjected to measurement change the naturalistic design tradition to mixed method. However, in studies that are primarily inductive and exploratory, the use of a structured set of questions or standardized scale represents a purposeful and focused approach to asking and is best introduced only when the investigator has been in the environment for some time and has developed rapport and "gained familiarity."

Four Components of Asking Strategies

Although we ask questions every day, posing clear questions that beget the answers we are seeking is not an easy task. We have all been in situations in which the answers to our questions seemed to come from "left field" until we realized that our questions were not understood as we had intended. Consider the following examples from our own experiences. A few years ago, we had the good fortune to travel to China. After going to the zoo to see the giant pandas, we were curious about what type of animals lived in the wild, so we asked several residents, all of whom spoke English. Each time we asked, we were told that pandas were wild and that the other animals also in the zoo lived in the wild. Clearly, we were not asking a precise question to get an unwanted answer. So while we may have been speaking the same words as our informants, we were not speaking the meaning that was intended.

A second experience, also from a country in which English is not the national language, further illustrates the importance not simply of asking questions but of reflecting on what was actually heard when a question is answered inaccurately. We were invited to Egypt to lecture at a university near Luxor.

Not speaking Arabic, we were reluctant until we were informed that the university held classes primarily in English. However, on arrival, we found that all classes were held in Arabic. Incredulous, we remarked, "I thought English was spoken here," to which our host replied, why would we speak English in a school in Egypt? At that point, we noticed ourselves becoming a bit annoyed with what seemed like a flip response. A few hours later, after some self-reflection we realized that the host perceived us as U.S.-centric, expecting English to be spoken in Egypt. Our intent was to ask why we had received misinformation about the university, but of course, the meaning or even the words in this example did not communicate what we were asking.

So now we turn to a more detailed discussion of asking. In naturalistic inquiry, there are four interrelated components of an asking strategy: access, description, focus, and verification.

Access

Asking begins with access. The investigator initially wants to meet and select one or more individuals who can articulate information about the people or a phenomenon that is the focus of the study. You may ask who would be willing to speak to a stranger about personal history, events, experiences, and feelings. It is important to know the reasons someone is willing to speak to you so that you have a context to understand what the person relates. Sometimes the first key informant is someone who is formally or informally designated by a cohesive group to speak to an outsider. At other times, the informant may be a person who is considered a "deviant" within the group or a person who has nothing to lose by "hanging out" with a stranger. In other cases, the informant may represent the person with the most knowledge, experience, or seniority in a group.

Regardless of the informant's group status, the investigator initially seeks to speak to a person or persons who can orient the researcher to the context or field of inquiry. As the research progresses, the investigator may want to select specific individuals to interview who possess distinct knowledge important to the study. Consider the following examples.

You are interested in developing an obesity prevention program for rural adult women. However, you want to learn from the women themselves what they would find relevant and compelling. You enter the study with broad criteria: women in a rural town adjacent to your own hometown who are willing and able to spend time in interview sessions over a period of a month. To establish rapport, you spend time "hanging out" in the grocery store, talking to women who shop there. After the rapport is established and you are trusted, you then focus a purposive recruitment of informants. •

In the classic ethnographic study of urban men by Liebow,[11] access was initially gained by "hanging out" on the street corner where men were likely to congregate. Liebow described his first entry into the social scene as occurring serendipitously. On his first day in the field, he noticed a commotion and immediately went to the site where it was occurring. As a result of being there, Liebow was able to introduce himself into the "culture of the street corner." •

Description

After access is obtained, the initial goal of asking is to describe. Description begins with asking broad questions that become more focused as trends, recurrent patterns, and themes emerge. Frequently the investigator begins the asking process with a broad probe such as, "Tell me about . . . ."

In Liebow's study, asking began informally when he invited a man whom he had met on the street corner to have coffee. Liebow clarified his task as a researcher and "sat at the bar for several hours talking over coffee."[11] •

Focus

On the basis of emerging descriptive knowledge, the researcher's asking becomes more focused and probing. Asking questions requires intense listening, a show of respect, and great interest in each aspect of what the informant is saying. The investigator wants to ask questions that yield answers that are detailed and go into depth about the phenomena of interest. If an informant shows or articulates lack of interest or boredom with the interview, the investigator should suspect that the questions are not salient or do not focus on the aspects of the experience or phenomenon important to the interviewee.

In developing an open-ended or semistructured interview in which you want to focus on details and elicit rich description, consider the guidelines listed in Box 18-2.

Verification

As the investigator gains an understanding of the context, asking strategies serve to verify impressions and clarify details of the setting. Verification is the process of checking the accuracy of impressions with informants.

Throughout a study, the interview process may occur in one session, several sessions, or many sessions. It is usually combined with one or more of the other primary data collection strategies of observation and review of existing materials. The decision about length and frequency of asking strategies depends on the nature and scope of the query, the purpose of the interviews, and the practical limitations that influence the conduct of the study.

Examining Materials

Examining source materials and images such as texts (records, diaries, journals, e-mails, articles, narratives, letters), images (photographs, logos, signs, spaces, architectures, and so forth), and objects is another essential data collection strategy in contemporary naturalistic research. This is particularly the case in health and human service research, in which textual records, objects, and images (e.g., charts, prostheses, progress notes, minutes, x-rays, pictures, brand identities) are routinely maintained and/or used as a natural part of the context.

Similar to looking, watching, listening, and asking, review of materials usually begins with a broad examination of items and images. Then the investigator moves to a more focused evaluation to explore recurring themes and emerging patterns. Knowledge about which materials are available may occur at any point in the process. For the most part, to access text documents that divulge personal information, the investigator should obtain appropriate consent, even if he or she is an insider. Exceptions to this principle include unobtrusive data collection in which the identities of the individuals studied will not be revealed and cases when consent may not be desirable or possible. The primary aim of unobtrusively collecting information will be to keep the research role covert, with the ethical boundaries of protection of human subjects.

Assume you are interested in determining the extent to which a supported employment program for persons diagnosed with Down syndrome improves successful employment in typical work environments. You may begin by observing workplace behavior. However, there are times throughout the day when you cannot observe. You may examine progress notes written by the employees and supported employment staff to obtain additional information about the behavior and performance of the individuals diagnosed with Down syndrome. You analyze the perceptions of employees and staff in light of your own observations and the other information you obtain. You also realize that positive attitudes and awareness of the nature of the Down syndrome diagnosis on the part of employees and employers are essential for job placement and maintenance. You find that a bulletin board in the workplace has photos of employees as well as advertisements for health and wellness. So you look at the images for signs that would indicate awareness and celebration of diversity as an important part of your data collection. ●

Consider the researcher who is asked to evaluate the impact of a community-based intervention designed to decrease drug abuse in a particular neighborhood. One indicator of drug abuse in the area is the presence of drug paraphernalia, such as the vials and needles strewn in a small, centrally located park. Examining the contents of the trash and the grounds of the community park may shed light on substance abuse patterns without causing harm to individual substance users. Further, unobtrusive approaches might be the most accurate method (or the only method) of obtaining data to ascertain the outcome of the intervention, especially in light of reluctance or refusal to self-report drug abuse behaviors. Positive changes in the environment may provide an important source of evidence that the intervention is having an impact. •

With the increasing reach of material and visual culture scholarship and its relevance to health and human services, object reading[19] has become increasingly used as a naturalistic data collection method. Although it is similar to examining physical materials, object reading has a specific purpose of understanding the meaning and influence of visuals through their design, placement, and use. This approach may be overt or covert (unobtrusive). An example of object reading is the work of Sobchack that we discussed in an earlier chapter, as she investigates the differential meanings of lower extremity prostheses.[19]

One example of unobtrusive data that is becoming central to research is big data.[20] Recall that we introduced big data in Chapter 17. Big data are those generated from the huge repositories of information whose capture and analysis are only made possible by contemporary computing. Big data can be used in all traditions. As an example of their use in naturalistic research, data from social networks is increasingly being used for inductive analyses and applications by health and human service researchers for visualizing trends and patterns across the globe.[18] We do not discuss these methods further here, as they are beyond the scope of the text. However, because big data collection and analysis are major contemporary methods, they may have much to contribute to researchers answering questions through strategies such as visual maps of health and economic disparities or drug abuse patterns.[18]

Recording Information

While in the research environment, an investigator can use several strategies to record the information that is obtained by looking, watching, and listening; asking; or reviewing materials. Recording information is an important aspect of collecting information. The record of information serves as a data set that is analyzed by the investigator in the process of doing a study and then more formally after leaving the environment. An investigator decides how he or she will record information while watching and listening, asking, and reviewing material. Usually, multiple recording strategies are used in a singe study. The decision about which strategy to use is based on the purpose of the study and the resources of the investigator. Let us examine three primary mechanisms for recording information.

Field Notes

Field notes have served as a staple, so to speak, to document data in naturalistic methods. Generally, field notes have two basic components: (1) recordings of what is observed (watching, listening, looking, and asking), and (2) recordings of the personal perspective of the observer. Different from historical field notes in which ethnographers would record copious notes and transcripts,[21] current descriptive notes include voice and video recording, photography, scanning, and even speech-to-text translation.[7]

Numerous formats are suggested in the literature for recording descriptive field notes regardless of the media used. A matrix design can be used to examine the interaction of persons, places, and objects.[1] Other formats are equally useful. Lofland and colleagues[12] suggested recording description and bracketing impressions and interpretation within the context of the description. We have found it useful to use a laptop computer, smartphone, or other handheld device with software that allows for the screen to be divided into two longitudinal columns either through the creation of a table or by using a template. Speech-to-text translation is also useful when typing or writing on a tablet or smartphone is not feasible. One side of the recording is used to describe, and the other side is used to document the investigator's immediate thoughts, impressions, hunches, and questions as the observation or interview occurs. The ability to separate a description from an interpretation is important to clarify and distinguish among observation, impression, one's emotive responses to the context of inquiry and what occurs within it, and thoughts and queries to guide future inquiry.

When to record has also been discussed in the literature. This decision is an important consideration in doing a study and will depend on the nature of the inquiry. Some investigators find it useful to keep a pencil and pad or electronic device available at all times during participant observation activities.

> Suppose you are studying homeless adolescents in a shelter setting as the basis for ascertaining their service, health, nutrition, and other support needs. To record your observations as you pass through the building, you carry a Bluetooth-compatible smartphone with a sensitive microphone to unobtrusively capture the informal interactions of the spontaneous shelter culture, which might give you important insights into the needs of the adolescents. •

Other investigators find any act of recording while participating in an event too intrusive and recommend documenting at the conclusion of the day and in privacy. Waiting until the end of the day carries the risk of depending on long-term memory and losing details that may later prove to be important. However, not recording also has its strengths, as people may be less comfortable and thus less forthcoming if they see the investigator actively documenting his or her observations.

Field notes are only one way to record information and are used in conjunction with other mechanisms.

Voice Recording

Voice recording is a fundamental data-recording strategy in naturalistic inquiry primarily used when conducting on-site or virtual interviews. To capture and retain communication as precisely as possible, it is especially important to use voice recording when conducting an open-ended interview. In such interviews, informants provide long, detailed accounts that are usually difficult for the investigator to write or type verbatim. Naturalistic investigators use digital recording, often with speech-to-text applications that automate transcription.

Audio recording requires the use of a microphone and digital or computer-embedded memory. When using an audio recording, remember to test the equipment before an interview to make certain that it will adequately record both your voice and that of the respondent. We have learned from experience that once you lose an interview, it cannot be recreated from memory. You should plan to have a backup memory source and another recording device in case there is equipment failure during the interview. You should plan for every contingency to avoid the risk of losing data.

Many researchers find digital recording extremely valuable and time efficient. Various types of recording equipment can be used, including cellular and smartphones and handheld devices that both record and digitally store information. Remember, digital recording glitches can occur, so make sure that you back up your data. After you record an interview, your next step is to label the data and backup files carefully. Of course, make sure that you use equipment and software applications that are compatible with your device platforms and that can be downloaded to your device or uploaded to the cloud for analysis and storage with ease. If using digital recording that cannot be automatically translated to text, you will need to transcribe the recording. If you do have a voice-to-text application such as Dragon Dictate, which is available free on tablet devices, make sure that the format for translation provides you with a useful, accurate, and well-structured transcript. Although speech to text is very valuable and can save much transcription time, "training" and correction of errors in translation are always part of the process. At least in the current technological context, computer applications are more accurate than tablet and smartphone apps, so if possible, purchase the application for your computer until the tablet apps are perfected.

Transcription is an important step that involves translating the entire recording to text, usually in a word-processing file. In transcribing, you will need to decide whether every utterance should be recorded, such as "uh hum" or laughter. You will need to decide how pauses and silences will be noted in the transcript. If you make a determination that all utterances and silences are important, you might want to type a transcript or at least augment an automated translation with manually inserted notations rather than relying exclusively on a computer application to create a text data file.

Typing a transcript takes time but often is worth the effort, and it is essential when you are searching for nuances of meaning beyond actual words. Every hour of dense interview can take 6 to 8 hours to transcribe. In any medium, after transcribing a voice recording, you need to compare the written record with the recording to ensure accuracy. Finally, you will want to listen to the voice recording to examine the nuances in vocalization, as well as read the transcript to analyze the narrative.

There are several considerations in using voice recording. First, decide whether recording will be intrusive in your setting and will prevent informants from expressing private thoughts. Second, when you are using voice recording, informants must be informed that their conversations with you are being recorded. In most cases, obtaining consent from study participants is not a problem. If you are studying issues that are highly sensitive, however, such as sexual practices of teenagers or drug use among business people, informants may express concerns. You will need to explain your plan for maintaining confidentiality and decide who will have access to the voice recordings and where they will be kept. Also, it is important to inform research participants that they can request that recording cease at any point in the interview process.

The third consideration in using voice recordings is their analysis. In the beginning phases of a study, some investigators find that it is important to transcribe voice to text immediately after completing an interview. Reviewing these early recordings often informs the initial development of analytical categories, subsequent data collection efforts, and type of follow-up questions that need to be pursued. As throughout all thinking and action processes in research, your study purpose is foremost in guiding your choice of voice-recording method and transcription. Practical considerations, such as cost, time, and available technological capacity, are other important factors in helping you decide how to proceed.

Imaging

Imaging, including both still photography and video, is another data-recording strategy that is being increasingly used in naturalistic inquiry. Imaging is particularly useful in studies that focus on environmental elements, objects, interactions between individuals, and person–environment activity, as well as observations of both nonverbal and verbal behaviors that are the focus of a research study. In participant observation, the investigator is involved with both nonverbal and verbal exchanges and may have difficulty monitoring the details of actions. Video imaging enables the investigator to record such details of spaces, images, and behaviors that may not be detected at the time of the observation. With imaging, the investigator obtains a permanent record that can be viewed and reviewed multiple times.

As in voice recording, many considerations and decisions are made when using imaging. Choice of and familiarity with the equipment and ability to manage it efficiently in the environment are clearly important. Imaging devices range from a simple camera on your cell phone or wristwatch to complex digital video camera equipment. Purpose and practical issues will help you decide the best technology and approach.

With imaging, the issue of "reactivity" needs to be considered. Do individuals monitor their appearance and behavior because of the camera? Investigators use various strategies to reduce discomfort and reactivity. Some recommend that the camera be introduced into the research environment before recording the events that are of interest. Having a camera present but not turning it on for several occasions can reduce fear or reluctance of participants to be filmed or photographed. A small, unobtrusive camera can also be used to create less interference in the natural setting. Another consideration is the angle of the setting and the behaviors that are captured by the camera. This approach is increasingly possible as powerful and precise equipment comes in smaller sizes. Remember, however, that all video images and still photos capture only the set of activities that are performed in front of the lens, and thus other movements and exchanges that occur simultaneously but outside its range of vision will be lost to visualization. However, voice recording can be done simultaneously to obtain peripheral but potentially important information.

As in voice recording, the investigator carefully reviews each still or video image many times for analysis and for planning subsequent data collection direction. Initial review of an image helps inform the investigator as to how to proceed in the environment and which questions to pursue. After leaving the research setting, formal analysis of the video images may proceed incrementally through the action captured on camera if the investigator has the appropriate equipment. The use and analysis of images can become quite complex, time-consuming, and expensive.

Imaging can be used in combination with other techniques, such as participant observation, interviewing, and voice recording.

Accuracy in Collecting Information

At this point, you may be asking how an investigator involved with naturalistic inquiry becomes confident that the information he or she has obtained is accurate and reflects empirically shared observations of the field. This concern has been labeled as the issue of "trustworthiness."[1] After all, the investigator wants to obtain information that most accurately captures the experiences, meanings, and events of the study environment. How are we to know whether the final description or interpretation is not simply a fabrication of the investigator or a reflection of his or her personal biases and presuppositions? A number of techniques in naturalistic inquiry are designed to enhance the "truth value" of the investigator's data collection and initial analytical efforts.

Multiple Data Gatherers

One technique used in naturalistic inquiry is the involvement of two or more investigators in the data-gathering and analytical process. The old adage "Two heads are better than one" is also true in naturalistic inquiry. If possible, two or more investigators should observe and record their own field notes or images independently. This technique checks the accuracy of the observations; more than one set of eyes and ears is examining and recording the same context. Careful training of both observers is essential to ensure that each observer practices skilled recording and reporting and that all investigators understand the purpose and intent of the study.

Consider an investigator who is studying the "culture" of a group of hospitalized adolescents. The purpose of such a study may be to determine the traditions and rituals of the culture as they emerge within the boundaries of the hospital unit. Using the technique of multiple observers, two or more investigators will record notes and images independently of one another and will initially analyze these data separately. The investigators will then meet to compare notes and impressions and reconcile any differences through in-depth discourse about the data set. Not only are multiple observers used, but multiple analyzers ensure accurate data collection as well.

Triangulation (Crystallization)

Another technique that increases the accuracy of information gathering is called *triangulation*.[1] To reflect the complexity of multiple approaches to obtaining information, some have suggested replacing triangulation with "crystallization."[22] To dispel the two-dimensional and linear image of a triangle, the metaphor of a crystal has become useful in depicting the multifaceted data collection methods and analysis in naturalistic inquiry.

However, because of the frequency of its current use, we refer to multiple methods of data collection with the traditional term "triangulation." By triangulation, we mean multiple approaches that bear on the same phenomenon. For example, pairing the use of observation with interviewing, including the examination of materials, or engaging the use of all three is characteristic of triangulation in traditional naturalistic research. More recently, quantitative measures and analytical techniques such as "content analysis" have also been introduced to provide the meaning of a phenomenon from a different angle.

However, we suggest once again that the introduction of strategies based on deductive logic shift the tradition to mixed methods. In triangulating, the investigator collects information from different sources to derive and validate a particular finding. The investigator may observe an event and combine observations with textual, narrative materials to develop a comprehensive and accurate description.

Saturation

Saturation is another way in which the investigator ensures rigor in conducting a naturalistic study. Saturation refers to the point at which an investigator has obtained sufficient information from which to obtain an understanding of the phenomenon under study. As previously discussed, when the information gathered by the investigator does not provide new insights or understandings, it is a signal that saturation has been achieved. If you can guess what your respondent is going to do or say in a particular situation, you have probably obtained saturation.[1,6] In Tally's Corner, Liebow's prolonged engagement in the study ensured that the investigator reached a point of saturation.[11]

However, lengthy immersion in a study environment may not be practical for service provider researchers, who may have limited time and funds to support such an endeavor.

> Suppose that you were constrained by time and money in conducting your study of the service and support needs of homeless adolescents. You would have to use other strategies such as triangulation to heighten the accuracy and rigor of your understandings and interpretations. •

You might also use random observation as a strategy to ensure saturation. In this technique, an investigator randomly selects times throughout the investigative period to increase the likelihood of obtaining a total picture of the phenomenon of interest. Recall the example of the student group examining the meaning of "hanging out" to teenagers. Or you might select random times during the week, including morning, afternoon, and night, to observe in the shelter. In this way, you could approximate full immersion in the culture of the shelter. Through random observation, it is theoretically possible to sample the total cycle of the phenomenon of interest.

Member Checking

Member checking is a technique in which the investigator checks out his or her assumptions with one or more informants.[1] For example, if your analysis identified that the adolescents in the shelter were in need of alternative high school settings, you might verify this with your informants by asking them whether your interpretations were accurate. This type of affirmation decreases the potential for the imposition of the investigator's bias where it does not belong. Member checking is used throughout the data collection process to confirm the truth value or accuracy of the investigator's observations and interpretations as they emerge. The informants' ability to correct the vision of their stories is critical to this technique.

> The importance of routinely using member checking is highlighted by our experience in conducting a needs assessment. We took on the task from a rural state health department to develop a grant proposal to obtain funding to restructure "personal care assistant" services. After a number of focus group interviews with diverse stakeholder groups, we analyzed our data and developed a series of principles to guide the preparation of a grant proposal. The primary principle that we identified was the need for adequate training and supervision of personal care assistants. However, when we submitted our preliminary ideas to the stakeholder groups, only the professionals agreed with our priority sequence. For families, consumers, and personal care assistants, the primary need was recruitment, because there were insufficient personnel to meet even basic service needs of the community. If we had not conducted member checks, we might have sought and obtained funding for training that would be unattended. •

Reflexivity

Dissimilar from experimental-type inquiry, the presence of investigator bias is expected and addressed through reflexivity. *Reflexivity* refers to the systematic process of self-examination. In reflexive analysis, the investigator examines his or her own perspective and determines how it has influenced not only what is learned but also how it is learned.[1,13] Using our needs assessment example, had we conducted reflexive analysis more rigorously when we initially examined the data set, we might have identified the bias toward training that we held as educators and researchers. Through reflection, investigators evaluate how understanding and knowledge are developed within the context of their own thinking processes.

In discussing the importance of reflexive analysis in their research on disability culture, Gilson and DePoy were interested in the difference in disability identity between those who had birth-based and those who had acquired diagnostic conditions. Gilson noted that he expected to find disability identity and camaraderie among all of his informants and a stronger disability identity among individuals with acquired conditions.[23] However, when he did not find this phenomenon in the interview transcripts, with the exception of a college student who had been exposed to the history and current status of disability rights movements, Gilson initially thought that he and his coinvestigator had not conducted a sufficient number of interviews. Yet even when they proceeded to recruit and interview more informants, the findings were consistent with the initial round of interviews. Had they engaged in reflexive analysis, they might have been able to identify their own bias and its influence on this method and findings.

A personal diary or method of noting personal feelings, moods, attitudes, and reactions to each step of the data collection process is a critical aspect of the process in naturalistic inquiry. These personal notes form the backdrop from which to understand how a particular meaning or analysis may have emerged at the data collection stage. Fetterman[24] suggested that keeping a personal diary is an effective quality control mechanism.

In Gilson and DePoy's study, a diary of their views of others through their personal lenses would have been purposive and important for analysis.

Audit Trail

Another way to increase rigor is to maintain an *audit trail* as the researcher proceeds analytically. Some suggest leaving a path of thinking and action processes so that others can clearly follow the logic and manner in which knowledge was developed. In this approach, the investigator is responsible not only for reporting results but also for explaining how the results are obtained. By explaining the thinking and action processes of an inquiry, the investigator allows others to agree or disagree with each analytical decision and to confirm, refute, or modify interpretations. In the final report, Gilson and DePoy clearly identified not only this method but also how the thinking and action processes unfolded to yield data, impressions, and theory. In this report, they discussed their reflexive analysis as well, indicating that they entered the study with expectations that were not met.[23]

Peer Debriefing

One technique to ensure that data analysis represents the phenomena under investigation is the use of more than one investigator as a participant in the analytical process. Throughout a coinvestigated study, researchers frequently conduct analytical actions independent of one another to determine the extent of their agreement. Synthesis of analysis and examination of areas of disagreement provide additional understanding on the research query. When only one investigator engages in a project, he or she will often ask an external analyzer to function in the capacity of a coinvestigator. In some cases, a panel of experts or advisors is used to evaluate the analytical process. This form of *peer debriefing* provides an opportunity for the investigator to reflect on competing interpretations offered in the peer review process, thus strengthening the legitimacy of the final interpretation. In Gilson and Cramer's study,[23] they recruited an external analyzer who provided important analysis, bringing them to the conclusion that disability identity was not universal but rather was a constructed phenomenon that emerged from awareness and exposure to disability activism or scholarship in disability studies.

Summary

The main purpose of the action process of data collection in naturalistic inquiry is to obtain information that incrementally leads to the investigator's ability to reveal a story—a set of descriptive principles or understandings, hypotheses, or theories. Each piece of information is a building block that the investigator inductively collects, analyzes, and puts together to accomplish one or more of the purposes just stated. The researcher begins with a broad query that gradually narrows, like a funnel, as data collection proceeds and the context becomes clearer to the investigator.

In naturalistic research, the organization and analysis of data collection go hand in hand. Data collection and data management continue to unfold dynamically (see Chapter 19) as analysis reveals further direction for information gathering (see Chapter 21). The investigator is the main vehicle for data collection, although the researcher's involvement may vary among design strategies. To enhance the accuracy of data collection, multiple observers and triangulation of collection methods are two action processes often used by naturalistic investigators.

The naturalistic researcher uses one or more of three basic methods to gather information: observing, asking, and examining visuals. Observing, consisting of looking, watching, and listening, ranges on a continuum from full to no participation in the context that is being observed. Asking also varies in structure, with interviewing as the primary asking process in naturalistic design. Examination of visuals occurs in an inductive way and is intended to reveal patterns related to the phenomena under study. Naturalistic data collection occurs along with analysis and moves from broad information gathering to more focused collection of information. The combination of these approaches is critical to obtain breadth and depth of analysis.

As descriptive data are collected to illuminate the answer to "what, where, and when," the next step in the process of many naturalistic designs is to focus data collection efforts based on the ongoing analytical process. The process of information collection continues with "why and how" questions. In ethnography, this effort is called "thick" description, or focused observation, in which meanings are sought.

Focused observation hones in on examining the patterns and themes that emerge from descriptive information. The investigator may choose to examine one pattern at a time or may focus on more than one. The investigator narrows the scope of inquiry to themes and the interaction between patterns and themes while remaining open to further discovery. In general, collection strategies provide information that answers the "where, who, how, when, and why" questions. Answers to these five questions yield description, understanding of the context, occurrences within the context, and timing.

EXERCISES

1. Select a public environment, such as a shopping mall, public transportation station, or Internet social networking site. Use unobtrusive methods first and then participatory observation to determine behavioral patterns that characterize the human experience in each setting. Compare your experiences using both forms of observation and what you learned from each.

2. Conduct an open-ended interview with a colleague to obtain an understanding of career choices and his or her career path. What other information-gathering techniques can you use to understand this phenomenon?

3. Select a research article that uses naturalistic inquiry. Identify the information-gathering techniques used and determine the ethical issues involved for each technique.

References

1. Denzin NK, Lincoln YS: *Sage handbook of qualitative research*, ed 4, Thousand Oaks, Calif, 2011, Sage.
2. Agar MH: *The lively science*, Minneapolis, 2013, Mill Press.
3. Goodley D, Lawthom R, Clough P, et al: *Researching life stories*, New York, 2004, Routledge.
4. Moustakas C: *Heuristic research: design, methodology, and applications*, Thousand Oaks, Calif, 1990, Sage.
5. Geertz C: *The interpretation of cultures*, New York, 1973, Basic Books.
6. Hillyard S: *New frontiers in ethnography*, Bingly, UK, 2004, Emerald Group.

7. Creswell JC: *Qualitative inquiry and research design: choosing among five approaches*, ed 3, Los Angeles, 2013, Sage.

8. Tashakkori A, Teddlie C: *Sage handbook of mixed methods in social and behavioral research*, ed 2, Thousand Oaks, Calif, 2010, Sage.

9. Shaffir W, Stebbins R: *Experiencing fieldwork*, Newbury Park, Calif, 1991, Sage.

10. Fielding NG, Lee RM, Blank G: *The handbook of online research methods*, Thousand Oaks, Calif, 2008, Sage.

11. Liebow E: *Tally's corner*, Boston, 1967, Little, Brown.

12. Lofland J, Snow D, Anderson L, et al: *Analyzing social settings*, ed 4, Belmont, Calif, 2006, Wadsworth.

13. Gilgun J: Reflexivity and qualitative research. *Curr Issues Qualitative Res* 1:2, 2010.

14. Rodwell M: *Social work constructivist research*, London, 1998, Routledge.

15. Gubrium JF, Holstein JA, Marvasti AB, et al: *The Sage handbook of interview research: the complexity of the craft*, Los Angeles, 2012, Sage.

16. Gubrium J: *Living and dying at Murray Manor*, New York, 1975, St. Martin's Press, pp x–xi.

17. Rubin H, Rubin IS: *Qualitative interviewing: the art of hearing data*, ed 3, Los Angeles, 2012, Sage.

18. Sicignano M: *Big data analysis and quality improvement in social services*, 2012. <http://www.socialjusticesolutions.org/2012/12/21/big-data-analysis-and-quality-improvement-in-social-services>.

19. Candlin F, Guins R: *The object reader*, London, 2009, Routledge.

20. Cukier K, Mayer-Schonberger V: *Big data: a revolution that will transform how we live, work, and think*, New York, 2013, Houghton Mifflin Harcourt.

21. Nanda S, Warms RL: *Cultural Anthrologogy*, Cenage, 2014, Belmont, CA.

22. Ellingson L: *Engaging crystallization in qualitative research*, Los Angeles, 2008, Sage.

23. Gilson S, DePoy E: Disability, identity, and cultural diversity. *Rev Disabil Stud* 1:16–23, 2004.

24. Fetterman DL: *Ethnography step by step*, ed 3, Thousand Oaks, Calif, 2010, Sage.

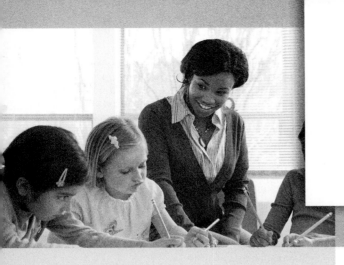

Chapter 19
Preparing and Organizing Data

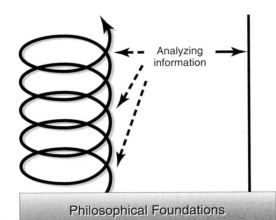

Analyzing information

Philosophical Foundations

After learning about various strategies that researchers use to collect information, you may be asking what exactly the investigator does with all of this collected information.

When you begin to collect information, you will find that you can quickly amass a massive amount of data, which you need to organize in a meaningful way. By meaningful we refer to the ability to organize a data set for ease of retrieval and analysis. In experimental-type research, even a small survey may yield multiple data points (single elements of data) for analysis. Think about all the information you may need to obtain, even if your study is small or a pilot. Information concerning a respondent's person's age, gender, other relevant personal characteristics, and living status may all be relevant and necessary to answer your research questions. Similarly, in naturalistic inquiry, a 1-hour interview may yield up to 50 or more pages of single-spaced typed narrative.

Organizing, or "managing," this information, whether the data take a numerical or narrative form, is a critical action process in all studies but is not typically included in study reports and until recently has not often made an appearance even in research texts. Many researchers learn to manage data through trial and error or by participating in the research process as mentored students or in graduate or postdoctoral training programs. However, with the explosion of information availability, the trends for professional accountability, the espousal of evidence-based practice by health and human services, and digital technology, the field of knowledge management has grown and has much to contribute to data management in health and human services research.[1,2] Knowledge management is a large and growing field that addresses and provides templates, so to speak, for organizing diverse types of data and knowledge for multiple purposes. In this chapter we discuss that what has been referred to as explicit knowledge management, or that which is generated by systematic inquiry. We will look at other types of knowledge management in Chapter 23 when we discuss sharing the analysis and reporting of findings from your research. We now enter the specific action processes of preparing and managing information in each of the research traditions.

Managing Data in Experimental-Type Research

In experimental-type research, because you will be primarily interested in obtaining a quantitative understanding of phenomenon, your data will be numerical. Recall the sequence of the research essentials. In this tradition, the analysis of numerical data is an action process that is performed after all the data have been collected for the study. That is, at the conclusion of collecting data, you will have many numerical responses to each of your questionnaires, interviews, and observations that you will then analyze.

> Consider a small study relying on survey methods involving a survey of 100 students in a college of health professions. Assume the survey is designed to examine student satisfaction with the quality of health profession education. The survey may include a number of background questions, such as gender, level of education, degree of financial assistance being received, marital status, and living arrangement. The survey will also include a scale that measures satisfaction with education, as well as a series of questions about other aspects of college life. This type of study may have 50 to 100 items or variables that will be measured. In a study involving 100 students, this may represent a total of 10,000 data points that will be submitted to statistical analysis. Thus, even in a relatively small study, the amount of information obtained can be enormous, requiring the assistance of computer technology. •

BOX 19-1   *Steps in Preparing Data for Statistical Analysis*

1. Check data for accuracy and completeness
2. Label each variable in a code book, on the instrument, or direct data entry program
3. Assign variable labels to computer locations using naming conventions of the particular statistical application you plan to use
4. Develop a comprehensive codebook
5. Enter data using double verification or implement other quality-control procedures
6. Clean raw data files to address missing information
7. Develop summative scores

The information may be collected through "paper-and-pencil" surveys (checksheets or bubble sheets) and then hand entered or scanned into a database for storage and analysis. Alternatively, the information may be entered directly as it is being collected on the Internet survey sites Survey Monkey[3] or Survey Gizmo.[4] If information is collected through interview, in experimental-type research, it is likely that the researcher will already have a scoring protocol and thus may use a mobile device or computer to score and enter responses to a database. Regardless of how the data are collected, the primary action is to prepare and organize the data for statistical analyses. The researcher follows seven basic steps (Box 19-1). If he or she is using a website that automates data entry and preparation for analysis, variable labels and code sheets are prepared in advance of data collection. However, the steps in Box 19-1 are still followed, albeit in a different sequence. We now discuss each step.

First, once data are obtained, the researcher examines each data set to check for missing information, double-coded responses, or unclear demarcations of responses. This information reflects possible errors that must be corrected before the numerical values are entered into a database. The researcher should attempt to address all missing data before data entry or shortly thereafter, as missing data may require contacting respondents and seeking answers to missed questions or clarification for double-coded responses.

TABLE 19-1 *Example of Raw Data Set*
LE 18-2
10291   1782312333828288384234343501293124224
10291   2221132000021231
10291   301924302 010212212736572524761
20822   1572122211272931888398479389842654746
20822   2634152346520012354365415142534 2563426234323
20822   368013223 654273242546546545212
12311   2234212352364246525641564265346235
12311   1812235552516617263555274354 41325423
12311   381726357 647652763674500000000
21071   1832112211253564562533413 24324342323
21071   2122242442424244231313322525 25251111122344
21071   318723648 723461987234687112333

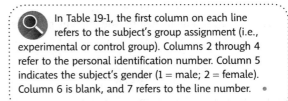

In Table 19-1, the first column on each line refers to the subject's group assignment (i.e., experimental or control group). Columns 2 through 4 refer to the personal identification number. Column 5 indicates the subject's gender (1 = male; 2 = female). Column 6 is blank, and 7 refers to the line number. •

Second, the researcher labels each variable on the data collection instrument and/or data entry application using a convention specified by the statistical package being used. Statistical Analysis Software (SAS), Statistica, or the Statistical Package for the Social Sciences (SPSS) are three of the most popular menu-driven, statistical computer applications that run on personal computers or on cloud sites. Each has a specific convention for labeling variables that is logical and straightforward.

Third, the researcher decides on the order in which the variables will be entered into a database. Usually, each subject or research participant is assigned a unique identification number located in the first 10 columns of a line or row, depending on the length of the "case identifier." If there is more than one line of data for a case, the subject identification number is repeated for each row of data. In Table 19-1, each number represents a response to a data collection instrument—in this case, a closed-ended questionnaire. These numbers are often referred to as a "raw data set" and form the foundation from which the experimental-type researcher performs statistical manipulations. A data set merely consists of all the numbers obtained through data collection, which are organized in the database according to the format designed by the researcher. Data are usually entered in the order in which the items are sequenced on the data collection protocol.

Figure 19-1 presents a screen capture of a small data set entered manually into SPSS. These data were generated in a class assignment in which 18 students completed a closed-ended response survey about their level of altruistic behavior.

In the fourth step, the researcher establishes a control file that consists of a list of the *variable labels*. Variable labels are names given to each variable by the researcher. Although these are arbitrary with the exception of the format required by the application, we suggest that the researcher select labels that are logical and transparent. For example, if one of your satisfaction items asks about cost of books and resources, you would choose a label that had the term or part of the term "course resources" contained in it. Doing so will save you time so that you do not have to look at the survey or scoring protocol each time you enter and/or analyze your data. Look at the names of each variable in Figure 19-1. The label "Gen" reminds you that the variable is gender, and "Age" reminds you that the variable is age.

Also, a written or, most often, electronic record can be generated, referred to as a *codebook* or "data definition record." This record is a copy of the variable labels and the range or values that that you have assigned. Some software statistical programs provide a separate window in which you can prepare a codebook simply by entering code information about your data set into menu-driven formats. Some direct entry and scanning systems generate a codebook for the researcher once the variables have been named.

The fifth step involves entering the numerical values into a computer-based program by a scanner, automatically from Web-based data collection protocols, or by manual entry. Although there are a variety of data entry programs, they are basically similar. For small data sets (e.g., those under 50 variables),

HELMN-I SAV (Dataset1) - IBM SPSS Statistics Data Editor

Visable: 24 of

	Gen	Age	Change1	Stranger2	Seat3	Carry4	Foodmoney5	lookedaft...	Borrow7	Charity8	Volunteer9	Blood10	Total	Change11	Change12	Seat13	Carry14	Foodmone...	Lookedafter6
1	1.00	23.00	2.00	1.00	.00	.00	5.00	.00	1.00	1.00	.00	.00	5.00	1.00	-	.00	.00	1.00	.00
2	1.00	41.00	1.00	5.00	.00	.00	2.00	4.00	.00	1.00	.00	.00	5.00	1.00	-	.00	.00	1.00	1.00
3	1.00	38.00	1.00	5.00	5.00	.00	3.00	.00	.00	1.00	2.00	.00	6.00	1.00	-	1.00	.00	1.00	.00
4	2.00	51.00	1.00	6.00	1.00	2.00	4.00	18.00	2.00	1.00	8.00	2.00	10.00	1.00	-	1.00	1.00	1.00	1.00
5	2.00	25.00	1.00	4.00	.00	.00	.00	.00	2.00	1.00	5.00	3.00	7.00	1.00	-	.00	.00	.00	.00
6	2.00	33.00	1.00	1.00	.00	1.00	.00	2.00	.00	1.00	.00	2.00	6.00	1.00	-	.00	1.00	.00	1.00
7	2.00	23.00	.00	15.00	6.00	.00	5.00	4.00	4.00	1.00	10.00	1.00	8.00	.00	-	.00	.00	.00	.00
8	2.00	23.00	1.00	5.00	.00	.00	2.00	.00	4.00	1.00	3.00	1.00	7.00	1.00	-	1.00	.00	1.00	1.00
9	2.00	36.00	1.00	1.00	1.00	.00	.00	.00	.00	1.00	1.00	.00	6.00	1.00	-	.00	.00	.00	.00
10	2.00	29.00	.00	5.00	.00	.00	2.00	.00	1.00	1.00	.00	.00	4.00	.00	-	.00	.00	1.00	.00
11	2.00	32.00	.00	5.00	2.00	1.00	.00	1.00	2.00	1.00	.00	.00	6.00	.00	-	1.00	1.00	.00	1.00
12	2.00	24.00	2.00	10.00	1.00	2.00	1.00	5.00	12.00	1.00	.00	.00	8.00	1.00	-	1.00	1.00	1.00	1.00
13	2.00	44.00	1.00	4.00	.00	1.00	1.00	6.00	2.00	1.00	2.00	.00	8.00	.00	-	.00	1.00	1.00	.00
14	2.00	37.00	.00	5.00	.00	3.00	1.00	.00	2.00	1.00	5.00	.00	6.00	.00	-	.00	1.00	1.00	.00
15	2.00	25.00	1.00	5.00	1.00	.00	.00	8.00	4.00	1.00	.00	.00	6.00	1.00	-	1.00	.00	.00	1.00
16	2.00	24.00	.00	1.00	.00	.00	.00	1.00	.00	1.00	.00	.00	3.00	.00	-	.00	.00	.00	1.00
17	2.00	26.00	1.00	5.00	5.00	.00	1.00	8.00	.00	1.00	5.00	.00	7.00	1.00	-	1.00	.00	1.00	1.00
18	2.00	22.00	3.00	7.00	8.00	2.00	.00	1.00	4.00	1.00	3.00	.00	8.00	1.00	-	1.00	1.00	.00	1.00

Figure 19-1 SPSS data view spreadsheet.

data entry can be conducted using a spreadsheet or *database management* program (e.g., Lotus 1-2-3, Microsoft Excel, FoxPro, Microsoft Access). For large data sets, it is preferable to use a computer-based program that has been specifically developed for the purpose of entering data. Most data entry computer programs enable the investigator to check for out-of-range codes, and some programs provide double verification. These are important quality-control features. Wild codes and out-of-range codes refer to errors in entering data in which characters or numbers entered in the program do not reflect the possible numerical scores assigned to the variable.

> 🔍 Assume the only responses to a question regarding marital status are 1 for "not married" or 2 for "married." The data entry operator, however, inadvertently types a 3. A data entry program can be created that will signal the operator that an error has been made or that will not permit the score of "3" to be entered. •

For manual entry, it is preferable to enter data twice, on two separate occasions. Then a comparative program can compare each numerical entry against itself, referred to as double verification. The program either alerts the key operator when a discrepancy between two entries occurs, or it allows the operator to inspect the two entries visually to determine discrepancies. For discrepant entries, the keyed responses must be manually checked against the original hard copy of the instrument to determine the correct value. Scanning data or direct entry of information at the moment it is being gathered eliminates the need for double verification. However, these approaches are not 100% accurate either, and the data that are entered still need to be checked to ensure accuracy.

The sixth step in preparing experimental-type data involves a process of "cleaning," regardless of how data entry occurs. Cleaning is an action process in which the investigator checks the inputted data set to ensure that all entries have been accurately transcribed from the instrumentation to the database. This action step (1) determines the extent of missing information, (2) ensures that each response has been

correctly coded, and (3) confirms that no errors were made in entering the numerical scores into the computer. For scanned or automated entry of data at time of data collection, computing basic checks such as calculating the range of data entered is one way to ensure accuracy.

For example, let's suppose you enrolled only individuals 70 years of age or older. Checking the range of ages entered in the data set would be one way to detect potential errors. If the lowest age of the full range of data entered into the age column was 27, you would know that an error was made and must be corrected. Just think of how the age of 27 rather than 72 would skew an understanding of the mean age and range of ages represented in the study sample.

A typical method used by researchers to inspect data for errors is computing the frequencies of responses for each variable in the data set. If "paper-and-pencil" instruments are used, in addition to checking frequencies, some researchers manually check a random number of lines of data against the original hard or electronic copy of the data collection instrument. Others use these methods in combination with printing or making a PDF copy of *raw data files* sorted both by line and subject identification numbers. These "printouts" allow the researcher to visually inspect for misaligned data, as well as for wild and out-of-range codes. However, this kind of quality check is not possible or necessary when data is directly entered into a Web-based or other data entry program. For example, online survey websites such as Survey Gizmo automate data entry and even allow you to select the format (e.g., .xls, .sav for importing into Excel or SPSS, respectively).

In Chapter 16, we discussed the possibility of having either random or systematic errors. Data entry can also serve as a possible source of random error.

Think about a particular study you plan to conduct or about which you have just read in a journal. Consider the way in which you will enter the information you collect. What are the possible data errors that might occur with the method you chose? How can the researcher address them? Researchers use many techniques to clean data and reduce sources of random error.

Assume you use a scale to ascertain the level of dependence in basic activities of daily living of the study sample. The possible responses for each self-care item range from 4 for "completely independent" to 1 for "completely dependent." When you compute the frequencies for each self-care item, you discover that "bathing" has two responses with a value of 5. You will immediately know by inspecting the ranges or frequencies of each variable that the entered data are not correct. You then need to identify the subject identification numbers of the two individuals with the out-of-range values and manually check their interview forms to determine the source of the error. The error may have been made inadvertently by the interviewer or data entry operator. •

As you can see, there are a number of ways to ensure the quality of the data that are collected and entered, and to minimize the possibility of random error at this stage of the research process. At minimum, it is important for the investigator to conduct a careful and systematic examination of the raw data set and the initial frequencies of key variables. Although this examination is often a time-consuming task at the beginning of the data analysis process, it minimizes random error and increases the accuracy of the data set. You should not perform any statistical manipulations until the data have been thoroughly cleaned and are error free. Unfortunately, not every researcher will spend time cleaning data, but we recommend that, as in every other thinking and action process, careful thought be given to this action process as well. Doing this task can make the difference between accuracy and inaccurate findings.

The seventh step and final action to prepare data for analysis involves reducing the vast quantity of information to general categories, summated scores, or single numerical indicators. As you can see from the small excerpt of a larger data set (see Table 19-1 and Fig. 19-1), most studies generate an enormous amount of information. One of the first statistical actions undertaken by experimental-type researchers is to summarize information. Index development (adding items together to form an index or scale) and descriptive statistical indicators, such as the mean,

mode, median, standard deviation, variance, and other statistically derived values, reduce and summarize individual responses and scores. This summary process is often referred to as *data reduction* and is discussed in greater detail in Chapter 20. These scores are submitted to other types of statistical manipulations to test hypotheses and make inferences and associations.

Before the popular use of desktop and mobile computing devices, only huge data sets were analyzed on mainframe computers. Since the late 1980s, however, superior hardware and software applications have made computer-aided data analysis available to most researchers. There are many statistical analytical programs on the market, several of which we have already mentioned and illustrated. Some are more "user-friendly" than others and some more capable of complex computations. Among the most popular and powerful are SPSS (McGraw-Hill, New York) and SYSTAT (SYSTAT, Evanston, Ill). SPSS is a software program that can run many types of statistical computations on large data sets. Both SPSS and SYSTAT are menu driven and relatively easy to use. In SPSS and SYSTAT, the user selects a statistical computation from a menu and is then prompted with a series of branches to perform the next step. Each program has its advantages and disadvantages. Sophisticated graphics are also created form data analysis.

For example, look at the graphs that were generated from the simple data set pictured in Figure 19-1.

These applications can be costly. In 2014, the student version of SPSS cost almost $80. But the good news is that there is freeware (PSPP) that has the analytical functionality of SPSS, without some of the high-end graphics and other features.

There are many other statistical programs. You can even find statistical software online for free. We advise that you carefully select one (with the assistance of a statistician) that fits your data analytical needs. Even with the use of computers, it is necessary to have a conceptual understanding of the range of available statistics offered in software programs.

Quantitative approaches to the analysis of data are well developed (see Chapter 20). Each statistical test has been developed and refined and new tools added as computer technologies and the field of

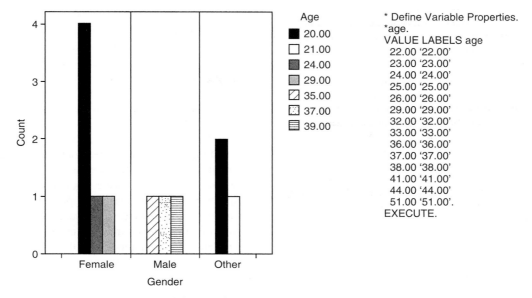

```
Age                * Define Variable Properties.
■ 20.00            *age.
□ 21.00            VALUE LABELS age
■ 24.00             22.00 '22.00'
■ 29.00             23.00 '23.00'
▨ 35.00             24.00 '24.00'
▣ 37.00             25.00 '25.00'
▤ 39.00             26.00 '26.00'
                    29.00 '29.00'
                    32.00 '32.00'
                    33.00 '33.00'
                    36.00 '36.00'
                    37.00 '37.00'
                    38.00 '38.00'
                    41.00 '41.00'
                    44.00 '44.00'
                    51.00 '51.00'.
                   EXECUTE.
```

Figure 19-2 SPSS automated definition of variable properties for age.

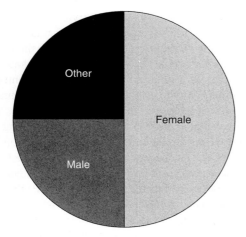

Figure 19-3 Pie chart—gender.

mathematics have advanced. There are clear and explicit rules as to when, how, and under what circumstances specific statistical analyses can be used. Because data must fit specific criteria for any analytical technique, you should be concerned with how you measure concepts and then proceed to prepare and organize your raw data. As discussed in Chapter 17, the measurement process will determine the type

of data you will obtain and, subsequently, the type of analyses you can perform.

Managing Data in Naturalistic Inquiry

As you can see, preparing a data set in experimental-type research involves a set of action processes that proceeds in a linear or step-by-step fashion and is somewhat independent from analytical actions. The overlap between preparation and analysis is in the formatting of the data necessary for using specific computer applications and for conducting specific statistical tests. This linear and prescribed sequence is not the case for naturalistic inquiry. In this tradition, organizing data is integral to the information gathering and analytical processes and is in fact an analytical action.[5] Thus, the separation of data setup from analysis, as we have shown here, is an instructional artifact that we use to clarify the process, rather than a representation of what actually occurs in the conduct of naturalistic inquiry. Therefore, we discuss aspects of organizing information and return to this action in Chapter 21, which focuses on analysis. Remember, however, that in contrast to the experimental-type separation of data collection, preparation, and analysis, these three action processes are integrated in most naturalistic designs, as we discussed in Chapter 18. Therefore, as you can surmise, if your research involves naturalistic inquiry, your approach to data management, cleaning, reduction, and analysis is vastly different from that used in experimental-type research. In what ways do you think naturalistic data management will differ from quantitative approaches?

First, although you may have some numerical data, for the most part the information that you obtain will be narrative, imagery, objects, concepts, video, and so forth. Second, the process of analysis will be ongoing and linked to collecting information. The integration of both actions is a critical aspect of naturalistic designs and is referred to as the "interactive process."[6] Third, you will have to attend to managing the enormous amounts of information that you obtain as you conduct fieldwork and engage in the process of collecting information. The type of analysis that you will conduct influences how the data are set up and managed.

The varied analytical strategies employed by researchers who use naturalistic inquiry are explored in Chapter 21. Most analytical strategies are designed to transform the volumes of interview transcripts, audio and video recordings, field notes, images, objects, and other electronic and observational information into meaningful categories, taxonomies, or themes that explain the essence, implications, and underlying patterns of the phenomenon of interest. Other analytical strategies are designed to explicate the substance of personal experiences as told to the investigator. As discussed in previous chapters, the information gathered in the various forms of naturalistic inquiry is not typically numerical but rather verbal and nonverbal manifestations that have been captured and recorded from a variety of information-gathering techniques and sources.

As shown in Chapters 16 and 18, there are many sources of data in naturalistic inquiry and, likewise, many analytical strategies. Furthermore, each source and technique requires a somewhat different approach to managing the information gathered. For example, information that is derived from

audio recordings is usually transcribed (by hand or through speech-to-text applications) into written text or narrative, whereas data involving video recordings or images are visually examined and usually coded or tagged[7] for repeated reviewing and interpretation.

Let us first examine the process of managing the voluminous amount of *narrative* information that is obtained in a naturalistic study. It is important to note that in naturalistic inquiry, managing data is also an essential part of the analytical process. As we discuss here, some of the steps in managing qualitative data involve applying analytical techniques. *Transcription* is the first step in analyzing narrative and involves transforming an audio recording into a verbatim written record. The interviewer, the investigator, or a professional transcriber may transcribe an interview if done by hand. If automated, an application such as Dragon Dictate can be used. In its current state of development, speech-to-text is improving in accuracy but certainly not perfected by any means. Thus, transcripts must be read and corrected by hand. One advantage of having the interviewer or investigator do the transcription by hand is that the act immediately immerses the researcher into the narrative and informs the analytical process. Transcribing can be tedious, however, and a slow typist or someone unfamiliar with the transcription process may find it difficult and not a good use of his or her time. You can expect an average of 6 to 10 hours of typing for each hour of interview recording, depending on the clarity of the recording, the density of the interview, and the typist's familiarity with the task, including, for example, names and subject matter. Explicit directions need to be given to a typist on how to handle the components of the voice recording. For example, you may want to record the number and length of pauses, silences, laughter, or repetitive phrases such as "uh huh." The decision as to what to transcribe will depend on the purpose of the study and represents an analytical decision concerning the importance of such utterances.

After the completion of a transcription, you check its accuracy; you will want to ensure that the typed version accurately represents the voice recording verbatim. In checking the transcription, you also need to resolve misspellings and missing sections attributed to poor sound reproduction.

After cleaning the transcription, the investigator becomes immersed in the data; that is, the transcription is read multiple times to begin the analytical process.[6] In the initial stages of any type of naturalistic narrative study, most investigators transcribe all voice recordings. As the study progresses, however, the investigator may transcribe a random selection from each voice recording or a sample for complete transcription.[8] Random selection is particularly useful for large-scale projects, such as in the tradition of classic ethnography in which the investigator increasingly selects which voice-recorded interviews are to be transcribed as the study unfolds.[9]

The short excerpt in Box 19-2 is taken from more than 50 pages of narrative derived from a transcription of a 1-hour voice recording with Aimee Mullins.[10] The voice recordings were generated from a face-to-face interview in which Mullins, a well-known model, actress, and athlete, was asked to discuss her views on contemporary and changing views and theories of disability. The excerpt is only the beginning of a lengthy interview in which Mullins was asked to reflect on how her career has been shaped by and facilitative of social change. The short 27-line excerpt is a precoded, corrected part of the transcript and illustrates one type of data in naturalistic inquiry. Consider this transcript and the other types of data that could have been collected from in-depth interviews and other sources of data. Also recall that investigator impressions could be included as part of the data set. Think about all these written words; you can quickly obtain an appreciation of the volume of information that is generated in this type of research. •

Transcription is only one aspect of preparing data for analysis. It is also critical to establish a system to organize information. On the most basic level, you can establish a log of each voice recording and the date of its recording. As you begin to identify categories of information, you establish a system for easy retrieval of key passages that reflect these categories. It is also important to keep track of coding and analytical decisions as you read and review materials. Researchers use a variety of organizational schemes,

depending on their personal style and preferences and the scope and needs of the research project. Some researchers use paper or electronic note cards or tagging. Others prefer to use word-processing programs or computer coding programs (e.g., ATLAS.ti or NVivo). Similar to experimental-type free ware, there is no-cost software for naturalistic analysis such as QDAP (The Qualitative Data Analysis Program).

In experimental-type research, computer-based statistical programs are a necessity and have facilitated the development of more sophisticated statistical tests. However, in naturalistic inquiry, computer-based coding programs assist the investigator in organizing, sorting, and manipulating the arrangement of materials to facilitate the analytical process. Also, programs can perform concept mapping, thematic coding, and content analyses. Obviously, the programs cannot develop an analytical scheme or engage in the interpretive process. Nothing can replace the need for the investigator to be immersed in reading and coding the narrative. Word-processing programs and specially designed qualitative software packages only enable the researcher to catalog, store, and rearrange large sets of information in various sorted files more efficiently. Even when computer assistance is used, many investigators also depend on other less sophisticated approaches (electronic log keeping), including "paper-and-pencil" organizing tools such as computerized or paper index cards or notebooks with tabs to separate and identify major topics and emerging themes. Files may also be electronic and color coded, a built-in option in most operating systems. Some investigators still work with multiple copies of narratives and cut and paste materials to organize and reorganize each written segment into meaningful categories.

In any case, researchers usually maintain a codebook in the form of paper or electronic index cards, word-processing files, or an electronic notebook that summarizes the codes that are used to describe major passages and themes and their location in a transcript. An index or codebook system can be developed in many ways and can even be located on an MP3 player or mobile device for quick reference.

BOX 19-2 *Excerpt From Interview Transcript With Preliminary Analytical Codes*

Line	Narrative
1	Being thought of as beautiful is new for me. I will take it as long as I have it.
2	It is a step up
3	A couple years ago, just to fess up, I was president of the women's sports
4	foundation. The black and white image taken by Harold Shotz of me in my
5	sprinting legs appeared in an issue of Sports Illustrated. I was away, before
6	internet was everywhere. When I returned I learned that there was this hubbub
7	from the leadership about some anonymous feminist blogger who wrote an attack
8	on the Sports Illustrated piece. She claimed that I was being objectified. Rather
9	than being lauded for my accomplishments she was distressed that the photo essay
10	was too sexy. Her concern was with the objectification of my body as sexy?
11	Wait a minute!!!!
12	That someone thought this photo was too sexy to be representative as an athlete
13	was a step up for me. That you can look at an image of a woman wearing two
14	prosthetic legs and see "too sexy" is a huge step up. It was only 5 years ago that
15	Aunt Millie and the massage therapist were saying, you would be so pretty if it
16	weren't for your legs. The women's foundation took the image off their website.
17	I was livid.
18	You can't have it both ways.
19	You cannot lambaste the idea that we have societally accepted conventions of
20	what is attractive and then at the same time throw darts at people you think fit that
21	vision.
22	The legs, the McQueen legs and glass legs are so beautiful. Now I am going the
23	other way from awww . . . so sorry to how beautiful. The man, a shoe designer, who
24	worked on my wooden legs came up totally emotional, for him it was a
25	touchstone in his career. It transformed what he thought about shoes as prosthetic.

Codes: A = Advancements in disability attitudes, O = Old stigma, AM = Ambivalence of Change.
A = 1, 2, 5-7, 16-18, 23-26
O = 3, 4, 8-15, 19
AM = 19-22

A code, its definition, and its line location in the transcript are recorded immediately below the numbered lines in Table 19-2. From this excerpt three broad analytical categories emerged from the beginning of the interview with Mullins[10]: advancements in disability attitudes, old stigma, ambivalence of change. Line numbering was used as the basis for identifying the location of thematic codes throughout the transcript. The text can then be sorted by codes, and smaller files can be created that reflect any category of interest (Box 19-2). Of course, there were many more codes that surfaced through inductive analysis. This tiny excerpt illustrates only three. •

Remember that narrative data are not the only sources of information in naturalistic inquiry. Codes and impressions are also relevant for images, objects and other types of data. Rose specifies a similar process of inductive coding for visual data.[7]

As mentioned earlier, as part of the information collection and storage process, the researcher may keep personal notes and diary-like comments and emerging insights that provide a context from which to view and understand notes at each stage of engagement in the study. This is an example of how data management and data analysis are interrelated in naturalistic research. In most forms of naturalistic inquiry, the investigator is an integral part of the

TABLE 19-2   *Excerpt From Codebook for Interview Transcripts*

Line	Narrative
1	Being thought of as beautiful is new for me.
2	I will take it as long as I have it. It is a step up.
3	A couple years ago, just to fess up, I was president
4	of the women's sports foundation. The black and white
5	image taken by Harold Shotz of me in my sprinting legs
6	appeared in an issue of Sports Illustrated. I was away,
7	before internet was everywhere. When I returned I
8	learned that there was this hubbub from some anonymous feminist blogger.
9	She claimed that I was being objectified. Rather than being
10	lauded for my accomplishments she was distressed that the
11	photo essay was too sexy. Her concern was with the objectification
12	of my body as sexy? Wait a minute!!!! That someone thought
13	this photo was too sexy to be representative as an athlete
14	was a step up for me. That you can look at an image of a woman
15	wearing two prosthetic legs and see "too sexy" is a huge step up.
16	It was only 5 years ago that Aunt Millie and the massage
17	therapist were saying, you would be so pretty if it weren't
18	for your legs. The women's foundation took the image off their website. I was livid.
19	You can't have it both ways. You cannot lambaste
20	the idea that we have societally accepted conventions
21	of what is attractive and then at the same
22	time throw darts at people you think fit that vision.
23	The legs, the McQueen legs and glass legs are so beautiful.
24	Now I am going the other way from awww . . . so sorry to how beautiful.
25	The man, a shoe designer, who worked on my wooden legs came
26	up totally emotional, for him it was a touchstone in his career.

Codes: A = Advancements in disability attitudes, O = Old stigma, AM = Ambivalence of Change.

A = 1, 2, 5-7, 16-18, 23-26

O = 3, 4, 8-15, 19

AM = 19-22

---

entire research process.[1,8] It is through the investigator and his or her interaction with informants, visuals, and so forth that knowledge emerges and develops. Thus, these personal comments are critical to the investigator's self-reflections, which occur as part of both the management and the analytical processes.

Through reflexivity[5] or reflecting on personal feelings, moods, and attitudes at each juncture of data collection and recording, the investigator can begin to understand the lens through which to interpret the cultural scene or slice of behavior at that point in the study. The organization of these notes and their emergent interpretations is an important technique. The investigator can develop questions to guide further data collection and to explain observations as they occur. Summarizing or *memoing*[5] as the researcher proceeds is both a management and an analytical technique that produces an "audit trail."[9] An audit trail indicates the key turning points of an inquiry in which the researcher has uncovered and revealed new understandings or meanings of the phenomenon of interest. Others can review the audit trail as a way to determine the credibility of the investigator's interpretations (see Chapter 18).

Some Words About Mixed Methods

Of course in mixing methods, if your data integrate strategies from both experimental-type and naturalistic traditions, you need to select management procedures that accomplish parsimony and purpose. Mixed method data management also will likely require that you have software applications for both approaches.

Practical Considerations

Another part of the action process of preparing data for analysis, whether for naturalistic, quantitative, or integrated-type research, involves practical considerations in managing data that can potentially affect the science of your investigation. One consideration is finding a safe place to store data in your office. Data (e.g., questionnaires, voice recordings, electronic databases, transcripts) should be stored in fireproof or metal cabinets that can be secured by lock and key. Locked filing cabinets or a locked office suite is essential because it is an ethical and legal responsibility to ensure the confidentiality of the information you have collected from human subjects; only members of the research team should have access to such information. Also, you should derive office policies as to who has access to your data (typically only those on the research team and listed on the institutional review board–approved protocol), whether the data can be accessed, and by whom. Identify a safe drop-in box, and establish a storage system for completed interviews and those that have been entered and cleaned. Be sure that all virus and spyware programs are up to date and that your computer is password protected so that no one can access electronic data. Some cloud-based storage mechanisms can be password protected, but it is important to ensure the adequacy of protection afforded. You may also encrypt files for extra security.

Another consideration is to develop a backup disaster plan. You should always have a backup of all data that have been entered or transformed. Cloud storage provides an excellent location for backup files.

Besides a backup and disaster recovery plan, you also must make sure that you keep any identifying information and informed consents (see Chapter 3) separate from and not traceable to the actual information or data that are collected. Your security procedures and spaces may in fact be audited by your institutional review board or research committee to make sure that you are compliant with all Health Insurance Portability and Accountability Act (HIPAA) and human subject regulations (see Chapter 3).

Although these are very practical considerations, they are part of the action of research. Consider the consequences for the analytical and reporting stages of your research if your completed audio recordings or interviews are mislabeled, misplaced, lost, not retrievable, or inaccurate. Although practical, these considerations reflect specific methodological procedures that the researcher and his or her team must put into place to ensure accuracy in data collection and storage. Adherence to strict management and security procedures reflects ethical actions: If you do not take the time and thought to develop and implement these safeguards, you are wasting the time and energy of your study participants and funders, if you have received grant monies for the conduct of your study, and possibly causing harm through violating confidentiality.

Summary

Organizing or managing the information collected in a study is an important research task that is not often explicitly discussed in research texts or other publications. Because they are not intuitive, techniques for effectively organizing data for analysis tend to be learned by novice researchers as you proceed through your studies and ask others for guidance. Nevertheless, data management represents a potential source of random error in experimental-type design or integrated research using that approach, and creates the potential for inaccuracy in both naturalistic inquiry. Preparation, management, and the practicalities of these action processes therefore warrant careful consideration.

Researchers in experimental-type research proceed with a series of actions to manage and prepare data for statistical analysis. As in all previous research steps, the approach in experimental-type research is linear; it follows data collection, precedes statistical testing, and involves a series of actions that occur in a stepwise fashion. In contrast, analysis is an ongoing and integral part of data collection actions in naturalistic inquiry. Likewise, the management of data and their cleaning and reduction into meaningful interpretive categories occur iteratively, first as part of data collection and then as part of a more formal analysis and report-generating process. In keeping with the different philosophical foundations that make up naturalist inquiry, researchers pursue diverse ways of storing, managing, and preparing information for ongoing analysis and final report writing. Mixing methods, particularly in data collection, requires attention to organization and management of data in both traditions.

EXERCISES

1. Contact two researchers at a university who work in the experimental-type tradition. Through interviewing, determine their data management

arrangements, data entry software, and types of codebook strategies.

2. Repeat Exercise 1 with two researchers who use naturalistic inquiry.
3. Repeat Exercise 1 with two researchers who use mixed methods.
4. Compare and contrast the different styles of managing information in the experimental-type and naturalistic research traditions, and then consider how styles would be integrated in mixed methods.

....

References

1. Leung ZC: Knowledge management in social work: towards a conceptual framework. *J Tech Hum Services* 43:179–196, 2007.
2. Booth A, Purdy R, Ward S, et al: *eLearning: managing knowledge to improve social care*, 2010, Social Care Institute for Excellence. <http://www.scie.org.uk/publications/elearning/knowledgemanagement/index.asp>.
3. *SurveyMonkey.com.*
4. *SurveyGizmo.com.*
5. Denzin NK, Lincoln Y: *Sage handbook of qualitative research*, Los Angeles, 2011, Sage.
6. Thyer B: *The handbook of social work research methods*, Los Angeles, 2010, Sage.
7. Rose G: *Visual methodologies*, Los Angeles, 2012, Sage.
8. Creswell J: *Research design: qualitative, quantitative, and mixed method approaches*, Los Angeles, 2014, Sage.
9. Fetterman D: *Ethnography: step by step*, ed 3, Thousand Oaks, Calif, 2009, Sage.
10. DePoy E, Gilson SF: *Disability design and branding*, London, 2014, Routledge.

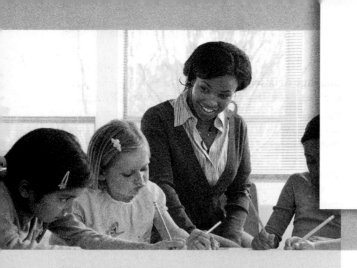

Chapter 20
Statistical Analysis for Experimental-Type Designs

KEY TERMS

Associational statistics
Confidence interval
Confidence level
Descriptive statistics
Dispersion
Frequency distribution
Inferential statistics
Interquartile range
Level of significance
Mean
Median
Measures of central tendency

Mode
Nonparametric statistics
Parametric statistics
Range
Standard deviation
Statistics
Sum of squares
Type I error
Type II error
Variance

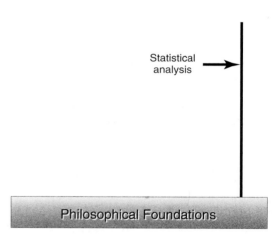

Statistical analysis →

Philosophical Foundations

Many newcomers to the research process often equate "statistics" with "research" and are intimidated by this phase of research. You should now understand, however, that conducting statistical analysis is simply one of a number of important action processes in experimental-type research. You do not have to be a mathematician or memorize mathematical formulas to engage effectively in this research step. Statistical analysis is based on a logical set of principles that you can easily learn. In addition, you can always consult a statistical book or website for formulas, calculations, and assistance. Because there are hundreds of statistical procedures that range from simple to extremely complex, some researchers and mathematicians specialize in *statistics* and thus provide another source of assistance if you should need it. However, except for complex calculations and statistical modeling, you should easily be able to understand, calculate, and interpret basic statistical tests.

The primary objective of this chapter is to familiarize you with three levels of statistical analyses and the logic of choosing a statistical approach. An understanding of this essential and its experimental-type action processes is important and will enhance your ability to pose appropriate research questions and design experimental-type strategies. Thus, our purpose here is to provide an orientation to some of the basic principles and decision-making processes in this action phase rather than to describe a particular statistical test in detail or discuss advanced statistical procedures. We refer you to user-friendly websites and the references at the end of the chapter for other resources that discuss the range of available statistical analyses. Also, refer to the interactive statistical pages at http://www.statpages.net and the large list of online statistical websites that are listed on Web Pages that Perform Statistical Calculations at http://www.geocities.com/Heartland/Flats/5353/research/statcalc.html.

What Is Statistical Analysis?

Statistical analysis is concerned with the organization and interpretation of data according to well-defined, systematic, and mathematical procedures and rules. The term "data" refers to information obtained through data collection to answer such research questions as, "How much?" "How many?" "How long?" "How fast?" and "How related?" In statistical analysis, data are represented by numbers. The value of numerical representation lies largely in the asserted clarity of numbers. This property cannot always be exhibited in words.[1]

> For example, assume you visit your physician, and she indicates that you need a surgical procedure. If the physician says that most patients survive the operation, you will want to know what is meant by "most." Does it mean 58 out of 100 patients survive the operation, or 80 out of 100? •

Numerical data provide a precise standardized language to describe phenomena. As tools, statistical analyses provide a method for systematically analyzing and drawing conclusions to tell a quantitative story.[2] Statistical analyses can be viewed as the stepping stones used by the experimental-type researcher to cross a stream from one bank (the question) to the other (the answer).

You now can see that there are no surprises in the tradition of experimental-type research. Statistical analysis in this tradition is guided by and dependent on all the previous steps of the research process, including the level of knowledge development, research problem, research question, study design, number of study variables, level of measurement, sampling procedures, and sample size. Each of these steps logically leads to the selection of appropriate statistical actions. We discuss each of these later in the chapter.

First, it is important to understand three categories of analysis in the field of statistics: descriptive, inferential, and associational. Each level of statistical analysis corresponds to the particular level of knowledge about the topic, the specific type of question asked by the researcher, and whether the data are derived from the population as a whole or are a subset or sample. Recall that we briefly discussed the implications of boundary setting for statistical choice. This last point, population or sample, will become clear in this chapter. Experimental-type researchers aim to predict the cause of phenomena. Thus, the three levels of statistical analysis are hierarchical and consistent with the level of research questioning discussed in Chapter 8, with description being the most basic level.

Descriptive statistics form the first level of statistical analysis and are used to reduce large sets of observations into more compact and interpretable forms.[1,2] If study subjects consist of the entire research population, descriptive statistics can be primarily used; however, descriptive statistics are also used to summarize the data derived from a sample. Description is the first step of any analytical process and typically involves counting occurrences, proportions, or distributions of phenomena. The investigator descriptively examines the data before proceeding to the next levels of analysis.

The second level of statistics involves making inferences. *Inferential statistics* are used to draw conclusions about population parameters based on findings from a sample.[3] The statistics in this category are concerned with tests of significance to generalize findings to the population from which the sample is drawn. Inferential statistics are also used to examine group differences within a sample. If the study subjects are a sample, both descriptive and inferential statistics can be used in concert with one another. There is no need to use inferential statistics when analyzing results from an entire population because the purpose of inferential statistics is to estimate population characteristics and phenomena from the study of a smaller group, a sample.

By their nature, inferential statistics account for errors that may occur when drawing conclusions about a large group based on a smaller segment of that group. You can therefore see, when studying a population in which every element is represented in the study, why no sampling error will occur and thus why there is no need to draw inferences.

Associational statistics are the third level of statistical analysis.[3,4] These statistics refer to a set of procedures designed to identify relationships between and among multiple variables and to determine whether knowledge of one set of data allows the investigator to infer or predict the characteristics of another set. The primary purpose of these multivariate types of statistical analyses is to make causal statements and predictions.

Table 20-1 summarizes the primary statistical procedures associated with each level of analysis. A summary of the relationship among the level of knowledge, type of question, and level of statistical analysis is presented in Table 20-2. Let us examine the purpose and logic of each level of statistical analysis in greater detail.

Some Words About Mixed Methods

Before we begin a more detailed discussion of statistics, we say a few words about statistical analysis in mixed methods. It is possible to use numbers throughout mixed methods, to quantify themes (content analysis discussed in Chapter 21), to count the number of informants, and so forth. Numbers, if

TABLE 20-1 Primary Tools Used at Each Level of Statistical Analysis

Level	Purpose	Selected Primary Statistical Tools
Descriptive statistics	Data reduction	Measures of central tendency: mode, median, mean Measures of variability: range, interquartile range, sum of squares, variance, standard deviation Bivariate descriptive statistics: contingency tables, correlational analysis
Inferential statistics	Inference to known population	Parametric statistics Nonparametric statistics
Associational statistics	Causality	Multivariate analysis Multiple regression Discriminant analysis Path analysis

TABLE 20-2 Relationship of Level of Knowledge to Type of Question and Level of Statistical Analysis

Level of Knowledge	Type of Question	Level of Statistical Analysis
Little to nothing is known	Descriptive, exploratory	Descriptive
Descriptive information is known, but little to nothing is known about relationships	Explanatory	Descriptive, inferential
Relationships are known, and well-defined theory needs to be tested	Predictive, hypothesis testing	Descriptive, inferential, associational

emerging inductively, remain in the naturalistic tradition. However, when used to examine the accuracy of theory, numeric data fall within the experimental-type tradition. Determining the logic structure that guides the use and interpretation of numeric data will tell you if a researcher is using numbers deductively, inductively, or abductively. When used deductively along with naturalistic strategies of analysis, we classify the study as a mixed methods design. We will come back to this point at the beginning of Chapter 21 and then again in Chapter 22. So master the language and action processes of statistics for use in experimental-type and mixed method designs.

Level 1: Descriptive Statistics

Consider all the numbers that are generated in a research study such as a survey (recall our illustrations in Chapter 19). Each number provides information about an individual phenomenon but does not provide an understanding of a group of individuals as a whole. Now reconsider the discussion in Chapter 17 of the four levels of measurement (nominal, ordinal, interval, and ratio). Large masses of unorganized numbers, regardless of the level of measurement, are not comprehensible and cannot in themselves answer a research question and thus tell a coherent and evidence-supported knowledge story.

Descriptive statistical analyses provide techniques to reduce large sets of data into smaller sets without sacrificing critical information. The data are thus comprehensible if summarized into a more compact and interpretable form. This action process, referred to as data reduction, involves the summary of data and their reduction to singular numerical scores.[2] These smaller numerical sets are used to describe the original observations. A descriptive analysis is the first action a researcher undertakes to understand the data that have been collected. Within this category of statistics, the techniques for reducing data include frequency distribution, measures of central tendency (mode, median, and mean), variances, contingency tables, and correlational analyses. These descriptive statistics involve direct measures of characteristics of the actual group studied.

Frequency Distribution

The first and most basic descriptive statistic is the *frequency distribution*. This term refers to both the distribution of values for a given variable and the number of times each value occurs. The distribution reflects a simple tally or count of how frequently each value of the variable occurs in the set of measured objects. As discussed in Chapter 19, frequencies are used to clean raw data files and to ensure

accuracy in data entry. Frequencies are also used to describe the sample or population, depending on which one has participated in the actual study.

Frequency distributions are usually arranged in table format, with the values of a variable arranged from lowest to highest or highest to lowest (depending on what makes the most sense to the researcher). Frequencies provide information about two basic aspects of the data collected: (1) allowing the researcher to identify the most frequently occurring class of scores and any pattern in the distribution of scores; and (2) producing "relative frequencies," which are the observed frequencies converted into percentages on the basis of the total number of observations. Relative frequencies tell us immediately what percentage of subjects has a score on any given value.

Assume you want to develop a drug abuse prevention program in a high school. To plan adequately, you need to know the ages of the students who will participate. You obtain a list of ages of 20 participants (Table 20-3); the ages are measured at the interval level (years) and are listed in the order in which the students register. However, the list is difficult to interpret. For example, the average age of the group, the age distribution among the categories, and the youngest and oldest ages of those who signed up for the program are not immediately apparent on the list. To understand the data, you can develop a simple frequency table (Table 20-4). This table organizes the ages (in years) of the sample in ascending order and indicates the number and percentage of students at each age. Only one variable is presented, and its level of measure is interval. This simple rearrangement of the data provides important information that you can immediately understand. From this table, it is readily apparent that ages range from 14 to 18 years and that the most frequently occurring ages are 15 and 17 years. You can reduce the data further by grouping the ages to reflect an ordinal or nominal level of measurement if you want to know how many students fall within the age range of 14 through 16 and 17 through 18 years (ordinal; Table 20-5) or young and old (categorical or nominal). •

Sometimes, for efficiency, researchers group data on a theoretical basis for variables with a large number of response categories. Frequencies are

TABLE 20-3	Ages of High School Students			
18	15	14	16	17
17	17	15	17	18
16	15	14	15	16
15	17	16	14	18

TABLE 20-4	Frequency Distribution of Ages of Students (N = 20)	
Age	Frequency	Percent
14	3	15
15	5	25
16	4	20
17	5	25
18	3	15

TABLE 20-5	Frequency Distribution by Age Interval (in years)	
Age Interval	Frequency	Percent
14 to 16	12	60
17 to 18	8	40

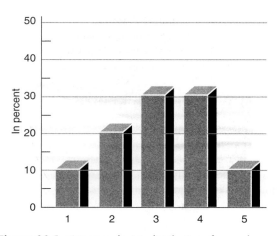

Figure 20-1 Histogram depicts distribution of scores by percentage of responses in each category.

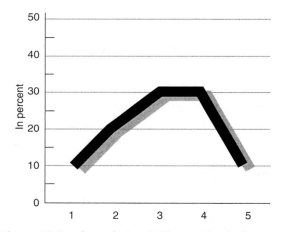

Figure 20-2 Polygon depicts distribution of scores by percentage of responses in each category.

typically used with categorical data rather than with continuous data, in which the possible number of scores is high, such as test grades or income. Simply looking at a table with a large distribution of numbers, it is difficult to derive any immediate understanding, so reducing data to a readily comprehensible format is warranted.

In addition to a table format, frequencies can be visually represented by graphs, such as a pie chart, histogram or bar graph, and polygon (dots connected by lines). Let us use another hypothetical data set to illustrate the value of representing frequencies using some of these formats. Assume you conducted a study with 1000 persons aged 65 years or older in which you obtained scores on a measure of "life satisfaction." If you examine the raw scores, you will be at a loss to understand patterns or ascertain how the group behaves on this measure. One way to begin will be to examine the frequency of scores for each

response category of the life satisfaction scale using a histogram. There are five response categories: 5 = very satisfied, 4 = satisfied, 3 = neutral, 2 = unsatisfied, and 1 = very unsatisfied. Figure 20-1 depicts the distribution of the scores by percentage of responses in each category (relative frequency).

You can also visually represent the same data using a polygon. A dot is plotted for the percentage value, and lines are drawn among the dots to yield a picture of the shape of the distribution, as well as the frequency of responses in each category (Fig. 20-2). The pie chart is often used as well to illustrate relative frequency (Fig. 20-3).

Frequencies can be described by the nature of their distribution. There are several shapes of distributions. Distributions can be symmetrical (Fig. 20-4, *A* and *B*), in which both halves of the distribution are identical. This distribution is referred to as a normal or bell-shaped distribution. Distributions can also be nonsymmetrical (see Fig. 20-4, *C* and *D*) and are characterized as positively or negatively skewed. A distribution that has a positive skew has a curve that is high on the left and a long tail to the right (see Fig. 20-4, *E*). A distribution that has a negative skew has a curve that is high on the right and a long tail to the left (see Fig. 20-4, *F*). A distribution can be characterized by its shape, or what is called kurtosis and is characterized by either its flatness (platykurtic; see

skew (a symmetry measure)

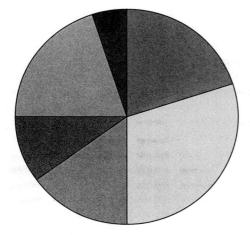

Figure 20-3 Pie chart.

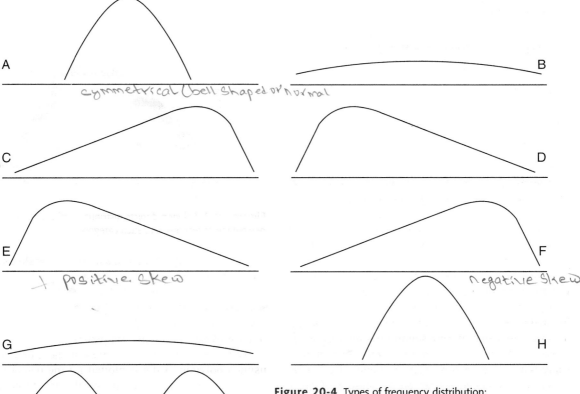

symmetrical (bell shaped or normal

+ positive skew

negative skew

Figure 20-4 Types of frequency distribution: A and B, symmetrical distribution; C and D, nonsymmetrical distribution; E, positively skewed distribution; F, negatively skewed distribution; G, platykurtosis (flatness); H, leptokurtosis (peakedness) **I,** bimodal.

Fig. 20-4, *G*) or its peakedness (leptokurtic; see Fig. 20-4, *H*). A bimodal distribution is characterized by two high points (see Fig. 20-4, *I*). If you plot the age of the 20 students who registered for the drug abuse prevention course (data shown in Table 20-4), you will have a bimodal distribution.

It is good practice to examine the shape of a distribution before proceeding with other statistical approaches. The shape of the distribution will have important implications for determining central tendency and the other types of analysis that can be performed.

Measures of Central Tendency

A frequency distribution reduces a large collection of data into a relatively compact form. Although we can use terms to describe a frequency distribution (e.g., bell shaped, kurtosis, or skewed to the right), we can also summarize the frequency distribution by using specific numerical values. These values are called *measures of central tendency* and provide important information regarding the most typical or representative scores in a group. The three basic measures of central tendency are the mode, median, and mean.

Mode

In most data distributions, observations tend to cluster heavily around certain values. One logical measure of central tendency is the value that occurs most frequently. This value is referred to as the "modal value" or the *mode*. For example, consider the data collection of nine observations, such as the following:

9 12 15 15 15 16 16 20 26

In this distribution of scores, the modal value is 15 because it occurs more than any other score. The mode therefore represents the actual value of the variable that occurs most often. It does not refer to the frequency associated with that value. Although the mode is frequently located within the middle of the possible range of scores, it does not always fall there, so you need to be careful in what statistics you choose for further analysis and in how you interpret your findings. The mode therefore can occur anywhere along the full range of possible scores and

thus, although referred to as a measure of central tendency, may be misleading if the researcher assumes it lies in the middle of a distribution.

As we noted earlier, some distributions can be characterized as "bimodal" in that two values occur with the same frequency. Let us use the age distribution of the 20 students who plan to attend the drug abuse prevention class (see Table 20-4). In this distribution, two categories have the same high frequency; 14 is the value of one mode, and 17 is the value of the second mode. So you can see how surmising that the mode is lies at the middle of a possible range of scores can be a problem.

In a distribution based on data that have been grouped into intervals, the mode is often considered to be the numerical midpoint of the interval that contains the highest frequency of observations. For example, let us reexamine the frequency distribution of the students' ages (see Table 20-5). The first category of ages, 14 through 16 years, represents the highest frequency. However, because the exact ages of the individuals in that category are not known, we select 15 as our mode because it is halfway between 14 and 16.

The advantage of the mode, except in a bimodal or multimodal (more than two modes) distribution, is that it can be easily obtained as a single indicator of a large distribution. Also, the mode can be used for statistical procedures with categorical (nominal) variables (numbers assigned to a category; e.g., 15 male and 25 female).

Median

The second measure of central tendency is the median. The *median* is the point on a scale above or below which 50% of the cases fall. Unlike the mode, the median is defined as the score that lies at the midpoint of the distribution. To determine the median, arrange a set of observations from lowest to highest in value. The middle value is singled out so that 50% of the observations fall above and below that value. Consider the following values:

22 24 24 25 27 30 31 35 40

The median is 27, because half the scores fall below the number 27 and half are above. In an odd number of values, as in the previous case of nine, the median is one of the values in the distribution. When an even number of values occurs in a distribution, the median may or may not be one of the actual values, because there is no middle number; in other words, an even number of values exist on both sides of the median. Consider the following values:

22 24 24 25 27 30 31 35 40 47

The median lies between the fifth and sixth values. The median is therefore calculated as an average of the scores surrounding it. In this case, the median is 28.5 because it lies halfway between the values of 27 and 30. If the sixth value had been 27, the median would have been 27. Look at Table 20-4 again. Can you determine the median value? Write out the complete array of ages based on the frequency of their occurrence. For example, age 14 occurs three times, so you list 14 three times; the age of 15 occurs five times, so you list 15 five times; and so forth. Count until the 10th and 11th value. What age did you obtain? If you identified 16, you are correct. The age of 16 years occurs in the 10th and 11th value and is therefore the median value of this group of students.

In the case of a frequency distribution based on grouped data, the median can be reported as the interval in which the cumulative frequency equals 50% (or midpoint of that interval).

The major advantage of the median is that it is insensitive to extreme scores in a distribution; that is, if the highest score in the set of numbers shown had been 85 instead of 47, the median would not be affected. Income is an example of how the median is a good indicator of central tendency because it is not affected by extreme values.

Mean

The *mean,* as a measure of central tendency, is a fundamental concept in statistical analysis used with continuous (interval and ratio) data. Remember that unlike the mode and median, which do not require mathematical calculations (with the exceptions discussed earlier), the mean is derived from manipulating numbers mathematically. Thus, the data must have the properties that will allow them to be subjected to addition, subtraction, multiplication, and division.

BOX 20-1 *Common Symbols for the Mean*

Mx = mean of variable x
My = mean of variable y
X = X bar or mean value of a variable
M = mu, mean of a sample

Suppose that you were doing a study in which you were interested in comparing how male and female young adults responded to a smoking prevention program. You assign the number "1" to code male gender and "2" to code female gender. It would not make sense to calculate a mean score for gender because 1 and 2 are nominal and used to "name" categories rather than magnitude. Similarly, if you coded ages as 1 = ages 18 through 21, 2 = ages 22 through 25, and 3 = ages 26+, you would not be able to subject your ordinal data (1, 2, 3) to the calculation of the mean because these numbers denote order, not mathematical magnitude. •

The mean serves two purposes. First, it serves as a data reduction technique in that it provides a summary value for an entire distribution. Second and equally important, the mean serves as a building block for many other statistical techniques. As such, the mean is of the utmost importance. There are many common symbols for the mean (Box 20-1).

The formula for calculating the mean is simple:

$$M = \frac{\Sigma X_i}{N}$$

where ΣX_i = sum of all values, M = mean, and N = total number of observations. You may recognize this formula as the one that you learned to calculate averages.

The major advantage of the mean over the mode and median is that in calculating the mean, the numerical value of every observation in the data distribution is considered and used. When the mean is calculated, all values are summed and then divided by the number of values. However, this strength can be a drawback with highly skewed data in which there are outliers or extreme scores, as stated in our discussion of the median. Consider the following example.

Suppose you have just completed teaching a continuing education course in cardiopulmonary resuscitation (CPR). You test your students to determine their competence in CPR knowledge and skill. Of a possible 100, the following scores were obtained:

100 100 100 95 95

To calculate the mean, you will add each value and divide the sum by the total number of values (100 + 100 + 100 + 95 + 95 = 490/5 = 98). The mean score of your group is 98. You are satisfied with the scores and with the high level of knowledge and skill. Now let us see what happens in the following distribution of test scores:

100 100 100 90 35

The mean is calculated as 100 + 100 + 100 + 90 + 35 = 425/5 = 85. The mean (85) presents quite a different picture, even though only one member of the group scored poorly. If only the mean were reported, you would have no way of knowing that the majority of your class did well and that one individual or outlier score was responsible for the lower mean. •

Which Measure(s) to Calculate?

Although investigators often calculate all three measures of central tendency for continuous data, they may not all be purposive. Their usefulness depends on the aim of the analysis and the nature of the distribution of scores. In a normal or bell-shaped curve, the mean, median, and mode are in the same (or a similar) location (Figure 20-5). In this case, it is most efficient to use the mean, because this score is the most widely used measure of central tendency and forms the foundation for subsequent statistical calculations.

However, in a skewed distribution, the three measures of central tendency fall in different places (Figure 20-6). In this case, you will need to examine all three measures and select the one that most reasonably answers your question without providing a misleading picture of the findings.

 Now consider another example that illustrates a limitation of the mean. Suppose the scores that were obtained on level of knowledge were:

100 100 100 66 66 66

You calculate the mean as 83 and, because it is close to the mean in the earlier example, surmise that the scores are similar. However, look at the bimodal distribution. What the mean cannot tell you is the shape of the distribution. •

Measures of Variability

So far, we have learned that a single numerical index, such as the mean, median, or mode, can be used to describe central tendencies in a large frequency of scores but cannot tell you how the scores are distributed. Thus, each measure of central tendency has certain limitations, especially in the case of a distribution with extreme or bimodal or multimodal scores. Most groups of scores on a scale or index differ from one another, or have what is termed "variability" (also called "spread" or "dispersion").[1] Variability is another way to summarize and characterize large data sets. By variability, we simply mean

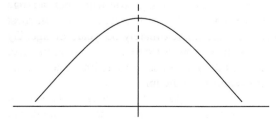

Figure 20-5 Normal curve, where mean, median, and mode are in the same location.

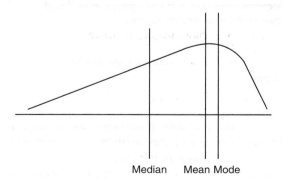

Figure 20-6 Skewed distribution, where the three measures of central tendency fall in different places.

TABLE 20-6	Life Satisfaction Scores for Two Groups*	
Group 1	**Group 2**
102	128
99	78
103	93
96	101
*See Figure 20-7.	

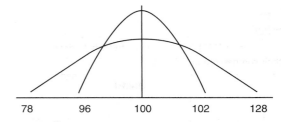

Figure 20-7 Dispersion of homogeneous and heterogeneous life satisfaction scores in two groups (see Table 20-6).

the degree of *dispersion* or the differences among scores. If scores are similar, there is little dispersion, spread, or variability across response categories. However, if scores are dissimilar, there is a high degree of dispersion.

Even though a measure of central tendency provides a numerical index of the average score in a group, as we have illustrated, it is also important to know how the scores vary or how they are dispersed around the measure of central tendency. Measures of variability provide additional information about the scoring patterns of the entire group.

Consider two groups of life satisfaction scores measured as continuous data, as shown in Table 20-6. In both groups, the mean satisfaction score is equal to 100. However, the variability, or dispersion, of scores around the mean is quite different. The scores in Group 1 are more homogeneous. In the second group, the scores are more variable, dispersed, or heterogeneous. The dispersion of scores for the two groups is shown in Figure 20-7. Therefore, knowing the mean will not help ascertain differences in the two groups, even though they exist. Let us assume you had to develop a support-group educational program for both groups. You would approach the focus of each group differently on the basis of your knowledge of the variability in scores. •

To describe a data distribution more fully, a summary measure of the variation or dispersion of the observed values is important. We discuss five basic measures of variability: range, interquartile range, sum of squares, variance, and standard deviation.

Range

The *range* represents the simplest measure of variation. It refers to the difference between the highest and lowest observed value in a collection of data. The range is a crude measure because it does not take into account all values of a distribution, only the lowest and highest. It does not indicate anything about the values that lie between these two extremes. In the Group 1 data listed in Table 20-6, the range is 96 to 103, or a range of 7 points. In the Group 2 data, the range is 78 to 128, or a range of 50 points.

Interquartile Range

A more meaningful measure of variability is called the *interquartile range* (IQR). The IQR refers to the range of the middle 50% of subjects. This range describes the middle of the sample or the range of a majority of subjects. By using the range of 50% of subjects, the investigator ignores the extreme scores or outliers. Assume your study sample ranges in age from 20 to 90 years, as follows:

20 20 21 34 35 35 35 38 39 45 85 90

If you only use the range, you will report a range of 20 to 90 with a 70-point spread. However, most individuals are approximately 35 years of age. By using the IQR, you separate the lowest 25% (ages 20, 20, and 21 years) and the highest 25% (45, 85, and 90 years) from the middle 50% (34, 35, 35, 35, 38, and 39 years). You report the range of scores that fall within the 50th percentile. In this way you ignore the outliers of 85 and 90. Usually, when reporting the median score for a distribution, the IQR is also used. To calculate the median, you count to the middle of the distribution. Similarly, with IQR, you count off the top and bottom quarters.

Sum of Squares

Another way to interpret variability is by squaring the difference between each score and the mean. Using squares ensures that positive and negative numbers, when added, do not cancel each other out and limit your ability to use the universe of scores that you obtain. These squared scores are then summed and referred to statistically as the *sum of squares* (SS). The larger the value of SS, the greater the variance. The SS is used in many other statistical manipulations. The equation for SS is as follows:

$$SS = \Sigma(X_M - X)^2$$

Variance

The *variance* (V) is another measure of variability and is calculated using the following equation:

$$V = \frac{\Sigma(X_M - X)^2}{N}$$

As the equation shows, variance is simply the mean or average of the sum of squares. The larger the variance, the larger the spread of scores.

Standard Deviation

The *standard deviation* (SD) is the most widely used measure of dispersion. It is an indicator of the average deviation of scores around the mean or, simply, the square root of the variance. In reporting the SD, researchers often use lowercase sigma (σ) or S. Similar to the mean, SD is calculated by taking into consideration every score in a distribution. The SD is based on distances of sample scores away from the mean score and equals the square root of the mean of the squared deviations. SD is derived by computing the variation of each value from the mean, squaring the variation, and taking the square root of that calculation. The SD represents the sample estimate of the population standard deviation and is calculated by the following formula:

$$S = \sqrt{\frac{\Sigma(y - y)^2}{n - 1}}$$

Examine the following calculation of the SD for these observations and a mean of 15.5 (or 16):

$$14\ 21\ 15\ 12$$

$$S = \sqrt{\frac{(16-14)^2 + (21-16)^2 + (16-15)^2 + (16-12)^2}{4-1}}$$

$$S = \sqrt{\frac{4 + 25 + 1 + 16}{4-1}}$$

$$S = \sqrt{\frac{46}{3}}$$

$$S = 3.9$$

The first step is to compute deviation scores for each subject. Deviation scores refer to the difference between an individual score and the mean. Second, each deviation score is squared. As we noted earlier, if the deviation scores were added without being squared, the sum would equal zero, because the deviations above the mean always exactly balance the deviations below the mean. The standard deviation overcomes this problem by squaring each deviation score before adding. Third, the squared deviations are added, the result is divided by one less than the number of cases, and then the square root is obtained. The square root takes the index back to the original units; in other words, the standard deviation is expressed in the units that are being measured.

The standard deviation is an index of variability of scores in a data set. It tells the investigator how scores deviate on the average from the mean. For example, if two distributions have a mean of 25 but one sample has an SD of 70 and the other sample an SD of 30, we know the second sample is more homogeneous because we know that the scores more closely cluster around the mean or that there is less dispersion (Fig. 20-8).

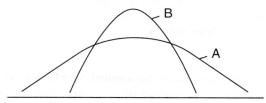

Figure 20-8 Comparison between small and large standard deviation. A, Large standard deviation. B, Small standard deviation.

Based on a normal curve, and by definition (see equation), approximately 68% of the means from samples in a population will fall within one standard deviation from the mean of means, 95% will fall within two standard deviations, and 99% will fall within three standard deviations.

The mean and standard deviation are often reported together in a data table and provide a powerful, descriptive, numeric story about a data set just from two numbers. These two measures of central tendency tell you about average and dispersion so that you understand fully the distribution that is presented.

Bivariate Descriptive Statistics

Thus far, we have discussed descriptive data reduction approaches for one variable (univariate); the procedures described are conducted for a univariate distribution. Another aspect of describing data involves looking for relationships among two or more variables. We describe two methods to do so: contingency tables and correlational analysis.

Contingency Tables

One method for describing a relationship between two variables (bivariate relationship) is a "contingency table," also referred to as a "cross-tabulation." A contingency table is a two-dimensional frequency distribution that is primarily used with categorical (nominal) data, although it can be used with all levels of data. In a contingency table, the attributes of one variable are related to the attributes of another.[2]

> Returning to an earlier example, you want to know the number of male and female students for each age category of the 20 high school students registered for a drug abuse prevention program. You can easily develop a contingency table that displays the number of male and female students for each age category (Table 20-7). •

Table 20-7 shows an unequal distribution, with more male than female students registered for the course. You can add a column on the table that indicates the percentage of male and female students for each age. Also, you can use a number of statistical

TABLE 20-7   Contingency Table of Age by Gender (N = 20)

Age	Gender Male	Female	Total
14	2	1	3
15	3	2	5
16	2	2	4
17	4	1	5
18	1	2	3
Total	12	8	20

procedures to examine the nature of the relationships displayed in a contingency table. You can determine whether the number of male students is significantly greater than the number of female students and not a chance occurrence. (This information would be particularly important in generalizing your sample findings to the population from which the sample was selected.) Such procedures are called "nonparametric statistics" and are discussed later in the chapter.

Correlational Analysis

A second method of looking at relationships among variables is correlational analysis. This approach examines the extent to which two variables are related to each other across a group of subjects. There are numerous correlational statistics. Selection depends primarily on the level of measurement and sample size. In a correlational statistic, an index is calculated that describes both the direction and magnitude of a relationship.

Three types of directional relationships can exist among variables: positive correlation, negative correlation, and zero correlation (no correlation). A positive correlation indicates that as the numerical values of one variable increase or decrease, the values for the other variable also change in the same direction. Conversely, a negative correlation indicates that numerical values for each variable are related in an opposing direction; as the values for one variable increase, the values for the other variable decrease.

The relationship between age and height in children younger than 12 years demonstrates a positive correlation, whereas the relationship between weight and hours of exercise represents a negative correlation. •

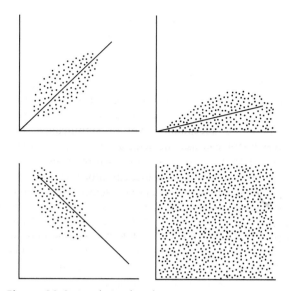

Figure 20-9 Correlational analyses.

To indicate the magnitude or strength of a relationship, the value that is calculated in correlational statistics ranges from −1 to +1. This value gives you two critical pieces of information: the absolute value denoting the strength of the relationship and the sign depicting the direction. The value of −1 indicates a perfect negative correlation, and +1 signifies a perfect positive correlation. By "perfect," we mean that the calculated values for each variable change at the same rate as another. Similarly, a value of +0.5 would be a moderate positive correlation (as one variable changed 1 unit the other changes ½ unit in the same direction) and −0.5 would denote a negative moderate correlation (as one variable changed 1 unit the other changes ½ unit in the opposite direction).

Assume you find a perfect positive correlation (+1) between years of education and reading level. This statistic will tell you that for each year (measured as a single unit) of education, reading level will improve 1 unit (as it is measured). •

A zero correlation is demonstrated in Table 20-6, which displays the relationship between life satisfaction and age. The closer a correlational statistical value falls to ~1 (absolute value of 1), the stronger the relationship (Fig. 20-9). As the value approaches zero, the relationship weakens.

Two correlation statistics are frequently used in social science literature: the Pearson product-moment correlation, known as the Pearson r, and the Spearman *rho*. Both statistics yield a value between −1 and +1. The Pearson r is calculated on interval level data, whereas the Spearman *rho* is used with ordinal data.

To illustrate the use of the Pearson r, suppose you were interested in investigating research productivity in health and human service faculty. You examine numerous variables measured with interval-level data to determine which were related to productivity in a sample of 200 faculty members. To ascertain the extent of the relationships among selected demographic variables and publication productivity, you would conduct a series of Pearson r calculations. Assume you find that the strongest correlation ($r = -0.38$) existed between hours spent in the classroom and productivity. Note the negative association. That is to say, more hours in the classroom are related to lower productivity. The weakest correlation ($r = 0.014$) existed between desire to publish and actual publication productivity. Note that the second correlation is positive.

If you had used ordinal data in your measurements, you would have used the Spearman *rho* to examine these relationships. •

Are these findings valuable? Could the relationships be a function of chance? Are these important in light of such seemingly low correlations? To answer these questions, the investigator must first submit the data to a test of significance, which determines the extent to which a finding occurs by chance. The investigator selects a *level of significance,* which is a statement of the expected degree of accuracy of the findings based on the sample size and on the convention in the relevant literature. The investigator examines a computer printout. If the computer presents an acceptable level of significance, the investigator can assume with a degree of certainty that the relationship was not caused by chance.

Consider how this statistical procedure is performed. Let us suppose that you select 0.05 as your confidence level. This number means the results will be caused by chance 5 times out of 100. If you were conducting this research before the ubiquity of statistical software, you would have located a table of critical values and found that the absolute value of your number of 0.38 exceeded the value you needed to determine that the finding was significant or not caused by chance. Therefore, you conclude that −0.38 is significant at the 0.05 level and report it to the reader as such. We mention this method because it illustrates the logic and reasoning that you need to make sense of significance. It is more likely, however, that you will conduct your analysis on a computer or mobile device using statistical software applications or a website. If so, you would search an electronically generated analysis to determine the corresponding level of significance, calculated for the value of $r = -0.38$. If it was 0.05 or smaller, you would conclude that this finding was significant. As you can see, the logic is the same as calculating the value of the correlation and then looking for a critical value, but the sequence of information presented is different from that in precomputer days.

Other statistical tests of association are used with different levels of measurement. For example, investigators often calculate the point biserial statistic to examine a relationship between a nominal variable and an interval level measure.[4] This statistic might be used to examine the relationship between gender and age expressed in years. When two nominal variables such as gender and rural or urban residency are calculated, the phi correlation statistic is often selected by researchers as an appropriate technique.[4] You can read about these tests and others in a text on statistical analysis.[1-4]

Level 2: Drawing Inferences

Descriptive statistics are useful for summarizing univariate and bivariate sets of data obtained from either a population or a sample. In many experimental-type studies, however, researchers also want to determine the extent to which observations of the sample are representative of the population from which the sample was selected. Inferential statistics provide the action processes for drawing conclusions about a population based on the data that are obtained from a sample.[3] Remember, the purpose of testing or measuring a sample is to gather and analyze data that allow statements to be made about the characteristics of the population from which the sample was obtained (Fig. 20-10).

Statistical inference, which is based on probability theory, is the process of generalizing from samples to populations from which the samples are derived. The tools of statistics help identify valid generalizations and those that are likely to stand up under further study. Thus, the second major role of statistical analysis is to make inferences. Inferential statistics include statistical techniques for evaluating many properties of populations, such as ascertaining differences among sets of data and predicting scores on one variable by knowing about others.

Two major concepts are fundamental to understanding inferential statistics: confidence levels and confidence intervals.

Because we are now interested in making estimates and predictions about a larger group from observations drawn from a subset of that group, we cannot be certain that what we observe in our smaller

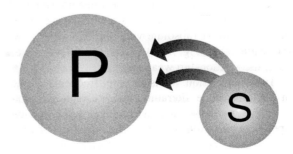

Figure 20-10 Relationship between sample (*S*) and population (*P*).

group is accurate for members of the larger group. This statement is the rationale for using probability theory to guide inferential statistical analysis. By specifying a confidence level and a confidence interval, we make a prediction of the range of observations we can expect to find and how accurate we expect our findings about the sample to be for the population. This set of predictions also specifies the degree of error that we are willing to accept, and it guides the researcher and consumer in the interpretation of statistical findings.

A *confidence interval* is defined as the range of values that we observe in our sample and for which we expect to find the value that accurately reflects the population. Consider the following example.

> You are interested in predicting the percentage of clients with mobility impairments on your rehabilitation unit who will use adaptive equipment after discharge. You randomly select a sample from your population of clients, and after surveying them for 3 months postdischarge, you find that 20% are still using their equipment. Should you expect that 20% of your population would follow the same pattern? This percentage would be your best guess, but it is derived from a subset of population members. Therefore, you need to expand your estimate to specify an interval of scores that you are confident will include the "true value" of the larger population—in this case, an interval of 15% to 30%. •

However, deriving a confidence interval is only the first step. Because we are now in the world of probability, specifying a confidence interval must contain a statement about the level of uncertainty as well. This is the point at which the confidence level comes into play. A *confidence level* is simply the degree of certainty (or expected uncertainty) that your confidence interval is accurate for your population. So you might be 50% confident or 99% confident that your findings will be accurate. In the previous example, if you specified a confidence level of 99%, you would be 99% certain that 15% to 30% of your population would use adaptive equipment 3 months after discharge from the rehabilitation unit. The degree of assuredness, or level of confidence,

that your sample values are accurate for the population constitutes the confidence level.

Before we discuss some of the most frequently used statistical tests and the sequence of action processes necessary to use them, consider another example.

> You are a mental health provider and are interested in testing the effect of a new intervention technique on the functional level of persons with schizophrenia residing in their own homes and attending your day program. In this study, you evaluate the rehabilitation technique for its effectiveness in achieving its outcome in a single group (experimental), and compare it to a group not receiving the intervention (control).
>
> Your research question is:
>
> *To what extent did the experimental intervention result in improving functional outcomes for persons diagnosed with schizophrenia living in their own homes?*
>
> Note that this question is articulated at level 3, and thus a true experimental design is warranted. The first step is to define your population carefully in terms of specific inclusion and exclusion criteria. You then randomly select a sample from your defined or targeted population using an appropriate random sampling technique. Next, you randomly assign the obtained sample to either an experimental or a control condition. You pretest all subjects, expose the experimental group to the intervention, and posttest all subjects. Hypothetically, the scores on your measure of functional status range from 1 to 10 in ascending order, with 1 denoting the least functional and 10 indicating the most functional. Now you have a series of scores: pretest scores from both groups and posttest scores from both groups. •

Let us assign hypothetical means to each group to illustrate the point. The experimental group has a pretest mean of 2 and a posttest mean of 6, whereas the control group has a pretest mean of 3 and a posttest mean of 5. In an actual study, you would calculate measures of dispersion as well, but for instructive purposes, we will omit this measure from our discussion. To answer your research question, you examine these scores at several levels. First, you will want to know whether the groups are equivalent before the intervention. You hypothesize that there will be no difference between the two groups before participation in the intervention. Also, you hypothesize that the groups adequately represent the population. Visual inspection of your pretest mean scores shows different scores. Is this difference occurring by chance, or as a result of actual group differences? To determine whether the difference in mean scores is caused by chance, you select a statistical analysis procedure (e.g., independent t-test) to compare the two sets of pretest data (e.g., experimental and control group mean scores). At this point, you hope to find that the scores are equivalent, and that therefore both sample groups represent the population.

Second, you want to know whether the change in scores at the posttest is a function of chance or what is anticipated to occur in the population. You will therefore choose a statistical analysis to evaluate these changes. The analysis of covariance (ANCOVA) is the statistic of choice for the true-experimental design. This statistic allows you to compare multiple groups of scores. In actuality, you will hope that the experimental group demonstrates change on the dependent or outcome variable at posttest time. You hypothesize that the change will be greater than that which may occur in the control group and greater than the scores observed at pretest time.

Thus, as a consequence of participating in the experimental group condition, you hope to demonstrate that the sample is significantly different from the control group and thus from the population from which the sample was drawn. In actuality, you will be testing two phenomena: inference, or the extent to which the samples reflect the population at both pretest and posttest time; and significance, or the extent to which group differences are a function of chance.

As you may recall, the "population" refers to all possible members of a group as defined by the researcher (see Chapter 14). A "sample" refers to a subset of a population to which the researcher wants to generalize. The accuracy of inferences from samples to populations depends on how representative the sample is of the population. The best way to ensure "representativeness" is to use probability sampling techniques. To use an inferential statistic,

---

BOX 20-2 *Steps in Using an Inferential Statistic*

Action 1: State the hypothesis.
Action 2: Select a significance level.
Action 3: Compute a calculated value.
Action 4: Obtain a critical value.
Action 5: Reject or fail to reject the null hypothesis.

---

you follow the five action processes introduced in Chapter 14, summarized in Box 20-2, and discussed now.

Action 1: State the Hypothesis

Stating a hypothesis is both simple and complex. In experimental-type designs that test the differences between population and sample, most researchers state an educated "hunch" of what they expect will occur. (Recall that this hunch is derived from theory underpinning the study.) This statement is called a working hypothesis. For statistical analysis, however, a working hypothesis is transformed into the null hypothesis. The null hypothesis is a statement of no difference between or among groups. In some studies or parts of studies, the investigator hopes to accept the null hypothesis, whereas in other studies or their parts, the researcher is hoping to fail to accept the null hypothesis.

Initially, as in the example of the experimental design given earlier, we hope to accept the null hypothesis between the pretest mean scores of both the experimental and control groups to ensure that our experimental and control groups are equivalent. We do not want our sample scores to differ from the population scores or the experimental and control groups to differ from one another at baseline (pretest) before the introduction of the treatment intervention. We pose and test the null hypothesis and hope that in testing it, the probability at which our statistical value is significant will be unacceptable (we describe significance in detail in the next section). For our posttest and change scores, however, we hope to "reject" (formally referred to in the language of probability theory as fail to accept) the null hypothesis. We want to find differences between the posttest scores of each group and a change between pretest and posttest scores only in the experimental group. These findings will tell us that the experimental group, after being exposed to the experimental condition (the intervention), is no longer representative of the population that did not receive the intervention. In other words, the intervention appears to have produced a difference in the scores of the individuals who participated in that group.

Why is the null hypothesis used? Theoretically, it is impossible to "prove" a relationship among two or more variables.[2] It is only possible to negate the null hypothesis of "no difference."[3] Nonsupport for the null hypothesis is similar to stating a double negative. If it is not "not raining," it logically follows that it is raining. Applied to research, if there is not "no difference among groups," differences among groups can be assumed, although not proven.

Action 2: Select a Significance Level

A level of significance defines how rare or unlikely the sample data must be before the researcher can fail to accept the null hypothesis. The level of significance is a cutoff point that indicates whether the samples being tested are from the same population or from a different population. This numeric value indicates how confident the researcher is that the findings regarding the sample are not attributable to chance. For example, if you select a significance level of 0.05, you are 95% confident that your statistical findings did not occur by chance. If you repeatedly draw different samples from the same population, theoretically you will find similar scores 95 out of 100 times. Similarly, a confidence level of 0.1 indicates that the findings may be caused by chance 1 of every 10 times.

As you can see, the smaller the number, the more confidence the researcher has in the findings and the more credible the results. Because of the nature of probability theory, the researcher can never be certain that the findings are 100% accurate. Significance levels are selected by the researcher on the basis of sample size, level of measurement, and conventional norms in the literature. As a general rule, the larger the sample size, the smaller the numerical value in the level of significance. If you have a small sample size, you risk obtaining a study group that is not highly representative of the population, and thus

your confidence level drops. A large sample size includes more elements from the population, and thus the chances of representation and confidence of findings increase. You therefore can use a stringent level of significance (0.01 or smaller).

One-Tailed and Two-Tailed Levels of Significance

Consider the normal curve in distribution of scores (see Fig. 20-4). Extreme scores can occur to either the left or the right of the bell shape. As we noted earlier, the extremes of the curve are called "tails." If a hypothesis is nondirectional, it indicates that the investigator assumes that extreme scores can occur at either end of the curve or in either tail. In this situation, the investigator uses a test to determine whether the 5% of statistical values that are considered statistically significant are distributed between the two tails of the curve. If, on the other hand, the hypothesis is directional, the researcher will use a one-tailed test of significance. The portion of the curve in which statistical values are considered significant is in one side of the curve, either the right or the left tail. It is easier to obtain statistical significance with a one-tailed statistical test, but the researcher will run the risk of a Type I error. A two-tailed test is a more stringent statistical approach.

Type I and II Errors

Because researchers deal with probabilities in statistical inference, two types of statistical inaccuracy or error (Type I and Type II) can contribute to the inability to claim full confidence in findings.

Type I Errors In a *Type I error*, also called an "alpha error,"[3] the researcher errs by failing to accept the null hypothesis when it is true. In other words, the researcher claims a difference between groups when, if the entire population were measured, there would be no difference. This error can occur when the most extreme members of a population are selected by chance in a sample. Assume, for example, that you set the level of significance at 0.05, indicating that 5 times out of 100 the null hypothesis can be rejected when it is accurate. Because the probability of making a Type I error is equal to the level of significance chosen by the investigator, reducing the level of significance will reduce the chances of making this type of error. Unfortunately, as the probability of making a Type I error is reduced, the potential to make another type of error (Type II) increases.

Type II Errors A *Type II error,* also called a "beta error,"[3] occurs if the null hypothesis is mistakenly accepted when it should be not be. In other words, the researcher fails to ascertain group differences when they have occurred. If you make a Type II error, you will conclude, for example, that the intervention did not have a positive outcome on the dependent variable when it actually did. The probability of making a Type II error is not as apparent as that of making a Type I error.[3] The likelihood of making a Type II error is based in large part on the power of the statistic to detect group differences.[4]

Determination and Consequences of Errors Type I and II errors are mutually exclusive. However, as you decrease the risk of a Type I error, you increase the chances of a Type II error. Furthermore, it is difficult to determine whether either error has been made because actual population parameters are not known by the researcher. It is often considered more serious to make a Type I error because the researcher is claiming a significant relationship or outcome when there is none. Because other researchers or practitioners may act on that finding, the researcher wants to insure against Type I errors. However, failure to recognize a positive effect from an intervention, a Type II error, can also have serious consequences for professional practice. For example, on the basis of an inaccurate finding, a valuable and productive intervention may be discarded.

Action 3: Compute a Calculated Value

To test a hypothesis, the researcher must choose and calculate a statistical formula. The selection of a statistic is based on the research question, level of measurement, number of groups that the researcher is comparing, and sample size. An investigator chooses a statistic from two classifications of inferential statistics: parametric and nonparametric procedures. Both are similar in that they (1) test

---

> **BOX 20-3** *Three Assumptions in Parametric Statistics*
>
> - Sample is derived from a population with a normal distribution.
> - Variance is homogeneous.
> - Data are measured at interval level.

hypotheses, (2) involve a level of significance, (3) require a calculated value, (4) compare the calculated value against a critical value, and (5) conclude with decisions about the hypotheses.

Parametric Statistics

Parametric statistics are mathematical formulas that test hypotheses on the basis of three assumptions (Box 20-3). First, your data must be derived from a population in which the characteristic to be studied is distributed normally (appearing as a bell shape or normal curve). Second, the variances within the groups to be studied must be homogeneous. Homogeneity is displayed by the scores in one group having approximately the same degree of variability as the scores in another group. Third, the data must be measured at the interval level.[3]

Parametric statistics can test the extent to which numerous sample structures are reflected in the population. For example, some statistics test differences between only two groups, whereas others test differences among many groups. Some statistics test main effects (i.e., the direct effect of one variable on another), whereas other statistics have the capacity to test both main and interactive effects (i.e., the combined effects that several variables have on another variable). Furthermore, some statistical action processes test group differences only one time, whereas others test differences over time. Most researchers attempt to use parametric tests when possible because they are the most robust of the inferential statistics. By "robust," we mean statistics that most likely detect a significant effect or increase power and decrease Type II errors.

Although we cannot present the full spectrum of parametric statistics, we examine three statistical tests frequently used in health and human service research[5,6] to illustrate the power of parametric testing: t-test, one-way analysis of variance (ANOVA), and multiple comparisons. These techniques are used to compare two or more groups to determine whether the differences in the means of the groups are large enough to allow the assumption that the corresponding population means are different.

t-Test The t-test is the most basic statistical procedure in this grouping. It is used to compare two sample means on one variable. Consider the following example.

> You want to compare the life satisfaction level of physical therapy (PT) students with occupational therapy (OT) students. You administer a general life satisfaction scale (scored such that ascending values indicate higher levels of satisfaction) to a randomly selected sample of students and obtain a mean score for each group. Assume the OT students have an average score of 125.6 and PT students an average of 120.3. At first glance it appears the OT group has the larger mean. However, it is not much larger than the mean derived from the PT group. The statistical question follows: To what extent are the two sample means sufficiently different to allow the researcher to conclude, with a high degree of confidence, that the population means are different from one another (even though we will never see the actual population means)? •

The t-test provides an answer to this question. If the researcher finds a significant difference between the two sample means, the null hypothesis will fail to be accepted. As a test of the null hypothesis, the t value indicates the probability that the null hypothesis is correct.[6]

Three principles influence the t-test. First, the larger the sample size, the less likely it is that a difference between two means is a consequence of an error in sampling. Second, the larger the observed difference between two means, the less likely it is that the difference is a consequence of a sampling error. Third, the smaller the variance, the less likely it is that the difference between the means is also a consequence of a sampling error.

The t-test can be used only when the means of two groups are compared. For studies with more than two groups, the investigator must select other statistical procedures. Similar to all parametric statistics, t-tests must be calculated with interval-level data and should be selected only if the researcher believes that the assumptions for the use of parametric statistics have not been violated. The t-test yields a t value that is reported as "$t = x, p = 0.05$"; x is the calculated t value, and p is the level of significance set by the researcher.

There are two types of t-tests. One type is for independent or uncorrelated data, and the other type is for dependent or correlated data. To understand the difference between these two types of t-tests, return to the example of the two-group randomized design to test an experimental intervention for patients with schizophrenia.

We stated that one of the first statistical tests performed determines whether the experimental and control group subjects differ at the first testing occasion, or pretest. The pretest data of experimental and control group subjects reflect two independent samples. A t-test for independent samples could be used to compare the difference between these two groups. However, let us assume we want to compare the pretest scores to posttest scores for only the experimental subjects. In this case, we would compare scores from the same subjects at two points in time. The scores are likely to be more similar than if the groups were constituted from different members because with subjects drawn from the same sample pretest scores often serve as good predictors of posttest scores. In this case, the scores are drawn from the same group and are apt to be highly correlated. Therefore, the t-test for dependent data will be used, which considers the correlated nature of the data. To learn the computational procedures for the test, we refer you to statistics texts.[1-4]

One-Way Analysis of Variance The "one-way" ANOVA, or "single-factor" ANOVA, serves the same purpose as the t-test. It is designed to compare sample group means to determine whether a significant difference can be inferred in the population. However, one-way ANOVA, also referred to as the "F-test," can manage two or more groups. It is an extension of the t-test for a two-or-more-groups situation. The null hypothesis for an ANOVA, as in the t-test, states that there is no difference between the means of two or more populations.

The procedure is also similar to the t-test. The original raw data are put into a formula to obtain a calculated value. The resulting calculated value is compared against the critical value, and the null hypothesis is not accepted if the calculated value is larger than the tabled critical value or accepted if the calculated value is less than the critical value. Computing the one-way ANOVA yields an F value that may be reported as "$F(a,b) = x$, $p = 0.05$"; x is computed F value, a is group degrees of freedom, b is sample degrees of freedom, and p is level of significance. "Degrees of freedom" refers to the "number of values, which are free to vary"[6] in a data set.

There are many variations of ANOVA. Some test relationships when variables have multiple levels, and some examine complex relationships among multiple levels of variables.

> Suppose you are interested in determining the effects of family support, acceptance of robotic assistive devices, and memory function on length of time that elders are able to remain in the community and age in place. Measuring the relationship between each independent variable and the outcome will be valuable. However, it will seem prudent to consider the interactive effects of the variables on the outcome. Several variations of the ANOVA (e.g., ANCOVA) should be considered. •

Multiple Comparisons When a one-way ANOVA is used to compare three or more groups, a significant F value means that the sample data indicate that the researcher should fail to accept the null hypothesis. However, the F value, in itself, does not tell the investigator which of the group means is significantly different; it only indicates that there is a difference in one or more groups.

Several procedures, referred to as multiple comparisons (post hoc comparisons), are used to determine which group difference is greater than the others. These procedures are computed after the occurrence of a significant F value and are capable of identifying which group or groups differ among those being compared.

Nonparametric Statistics

Nonparametric statistics are formulas used to test hypotheses when the data violate one or more of the assumptions for parametric procedures (see Box 20-3). If variance in the population is skewed or asymmetrical, if the data generated from measures are ordinal or nominal, or if the size of the sample is small, the researcher should select a nonparametric statistic.[7]

Each of the parametric tests mentioned has a nonparametric analogue. For example, the nonparametric analogue of the t-test for categorical data is the chi-square. The chi-square test (chi^2) is used when the data are nominal and when computation of a mean is not possible. This test is a statistical procedure that uses proportions and percentages to evaluate group differences. Thus, in computing it, differences between observed frequencies and the frequencies that can be expected to occur if the categories were independent of one another are calculated. If differences are found, however, the analysis does not indicate where the significant differences are. Consider the following example.

> You want to know whether 100 men and 100 women differ with regard to their views on prenatal testing for Down syndrome (in favor or not in favor). Your first step will be to develop a contingency or "cross-tab" table (a 2 × 2 table) and carry out a chi-square analysis. If there are no differences, you will expect each cell to have an equivalent number of observations. The same number of men and women will have indicated the same views (e.g., 50 men indicate in favor, 50 men indicate not in favor; likewise, 50 women indicate in favor, and 50 women indicate not in favor). However, the actual data look somewhat different, with unequal cells. The chi-square evaluates whether differences in cells are statistically significant—that is, whether the differences are not attributable to chance—but it will not tell you where the significance lies in the table. •

The Mann-Whitney U test is another powerful nonparametric test. It is similar to the t-test in that it is designed to test differences between groups, but it is used with data that are ordinal.

Suppose you now ask male and female respondents to rate their favorability toward prenatal testing for Down syndrome on a four-point ordinal scale from "strongly favor" to "strongly disfavor." The Mann-Whitney U would be a good choice to analyze significant differences in opinion related to gender. Many other nonparametric tests are useful as well, and you should consult texts that detail nonparametric procedures to learn about these techniques (see the references at the end of this chapter).

For some of the nonparametric tests, the critical value may have to be larger than the computed statistical value for findings to be significant.[7] Nonparametric statistics, as well as parametric statistics, can be used to test hypotheses from a wide variety of designs. Because nonparametric statistics are less robust than parametric tests, researchers tend not to use nonparametric tests unless they believe that the assumptions necessary for the use of parametric statistics have been violated.[6]

strong & creative

Choosing a Statistical Test

The choice of statistical test is based on several considerations (Box 20-4). The answers to these questions guide the researcher to the selection of specific statistical procedures.

BOX 20-4 *Questions to Consider in Choosing a Statistical Test*

1. What is the research question?
   - Is it about differences?
   - Is it about degrees of a relationship between variables?
   - Is it an attempt to predict group membership?
2. How many variables are being tested, and what types of variables are they?
   - How many variables do you have?
   - How many independent and dependent variables are you testing?
   - Are variables continuous or discrete?
3. What is the level of measurement? (Interval level can be used with parametric procedures.)
4. What is the nature of the relationship between two or more variables being investigated?
5. How many groups are being compared?
6. What are the underlying assumptions about the distribution of a measurement in the population from which the sample was selected?
7. What is the sample size?

The discussion of the tests frequently used by researchers that follows should be used only as a guide. We refer you to other resources to help you select appropriate statistical techniques.[1-4,6,7]

Action 4: Obtain a Critical Value

As we have noted previously, before the widespread use of computers and mobile devices, researchers located critical values in an appropriate table in the back of a statistics book. Recall that the "critical value" is a criterion related to the level of significance and tells the researcher what number must be derived from the statistical formula to indicate a significant finding. However, as we noted, although using the same logic, electronic statistical analysis venues report your findings differently than they were rendered before computerized calculation. Rather than identifying your probability level and then examining the critical value you need to use as your criterion for determining significance, the computer printout will tell you at what probability your calculated value is a critical value. So rather than looking at the calculated value of your statistic, you identify significant findings by searching for levels of probability that are smaller in value than the value that you have chosen.

Suppose you are interested in testing the degree to which an obesity prevention program resulted in knowledge acquisition about nutrition and exercise. Table 20-8 presents a hypothetical computer-generated analysis for your inquiry. Using a pretest-posttest quasi-experimental design, you test your sample of 50 participants before the intervention on a knowledge test scored from 0 to 100, with higher scores indicating greater knowledge. You then deliver the intervention and administer the posttest to determine the degree to which knowledge increased. To test your working hypothesis that knowledge will significantly increase, you formulate the null hypothesis of no difference between the mean pretest and posttest scores, then test it using a one-tailed t-test for dependent samples. (Remember that one-tailed tests are used if you hypothesize the direction of change, and dependent t-tests are used when a single sample tested on two occasions generates the two data sets to be compared.) •

TABLE 20-8 *Hypothetical Data From Analysis of Knowledge Acquisition*

Pretest Mean/SD	Posttest Mean/SD	t Value	P
67/9.75	89.6/2.63	10.56	.004

P, Probability; *SD,* standard deviation.

Action 5: Reject or Fail to Reject the Null Hypothesis

The final inferential action process is the decision about whether to accept or fail to accept the null hypothesis. Thus far, we have indicated that a statistical formula is selected along with a level of significance. The formula is calculated, yielding a numerical value. How do researchers know whether to accept or fail to accept the null hypothesis based on the obtained value?

Once again, before the use of electronic statistical calculation, the researcher would set a significance level and calculate degrees of freedom for the sample or number of sample groups (or both). Although it is not likely that you will use a printed table, once again we discuss this action process here for instructive purposes. Degrees of freedom are closely related to sample size and number of groups and refer to the scores that are "free to vary." Calculating degrees of freedom depends on the statistical formula used. By examining the degrees of freedom in a study, the researcher can closely ascertain sample size and number of comparison groups without reading anything else. In the t-test, for example, degrees of freedom are calculated only on the sample size. Group degrees of freedom are not calculated because only two groups are analyzed, and therefore only one group mean is free to vary. When degrees of freedom (DF) for sample size are calculated, the number 1 is subtracted from the total sample (DF = $n - 1$), indicating that all measurement values with the exception of 1 are free to vary. A simple way to think about degrees of freedom is to consider 5 scores when summed that equal 10. The first four scores $(1 + 2 + 3 + 4)$ can vary, but once the four scores are generated, the fifth score is fixed as $10 - (1 + 2 + 3 + 4)$. Thus in this example there are 4 degrees of freedom of one less that the total number of scores.

For the F ratio, degrees of freedom are also calculated on group means because more than two groups may be compared. So, using the same logic as before, if there are 3 groups, there are 2 "group" degrees of freedom. Calculating degrees of freedom is not always as simple as our illustration. However, we provided the example to give you a conceptual picture of the meaning of degrees of freedom. We refer you to references to read more about calculating degrees of freedom for more advanced statistics.[4]

After the researcher has calculated the degrees of freedom and the statistical value, he or she locates the table that illustrates the distribution for the statistical values that were calculated. The critical values are located by observing the value that is listed at the intersection of the calculated degrees of freedom and the level of significance. If the critical value is larger than the calculated statistic, in most cases the researcher accepts the null hypothesis (i.e., no significant differences between groups). If the calculated value is larger than the critical value, the researcher rejects the null hypothesis, and within the confidence level selected, accepts that the groups differ.

Statistical software on the computer or mobile device is capable of calculating all values and further identifying the p value at which the calculated statistical value will be significant. In the hypothetical data in Table 20-8, the means and standard deviations are presented for both pretest and posttest scores. The calculated value of t is 10.56, and the probability value at which the calculated value would be a critical value is .004. You would therefore accept the null hypothesis because the probability is smaller than your selected level of .05. Therefore, using a computer to calculate statistics presents the information so that you can immediately determine whether your findings are significant simply by examining the probability values.

Level 3: Associations and Relationships

The third major role of statistics is the identification of relationships between variables and whether knowledge about one set of data allows the researcher to infer or predict characteristics about another set of data. These statistical tests include factor analyses, discriminant function analysis, multiple regression, and modeling techniques. The commonality among these tests is that they all seek to predict one or more outcomes from multiple variables. Some of the techniques can further identify time factors, interactive effects, and complex relationships among multiple independent and dependent variables.[8]

To illustrate this level of statistical analysis, let us consider a hypothetical study in which you are interested in investigating predictors of outcome of marital counseling.

Given the complexity of the topic marital counseling, you have identified 22 variables from the literature that have the potential to predict outcomes on two variables: length of counseling and degree of reported improvement in the marital relationship. Included among the independent or predictor variables are the extent of investment in the counseling process on the part of the couple, degree of communication difficulty, current living arrangements of the couple, perceived equality of shared responsibility, and future expectations for success expressed by the couple. To analyze your complex data set, you choose an analysis technique called "automatic interaction detector," a statistical procedure that can reveal predictive relationships and the strength of those relationships to examine the effect of the 22 variables on both outcomes.[6] As you can see, predictive statistics are extremely valuable in that they suggest what might happen in one arena (outcome in counseling), based on knowledge of certain indicators (22 predictive variables). •

Multiple regression is used to predict the effect of multiple independent (predictor) variables on one dependent (outcome or criterion) variable. Multiple regression can be used only when all variables are measured at the interval level. Discriminant function analysis is a similar test used with categorical or nominal dependent variables.[4]

In the previous example of an examination of research productivity in health and human service faculty, suppose, as the basis for making decisions about tenure and promotion, you were interested in

determining the predictive capacity of hours spent in the classroom, desire to publish, university support for publication, and degree of job satisfaction on publication productivity, the four variables as illustrated. Multiple regression is an equation based on correlational statistics in which each predictor variable is entered into an equation to determine how strongly it is related to the outcome variable and how much variation in the outcome variable can be predicted by each independent variable. In some cases, a stepwise multiple regression is performed in which the predictors are listed from "least related" to "most related" and the cumulative effect of variables is reported. In your study, it was found that all four predictor variables were important influences on the variance of the outcome variable.

Other techniques, such as modeling strategies, are frequently used to clarify complex system relationships.[6] Assume you are interested in determining why some persons with chronic health conditions live independently and others do not. With so many variables, you may choose a modeling technique that will help identify mathematical properties of relationships, allowing you to determine which factor or combination of factors will best predict success in independent living. (See the list of references for further information about these more advanced statistical techniques.)

Geospatial Analysis: GIS

As we have presented in Chapter 16, geospatial analysis is growing in popularity. A geographic information system (GIS) is a computer-assisted action process that has the capacity to handle and analyze multiple sources of data, providing that they are relevant to spatial depiction. Remember that GIS relies on two overarching spatial paradigms, raster and vector. Raster GIS carves geography into mutually exclusive spaces and then examines the attributes of these. This type of analysis would be relevant to questions of comparative attributes to specific locations. Vector GIS is relevant to determining characteristics of a space that is defined by points and the lines that "connect the dots."[8]

GIS maps are constructed from data tables, and because GIS software allows the importation of data from frequently used spreadsheets and data bases such as Excel, Access, and even SPSS, combining visual and statistical analytic techniques is a relatively simple and powerful action process. We refer you to the multiple texts on GIS for specific techniques. Here we consider an example. Suppose you were interested in looking at the need for health promotion and illness prevention programs in the state of Maine. Figure 20-11 depicts the density of these programs within the state. To create this visual map, the addresses of each program were entered into a database and analyzed with GIS software. The minor civil divisions are used to carve up locations into smaller areas for census procedures but do not tell you how many people live in each division. Thus, this vector approach describes the distribution of programs but cannot tell you about the relationship between population density and program density. Figure 20-12 answers that relational question by mapping two layers, population and program distribution.

Other Visual Analysis Action Processes

Mapping is only one type of visual analysis. In statistical analysis, image is primarily used to represent numeric data. Visuals such as graphs and charts have been used to display and analyze information since the inception of statistics in the mid-17th century. Similar to numeric analysis, visuals reduce data to comprehensible forms. Consider the normal curve, polygons, and bar charts. Each tells an analytic story, translating statistical analysis into a visual form. According to Tufte, "Of all methods for analyzing and communicating statistical information, well-designed data graphics are usually the simplest and at the same time, the most powerful."[9]

Figure 20-13 depicts the gender composition of students taking an undergraduate disability studies class. Figure 20-14 is an image of the bivariate relationship between height and weight.

In addition to description, visual analysis is often used in intervention research. We discuss how visual data analysis can be used in a case study in Chapter 12 and here provide an example.

Suppose you are interested in measuring change in a child's socialization frequency following a social skills intervention. To obtain a baseline level of socialization, you count how many times per hour that you observe the child engaging with another child on the playground. You then provide the intervention and measure socialization frequency for 1 week following the intervention. Figure 20-15 presents no change, because the slope or trajectory of the line following the intervention does not change. However, if your findings are displayed in Figure 20-16, you can assume that there was a change.

Before we leave visual analysis, we bring your attention to several areas of critical use. First is your own inspection of data points and distributions to decide on what further statistical tests to use. Remember that we distinguished between parametric and nonparametric statistics, indicating that one of the three criteria for selection is the shape of the distribution. Visualizing the values of each variable by creating a scatterplot can quickly tell you whether your distributions are normal. Figure 20-17 presents a univariate scatterplot. Scatterplots can also be helpful in determining the nature of bivariate relationships as shown in Figure 20-18.

Second, visuals can clarify complex, multivariate relationships. An example of this point is the presentation of mapped data with multiple layers of information presented in the previous section on GIS mapping. Of course, there are many options for visual data analysis and representation in experimental-type design.

Finally, recall that we introduced big data. Network and similar analyses of huge data sets are often presented as interactive visuals on which nonlinear relationships are mapped and put into action. Figure 20-19 is a graphic depiction of a communication network on a Facebook group.

Visuals can be used for many levels of analysis, from simple univariate descriptive through multivariate prediction. They complement and sometimes supplant text and numeric displays. Choice of presentation method should be purposive and consider the audience with whom the data analysis will be shared.

Remember that statistical analysis is a method that is used in experimental-type designs. As we illustrate in Chapter 21, when used with naturalistic analysis, the study design turns to mixed methods.

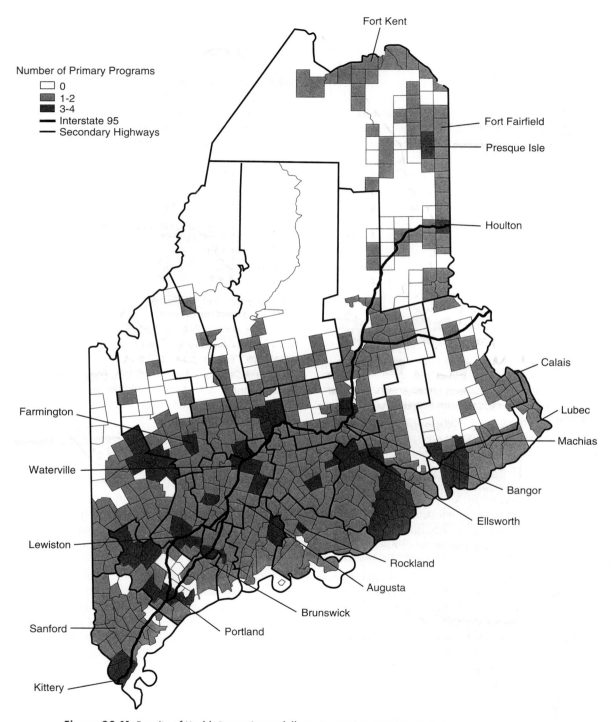

Figure 20-11 Density of Health Promotion and Illness Prevention Programs in Maine.

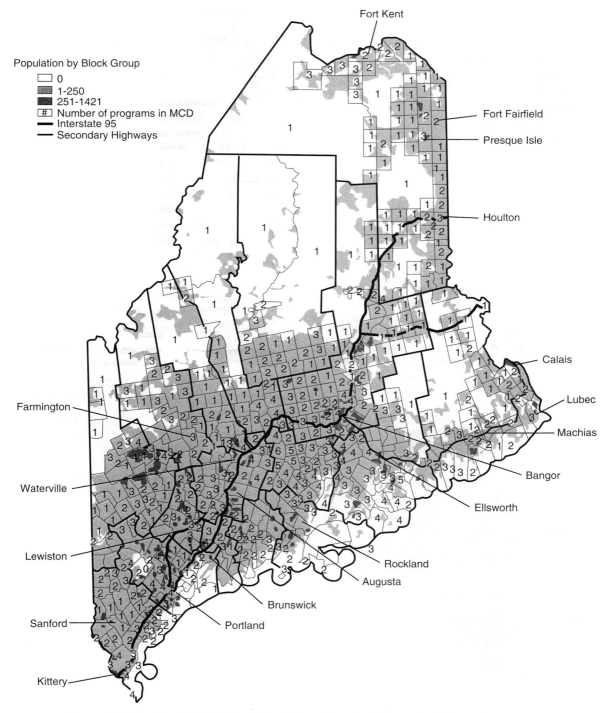

Figure 20-12 Density of Health Promotion and Illness Prevention Programs in Maine.

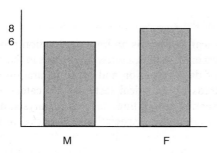

Figure 20-13 Gender composition of students.

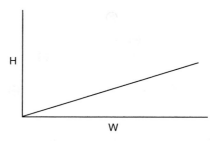

Figure 20-14 Bivariate relationship between height and weight.

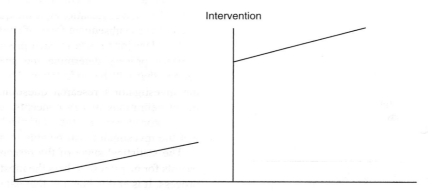

Figure 20-15 No change following intervention.

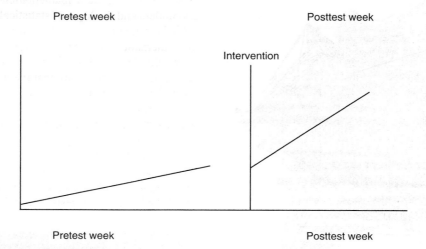

Figure 20-16 Change following intervention.

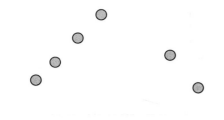

Figure 20-17 Univariate scatterplot.

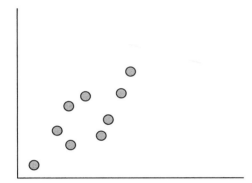

Figure 20-18 Bivariate relationships.

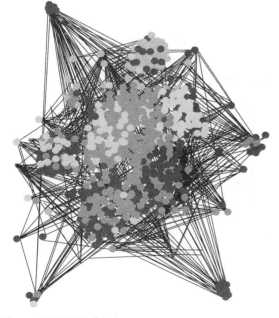

Figure 20-19 Big data image.

Summary

Statistical analysis is an important action process in experimental-type research that occurs at the conclusion of data collection and data preparation efforts. Hundreds of statistical tests can be categorized as representing one of three levels of analysis: descriptive, inferential, or associational. The level of statistical analysis used depends on many factors, especially the research question, level of measurement of study variables, sample size, and distribution of scores. Each level of analysis builds on the other. Descriptive analyses are always conducted first, followed by inferential and associational, if the question and data warrant each subsequent form of analysis.

The decisions made in each previous step of the research process determine the specific statistical actions that will be undertaken. Thus, embedded in the investigator's research question, in the operational definitions of key concepts, and in the sampling procedures are the statistical manipulations that the investigator will be able to use.

The statistical stage of the research process represents for many researchers the most exciting action process. It is at this juncture that data become meaningful and lead to knowledge building that is descriptive, inferential, or associational. The researcher does not have to be a mathematician to appreciate and understand the logic of statistical manipulations. If the investigator does not have a strong background in mathematics, geographic analysis, or graphics, he or she should consult an expert or a statistician at the start of the study to ensure that the question and data collection methods are compatible with the statistical approaches that best answer the research question. When statistics are used in concert with naturalistic analysis, we then classify the study as mixed method.

The purpose of this chapter is to "jump-start" your understanding of this action research process. Many guides and statistical resources describe in detail the hundreds of tests from which to choose.

EXERCISES

1. Select a research article that uses statistical procedures: (a) determine the level of statistical techniques used; (b) ascertain the rationale behind

the selection of the specific statistics used; and (c) critically analyze the statistical tests and determine whether they were appropriate to answer the question the investigator initially posed and appropriate to the level of measurement and sample size.

2. Given the following scores, develop a frequency table and find the mode, median, mean, range, and standard deviation: 12 35 34 26 26 13 21 22 22 22 24 35 36 37 39 51 23 42 41 21 21 22 25 26 27 44 42 13 35 43 12 3. Identify a research article that reported in table format mean and standard deviation scores to describe the basic characteristics of the study sample. Examine the table; in your own words, write a description of the study based on the numbers presented. Compare your description with that of the study authors.

3. Find examples of GIS mapping and big data in visual format.

References

1. Gould R, Ryan C: *Introductory statistics*, Saddle River, NJ, 2014, Pearson.
2. Frankfort-Nachmias C, Leon-Guerrero A: *Social statistics for a diverse society*, Los Angeles, 2014, Sage.
3. Trochim W: *Inferential statistics*, 2006. Retrieved from Research Methods Knowledge Base: <http://www.social researchmethods.net/kb/statinf.php>.
4. Pelham B: *Intermediate statistics*, Los Angeles, 2013, Sage.
5. DePoy E, Gilson S: *Evaluation practice*, Belmont, Calif, 2002, Brooks-Cole.
6. Healey JF: *The essentials of statistics: a tool for social research*, ed 2, Belmont, Calif, 2009, Wadsworth.
7. Wasserman L: *All of nonparametric statistics*, New York, 2007, Springer.
8. ESRI: *What is GIS?* n.d. <http://www.esri.com/what-is-gis>.
9. Tufte E: *The visual display of quantitative information*, Cheshire, Conn, 2001, Graphics Press.

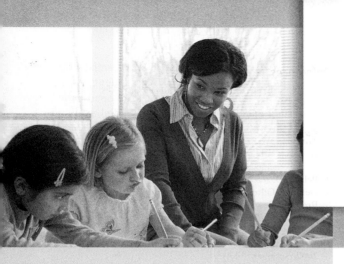

Chapter 21
Analysis in Naturalistic Inquiry

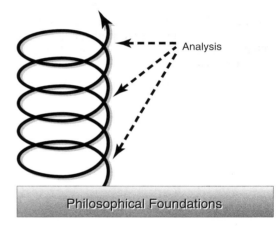

We now turn our attention to the way in which researchers approach the analysis of data in naturalistic inquiry. As you probably surmise at this point, the action process of conducting analyses in naturalistic inquiry is quite different from the actions undertaken during statistical decision making and enactment in experimental-type research. Although there are diverse approaches to working with data, for the most part, analysis in naturalistic research is a dynamic and iterative process. That is to say, in its most inductive form, analysis is interwoven with data collection, is fluid, and is constantly occurring in response to new data throughout your study. Also, as noted in Chapter 17, keep in mind that organizing information in naturalistic inquiry is an analytical action, and it is difficult to separate the actions

311

involved in organization and management from the analytical actions.

Although all analytical strategies are systematic, there is no step-by-step, recipe-like set of rules that can be followed by an investigator in naturalistic inquiry. Many organizational and analytical tools can be used at different points in the process of the study. The analytical process also is shaped by the type of data that are collected, and it will vary depending on whether the data are narrative, observational, visual, musical, diaries, email text, tweets, blogs, objects, historical documents, or any other data formats.

After you read this chapter, you may want to refer to other literature sources to obtain more in-depth and specific understanding of particular analytical approaches in naturalistic inquiry.[1-4] Here, we cannot address analysis in each design, but rather provide an introduction to and overview of the basic principles that underlie the general thinking and action processes of researchers involved in various forms of analysis across the traditions of naturalistic inquiry. Specifically, we address uncovering themes (thematic analysis) and understanding relationships among the themes as the basis for theory development.

Some Words About Mixed Methods

Similar to our statements in Chapter 20, we remind you here that naturalistic analysis is inductive and abductive. So even if open-ended interviews are the source to be analyzed, in order to be considered naturalistic, knowledge must be emergent rather than imposed in naturalistic traditions. If a deductive approach is used to analyze narrative data, for example, then we would classify the study as mixed methods. Consider this example. One of our students just completed a project in which people receiving mental health counseling from clinical social workers were interviewed to determine their experience in therapy. This broad query, if answered inductively with all essentials proceeding in the naturalistic tradition, would have been classified as such. However, the student had a theory for use in mind as well as a research question. In carrying out the analysis, the student imposed the theory of treatment satisfaction[1] on unstructured interview data and ultimately answered the question, "What level of satisfaction was attained by clinical social work clients?" The integration of deductive analysis with open-ended data was an excellent although unintended example of mixed methods design.

Although many students often think that naturalistic analysis is a process that is more akin to nonresearch thinking because it does not involve numbers and formulas, we suggest that when done correctly, induction is not an easy task. Using naturalistic analysis in mixed methods should be done in a purposive fashion. If indicated by the level of theory development, research questions/queries, purposes, and constraints of your study, mixing analytical strategies can lead to the production of new knowledge, at the same time testing existing theory.[2] So let us begin our exploration of the essential of analysis in naturalistic inquiry.

Strategies and Stages in Naturalistic Analysis

As we have emphasized throughout, the selection of a particular approach to analysis depends on the primary purpose of the research study, the scope of the query, the particular design, and the constraints of the study context. Table 21-1 summarizes the basic purpose and analytical approach used by naturalistic designs that we have discussed previously.

Some analytical strategies in naturalistic inquiry are extremely unstructured, such as in phenomenology, heuristic designs, object reading, and several contemporary approaches to ethnography. Other analytical strategies are highly structured, as in grounded theory. Still other analytical tools may incorporate numerical descriptions and may vary in the type of analysis used, as in certain forms of ethnography, endogenous designs, and participatory action research. There is also a large continuum of researcher interpretation, from none to extensive. Each analytical approach provides a different understanding of the phenomenon under study. Furthermore, in any given study, a researcher may use a combination of analytical strategies at different points in the course of the investigation. Even when using multiple analytical tools, if the analysis is inductive or

TABLE 21-1   *Purpose and Analytical Strategy of Naturalistic Study Designs*

Study Design	Main Purpose	Basic Analytical Strategy
Endogenous	Varies	Varies
Participatory action research	Varies	Varies
Phenomenology	Identifies essence of personal experiences	Groups statements based on meaning; develops textual description
Heuristic	Discovers personal experiences	Describes meaning of experience for researcher and others
Life history	Provides biographical account	Describes chronological events; identifies turning points
Ethnography	Describes and explains cultural patterns	Identifies themes and develops interpretive schema
Grounded theory	Constructs or modifies theory	Provides constant comparative method to name and frame theoretical constructs and relationships
Critical theory	Social change	
Narrative inquiry	Describes and explains patterns and experiences	
Object reading	Provides a form to understand meaning in nonhuman artifacts[6]	

abductive in nature, we would still classify a design as naturalistic.

> Assume you are conducting an ethnographic study of the meaning of "good" daily life in an assisted-living facility for residents. You decide to use several data collection strategies, such as interviewing residents and family members, observing daily activities, and video-recording staff interactions with residents. The initial purpose of your analysis is to describe daily routines and behaviors of the residents. One analytical strategy may involve counting the number of activities in which residents are engaged, then grouping activities by the categories they represent (e.g., self-care, leisure, social, cognitive, physical). Another purpose of the analysis is to identify themes that explain the meanings attributed by residents to their daily life in the facility. Analysis will involve an interpretive process to identify statements that reflect core meanings of the experience of a good life in assisted living. On the basis of these two analytical steps, suppose you discover that staff relationships are a salient factor in "good" experiences of residents. To better understand this particular finding, you may add another analytical strategy, such as frame-by-frame video analysis of staff-resident verbal interactions. •

Therefore, you would need to use three analytical approaches in this study. Each approach would reflect a specific purpose and yield a particular understanding of the phenomenon of interest. The findings from each approach would then be integrated to contribute to a comprehensive and synthetic understanding of the initial research query (e.g., "What is the nature of a good daily life in assisted living?").

Although each type of naturalistic design uses a different analytical strategy, the basic process in naturalistic design for the most part can be conceptualized as occurring in two overlapping and interrelated stages. The first stage of analysis occurs at the exact moment the investigator enters the virtual, conceptual, or physical context of the study. It involves the attempt to make immediate sense of what is being observed, heard, or read—what we have referred to as "gaining familiarity." At this stage, the purpose of analysis is primarily descriptive and yields "hunches" or initial interpretations that guide data collection decisions made in the physical, virtual imaged, and/or conceptual environments in which the study occurs. The second stage follows the conclusion of data collection and involves a more formal review and analysis of all the information that has been obtained. The investigator refines or evolves an interpretation (if warranted by the design) that is recorded for dissemination to diverse communities.

At each stage, the researcher may use a different analytical approach. The actions during each stage are best conceptualized as a "spiral," each loop of which involves a set of analytical tasks that lead to the next loop in successive fashion until a complete understanding of the field or phenomenon under study is derived.

Stage One: Inception of a Study

As shown in previous chapters, the process of naturalistic inquiry is iterative. Let us examine what this means in the initial analytical stage. First, data analysis occurs immediately as the researcher enters the study environment, and analysis continues throughout the investigator's engagement in the field. Analysis is the basis from which all subsequent decisions are made: whom to interview, what to observe, and/or which piece of information to read and explore further. Data collection efforts are inextricably connected to the initial impressions and hunches that are formulated by the investigator; that is, an observation, or datum, gives rise to an initial understanding of the phenomenon under study. This initial understanding informs or shapes the next data collection decision. Each decision and collection-analytical action builds successively on the previous action and shapes the subsequent action.

Thus, during the research process, the investigator begins by systematically examining data—notes, recorded observations, readings, videos, images, objects, and transcriptions of interviews—to obtain initial descriptions, impressions, and hunches. (It is important to note that transcriptions are usually completed immediately or shortly after the completion of an interview, observation, or readings of documents to enable the investigator to evaluate the data and make subsequent decisions to further the data collection efforts.) The investigator also keeps careful records of his or her perceptions, biases, or opinions in the form of reflexive notes and begins to group information into meaningful *categories* that describe the phenomenon of interest. This descriptive analysis is especially critical in the early stages of a study. It is essential to the process of reframing the initial query and setting limits or boundaries as to whom and what should be investigated and when.

This initial set of analytical steps involves four interrelated thinking and action processes (Box 21-1). Keep in mind that these are dynamic. That is,

---

> **BOX 21-1** | *Analytical Thinking and Action Processes*
>
> ....
>
> - Engaging in inductive and abductive thinking
> - Developing categories
> - Grouping categories into higher levels of abstraction
> - Discovering meanings and underlying themes

---

the four processes are not neat, separate steps or entities that occur in sequence at a particular time in a study. Rather, they are ongoing, overlapping processes that lead to refinement of observations and/or interpretations throughout the data-gathering effort.

Investigators, particularly those new to this type of inquiry, initially may feel overwhelmed by process. The sheer quantity of information generated in a short time can also make the investigator feel inundated. However, these feelings are a natural part of the experience of conducting naturalistic inquiry. The researcher must be able to feel comfortable with being in "limbo" at first—that is, not knowing the whole story and letting it unfold.

Engaging in Thinking Process

Naturalistic inquiry is based on either an inductive or an abductive thinking process (see Chapter 1). These logic structures are key to all the analytical approaches of naturalistic inquiry. One of the first analytical efforts of the researcher is therefore to engage in a thoughtful process. This point may seem basic to any research endeavor, but the active engagement of the investigator in thinking about each datum in naturalistic inquiry assumes a quality that is different from experimental-type endeavors. Fetterman described this basic analytical effort in ethnographic research as follows:

> *The best guide through the thickets of analysis is at once the most obvious and most complex of strategies: clear thinking. First and foremost, analysis is a test of the ethnographer's ability to process information in a meaningful and useful manner.[5] (p 93)*

More specifically, an inductive and abductive thinking process is typically characterized by the development of an initial organizational system and the review of each datum. The organizational system therefore emerges from the data. The investigator avoids imposing constructs or theoretical propositions before becoming involved with the data. For example, in the case of data collected through an interview, the researcher will read and reread the transcriptions. Similarly, if text from emails or tweets is the source of data, an initial analytical step involves reading and rereading the initial set of emails and tweets that is identified. From these initial readings, ideas and hunches will be formulated. In a phenomenological, heuristic, or life history approach, the investigator will continue working inductively until all meanings of an experience are explicated. Object analysis involves similar processes, but with "things" or descriptions of artifacts.[6,7]

In an abductive approach, the thinking process begins inductively with an idea. The investigator explores information or behavioral actions and formulates a working hypothesis, which is then examined in context to see whether it fits and/or requires additional data collection. Even within the inductive process, the investigator sometimes works somewhat deductively to draw implications from the working hypothesis as a way of verifying its accuracy. This process characterizes the actions of the investigator throughout the study, especially for grounded theory[8] and ethnography.[5]

In ethnography, Fetterman labeled this process "contextualization," or the placement of data into a larger perspective.[5] While in the study environment, the investigator continually strives to place each piece of data into a context to understand the "bigger picture" or how the parts fit together to make the whole. One way the investigator strives to understand how a datum fits into the larger context is by grouping information into categories. Although not always used (for example, in designs that do not rely on investigator interpretation), category development is fundamental to much of analysis in the naturalistic tradition. We turn to that process now.

Developing Categories

In many naturalistic studies, a voluminous amount of information is gathered within a short period of time. The researcher needs to manage the immense amount of data so that the study proceeds systematically and does not get out of hand. Consider when you have had to review a large body of literature for a course. Perhaps you first went to the library website to search for and find information from the literature. You probably soon realized that your notes from the readings had become overwhelming and that you needed to develop some organization to make sense of the information you gathered. The same principle applies in the initial stages of analysis in naturalistic inquiry. The researcher must find an organization that will serve the remainder of the work.

One of the first meaningful ways in which the investigator begins to organize information is to develop categories that are common in a data set. Northcutt and McCoy[9] noted the similarities between categories and variables, indicating that categories are single phenomena that can be named and in which multiple elements must occur. This categorization process represents a major step in naturalistic analysis.[10] How do categories emerge? As Wax eloquently described in a classic work:

> *The student begins "outside" the interaction, confronting behaviors he finds bewildering and inexplicable: the actors are oriented to a world of meanings that the observer does not grasp ... and then gradually he comes to be able to categorize peoples (or relationships) and events.*[11]

The researcher enters the research environment to see and understand phenomena without imposing concepts, labels, or meanings a priori. Thus, categories emerge from researcher-environment interactions and the initial information that is obtained and synthesized. Preliminary categories are developed and become the conceptual tools used to sort and classify subsequent information as it is received. Thus, categories represent the initial attempt to group observations or phenomena in a meaningful way.[12] Categories such as "student," "provider," and "client" make it easier to anticipate the behavior of individuals in these groups and to identify the contextual rules that govern their behavior. Categories are basic elements that enable people to organize experiences, objects, and images and to craft and follow social conventions. These groupings change from environment to environment, time to time, and context to context. Categories can also reflect ways people describe their own experiences.

Let us look at an example of how contemporary naturalistic researchers conduct this first level of analysis. One of the first seminal naturalistic studies to examine mobility device use and nonuse was conducted by Gitlin and colleagues,[13] who sought to understand the meanings attributed to mobility aids and other assistive devices by people who were undergoing rehabilitation for stroke and were first-time users of the equipment. The initial analytical strategy involved using a pile-sorting technique[14] in which two members of the research team independently read each statement about the devices, as generated by patients during brief interviews. These comments were independently sorted by each researcher into basic categories based on perceived similarities and differences. The categories reflected the underlying topics expressed in patient statements. (A statement about a "reacher" device, such as "It's good for picking up things," was categorized as representing a comment that explicitly focused on instrumental utility and the patient's attitude, which in this case was positive toward the device.) Next, the two researchers compared their summary lists of the categories they had generated. Differences were discussed, and the categories were refined. A final comprehensive list was prepared and reviewed by all investigators. This process yielded 11 basic topics or categories of meaning.

As the data collection activity proceeds, the naturalistic investigator uses the original categories as the basis for analyzing new data. New data either are classified into existing categories or may serve to modify or create new categories to depict the phenomenon of interest accurately. Data can then be placed into categories on the basis of characteristics that they share. The researcher decides on the placement scheme, referred to by Lofland and colleagues as "filing,"[15] and considers both descriptive and analytical cataloguing. Data placed in the descriptive categories answer "who, what, where, and when" queries and are not subjected to further investigator interpretation. Analytical or more interpretive categories answer "how and why" queries. Because any one datum can be categorized in several ways, one datum can therefore belong to more than one group

(when indicated), adding another level of complexity to the analytical process.

A number of methods to identify categories can be used, depending on the investigator's personal style and preferences for working. For example, some researchers generate multiple copies of a data set (e.g., transcription from an interview) and literally cut sections from the transcript that reflect the identified groupings. Each cut section is pasted in a paper or electronic notebook or on a paper or digital index card and filed by the category it represents. Most researchers, however, use qualitativeal data software programs to manage this analytical stage. Software and applications such as Atlas.ti and NVivo, among others, are becoming very popular among researchers who work in naturalistic traditions. Although software applications differ in structure and function, they contain similar sorting, categorizing, concept mapping, and coding functions and facilitate multiple coding and categorizing of data.

This inductive approach can be used with forms of data other than interview. For example, the development of categories may also involve repeated review and examination of narrative, video, object, image or other types of information that have been obtained. Consider the study currently being conducted of mobility devices in the gilded age. As a basis for informing the design of new mobility devices, this retrospective study builds on the seminal work done by Gitlin and colleagues[13] involving the examination of artifacts, images, and narratives about mobility devices used following the Civil War.[16]

Coding

Once categories are established, codes are assigned to each such that diverse analytical methods can be used if indicated by the query and level of development within the data set.[10] As we introduced earlier, computer software programs (e.g., NVivo, Atlas.ti) are particularly useful in facilitating the *coding* process for large data sets. These programs automatically assign codes to similar passages or keywords first identified by the analyzer. The code is developed initially by the investigator, and then the software goes to work. For example, the investigator may configure the computer application to search for and assign the code "descriptive appearance barrier" to every reference to unpleasing appearances of mobility devices. Keywords and even images (in some applications such as Atlas) can be selected based on categories that arise from the data set, and the computer can be programmed to assign codes automatically based on a key word or image list.

Developing Taxonomies

A *taxonomy* is a system of categories and relationships. Taxonomies have also been called "typologies" and "mindmaps."[4] Developing a taxonomy represents the next level of organizing information. In this analytical process, the investigator uncovers the threads or inclusionary criteria that distinguish and link categories. For example, basic categories such as "whales" and "dogs" belong to the larger category of "animals"; basic categories such as "blocks" and "dolls" belong to the larger category of "toys." In taxonomy, sets of categories are grouped on the basis of similarities. Taxonomic analysis is therefore an analytical procedure that results in an organization of categories and that describes their relationships. In a taxonomic analysis, the focus is on identifying the relationship between wholes and parts.

Taxonomic analysis involves three processes: (1) organizing or grouping similar or related categories into larger categories, (2) identifying differences between sets of subcategories and larger or overarching categories, and (3) representing the relationships among the categories and subcategories[4] (discussed later). The taxonomy is most frequently depicted in visual form as a "map" of related concepts and constructs.

> In the Gitlin and colleagues study[13] of people who recently experienced strokes, the 11 initial categories identified were further grouped into six broader dimensions to reflect the experience of device use among first-time users. For example, one dimension was labeled "issues posed by device use." This dimension included four subcategories that reflected concerns ranging from the physical interface between the equipment and the user to the social consequences of being a device user. •

Discovering the Whole

One of the main purposes of analysis in naturalistic research is to understand how each observation or part fits into the whole to make sense of and interpret the layers of meanings and the multiple perspectives contained therein. While different according to design, the processes used in "discovering the whole" have commonalities. The major methods to accomplish this task involve searching for relationships among categories, revealing the underlying *themes* or meanings in categories and their components beyond what is immediately visible. The researcher engages in the thinking process of "integrating," in which he or she finds relationships (recall the third aim of taxonomic analysis listed earlier) among categories and further searches for overlap, exclusivity, or hidden meanings among categories. These rigorous methods are part of an inductive approach to analysis, and they move the researcher up each loop of the spiral toward understanding and interpretation. Each analytical step from category and taxonomy to thematic identification allows the researcher to uncover the multiple meanings and perspectives of individuals and to develop complex understandings of their experiences and interactions.

In his seminal work on ethnography, Agar suggested that it is from the "simple" process of first establishing topics, categories, and codes that "you begin building a map of the territory that will help you give accounts, and subsequently begin to discuss what 'those people' are like."[17] Thus, in ethnography, the researcher uses these analytical processes to uncover patterns of behavior by examining repeated actions.[5] Have[18] reminded us that we are not seeking to interpret intrapsychic phenomena; rather, in "ethnomethodology," we focus on activity as the basis for analysis and meaning.

Investigators proceeding with grounded theory methods use the term "theoretical sensitivity" to refer to the researcher's sensitivity and ability to detect and give meanings to data, to go beyond the obvious, and to recognize what is important in a context.[18]

In naturalistic analysis, categories and taxonomies are compared, contrasted, and sorted until a discernible thought or behavioral pattern becomes identifiable and the meaning of the pattern is revealed. As exceptions to rules emerge, variations on themes are detectable. Using an iterative process, as themes are developed on the basis of abstractions (categories and taxonomies), they are examined in light of ongoing observations. At this point, the investigator may use a literature review or other theoretical concepts to derive an understanding and explanation of the categories based on what has already been investigated or theoretically posited.[11]

Stage Two: Formal Report Preparation

Analysis is a critical and active component of the data collection process. As noted, it begins early in the action process of data collection and continues after the investigator formally leaves the study environment and has completed collecting information. This final stage of the process is a more formal analytical step in which the investigator enters into an intensive report-preparation effort that furthers the interpretive process. The main objective is to consolidate the investigator's understandings and impressions by writing one or more manuscripts, a final report, or even a book. Except in designs that do not include deliberate investigator explanation (e.g., endogenous, some forms of phenomenology), the reporting effort involves a self-reflective and highly interpretive process, the ease of which often depends on how well the investigator initially organizes and cross-references the voluminous records and notes. In the second and more formal analytical stage, the investigator reexamines materials and refines categories, taxonomies, and themes and derives an *interpretation*. The investigator purposely and carefully selects quotes and examples to illustrate and highlight each aspect of the refined interpretation. Selections are carefully made to (1) ensure adequate representation of the interpretation or themes the investigator wants to convey, (2) remain "true" to the voices and experiences being referenced, and (3) depict accurately the context in which the study occurred.

In the final interpretation, the investigator moves beyond each datum or piece of information to suggest a deeper understanding of the "whole" through

theory development, explication of the themes and general principles that emerge from the study of the phenomenon of interest, or the application of theoretical constructs.

Examples of Analytical Processes in Diverse Naturalistic Designs

As we have stated, researchers use the basic analytical processes somewhat differently and often label these activities distinctly. In this section, we examine these similarities and differences in two naturalistic approaches; grounded theory to demonstrate its highly structured approach, and ethnographic approaches to illustrate the combination of less structured approaches.

Grounded Theory

One of the most formal and systematic analytical approaches in the naturalistic tradition occurs in grounded theory.[12] As we discussed in Chapters 4, 7, 10, the primary purpose of this approach is to develop theory from observations, interviews and other sources of data. Corbin and Strauss[19] suggested specific procedures to examine data. Their approach to grounded theory systematizes the inductive incremental analytical process and the continuous interplay between previously collected and analyzed data and new information. These authors labeled their analytical approach the *constant comparative method*. As information is obtained, it is compared and contrasted with previous information to fit all the pieces inductively together into a larger puzzle. Patterns emerge from the data set and are then coded (placed in a category). Data filing[15] occurs by categorizing and coding. In the constant comparative method, researchers not only search for themes to emerge but also code each piece of raw data according to the categories in which it belongs.

Initially, codes are open, which refers to a "process of breaking down, examining, comparing, conceptualizing and categorizing data." Axial coding then occurs, which refers to "a set of procedures whereby data are put back together in new ways after open coding by making connections between categories." Selective coding occurs next, which is the "process of selecting the core category, systematically relating it to other categories."[19] Codes reflect the similarities and differences among themes and continue to test the category system through analysis of each datum and categorical assignment as data are collected. In this way, the analysis is grounded in and emerges from each datum. Theory emerges from the data, is intimately linked to the field reality, and reflects a synthesis of the information gathered.

Grounded theory may be the most systematic and procedure-oriented process in naturalistic inquiry. In various books, Corbin and Strauss[19] and Glaser[20]—together, individually, and with other authors—systematically walk the researcher through each analytical step of coding and categorizing and use a prescribed language to identify each procedure and task (see References).

Ethnography

Most ethnographic field studies use a range of analytical approaches, based on the specific purpose and nature of the study. The researcher may borrow techniques from grounded theory or use a more general thematic analysis, depending on the particular philosophical stance and analytical orientation of the researcher. Consider how you might proceed to use ethnography if you wanted to learn the health practices and beliefs of a group of people who recently immigrated from Somalia to your rural state.

Because of the absent theory that explained health practices and beliefs in these new residents of your state, you initially chose a qualitative approach to address their research query. You begin by examining the geographic environment where the group currently lives in order to gain access to people who may be able to act as informants. After a period of observation, you identify the boundaries of the community and any health facilities in it that serve the Somalian residents. From these observations, you are able to develop two categories: the human health environment and the physical health environment. Continuing to collect additional data, you find that the physical health environment has two major subcategories, the formal provider offices and the home environment. You therefore have developed a descriptive taxonomy with two subcategories of physical health environment. As you proceed to observe and interview key informants in each of the physical settings, you find that home and provider health environments differ in both practices and thus are in conflict. Through prolonged engagement, you are able to observe behaviors, spaces, images, and artifacts in the home and interview the residents to describe their health practices. Further immersion provides enlarged opportunity for you to speak to adults about their health beliefs. After reading and rereading your notes and listening to transcripts, you find patterns of health behaviors and beliefs of residents. This analysis provides greater insight as to the reasons that the immigrant residents avoid health facilities even when there is a nominal or no charge for services.

Figure 21-1 depicts the simple taxonomy that inductively emerges from your data set. As you can see, some lines demonstrate bidirectional connections among categories of findings while others are unidirectional. The categories that you hope would be connected are not.

Accuracy and Rigor in Analysis

In naturalistic research, a major concern is obtaining an in-depth, rich description and explanation of phenomena. Unless you are conducting a mixed method study, generalizability or external validity of study findings is not relevant. Rather, the primary focus is obtaining a comprehensive and accurate representation of a particular context. At this point, however, you may be wondering how you, as a consumer of naturalistic research, can trust an investigator's interpretations. How can you determine the accuracy or the *truth value* of an investigator's interpretation of data? How can you be assured that the experiences of research participants are "accurately" represented in a final report? Of concern is whether the findings of naturalistic inquiry reveal meanings that would have emerged if another researcher had conducted the same set of interviews, observations, and analytical orientation. That is, do findings reflect the realities of the culture, community, individuals, or context studied, or rather that of the investigator? The issues of validity and truth are not only important but critical in ethical consumption and application of knowledge, as we discussed in Chapter 3. Suppose in the example earlier, another investigator reinterpreted

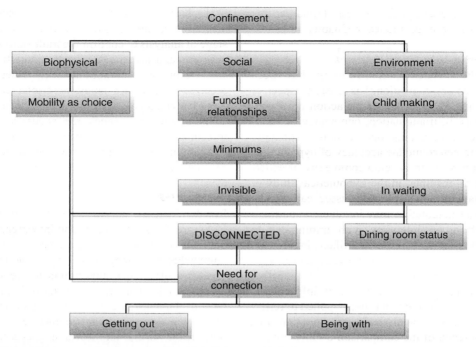

Figure 21-1 Taxonomy for study of health behaviors and beliefs.

your data to theorize noncompliance with health care providers on the part of the immigrants? This interpretation would inform different actions than your conclusions. Based on your study, the health care providers might seek to understand the nature and outcomes of folk and herbal remedies and perhaps integrate those practices into their services. Yet if noncompliance were the conclusion, education and incentives might be warranted.

In naturalistic research the debate continues over how best to construct standards for conducting and evaluating data-gathering and analytical efforts. Denzin and Lincoln labeled this as a concern with the trustworthiness or *credibility* of an account.[4,8] Using a rather structured approach, these authors and others have identified a number of strategies by which an investigator can enhance the confidence in the truth value of the findings from naturalistic inquiry.[8] The concern with credibility of an account or interpretive scheme is similar to the issue of internal validity in experimental-type research. In reading a report involving naturalistic inquiry, the critical

---

BOX 21-2 *Techniques to Enhance Credibility of Analysis*

....

- Triangulation (crystallization)
- Saturation
- Member checking
- Reflexivity (self-examination)
- Audit trail
- Peer debriefing

---

reader needs to ask two primary questions: (1) To what extent are the biases and personal perspectives of the investigator identified and considered in the data analysis and interpretation? and (2) What actions has the investigator taken to enhance the credibility of the investigation?

To enhance the accuracy of representation of data and the credibility of interpretation, researchers often use six basic actions (Box 21-2). When reading a published study that employed naturalistic inquiry, check whether the investigator has used any of these strategies. Let us review each approach to see how it applies to the analytical process. (Also see the discussion of these techniques in Chapter 18.)

Triangulation (Crystallization)

Triangulation, which more recently has been referred to as crystallization,[21] is a basic aspect of data gathering that also shapes the action process of data analysis. In triangulation, one source of information is checked against one or more other types of sources to determine the accuracy of hypothetical understandings and to develop complexity of understanding. For example, in the hypothetical study of health behaviors and beliefs discussed earlier, one approach to triangulation may involve comparing a narrative from an interview with immigrants to object reading of health-related artifacts in a household.[14] Triangulation enables the investigator to validate a particular finding by examining whether different sources provide convergent information. The term "crystallization" has been applied to reflect the comprehensive analytical understanding that occurs as a result of the comparison of different and diverse sources to explain a phenomenon.[21]

Saturation

Saturation refers to the point at which an investigator has obtained sufficient information from data collection.[4] As you may recall, there are several indicators that data collection can be terminated (see Chapter 18). For example, the investigator has reached saturation when the information gathered does not provide additional insights or new understandings. Another indication that saturation has been achieved is when the investigator can guess what a respondent is going to say or do in a particular situation. If saturation is not achieved, the investigator reports only partial information that is preliminary, and a credible and comprehensive account or interpretive schema cannot be developed.

Member Checking

Member checking is a technique in which the investigator checks an assumption or a particular understanding with one or more informants. Affirmation of a particular revelation from a research participant strengthens the credibility of the interpretation and decreases the potential for introducing investigator bias. This technique is often used throughout the data collection process. It is also introduced in the formal stage of analysis to confirm the truth value of specific accounts and investigator impressions. If you were going to use this technique in the hypothetical health behavior and belief study described earlier, you would develop your impressions and draft your final analysis and then check the accuracy with your informants. This approach would decrease the chance that you are reflecting your own opinions instead of the "culture."

Reflexivity

In naturalistic inquiry it is not considered possible to eliminate "bias." Thus bias and investigator opinion are not considered fundamental limitations on knowledge development, as long as the investigator identifies his or her fingerprints in the knowledge process. In the final report or manuscript, it is important for the researcher to discuss his or her personal biases and assumptions in conducting the study and how these affect the research process. Personal biases are revealed in the course of collecting data and during the active process of reflexivity (self-examination). The investigator purposely engages in a reflexive process to examine his or her perspectives and personal biases to determine how these may have influenced not only what is learned but also how it is learned.[4]

Audit Trail

Another way an investigator can increase truth value is by using an audit trail. Denzin and Lincoln[4] suggest that an investigator should leave a path of his or her thinking and coding decisions so that others can review the course of logic and decision making that was followed. The principle here is that the investigator needs to be able to clearly articulate the analytical pathways so that others can agree, disagree, and/or question the decisions that have been made. Remember that research is a critical thinking process in both experimental-type and naturalistic traditions.

Peer Debriefing

Peer debriefing is another strategy that can be used to affirm emerging interpretations. In this approach the investigator purposely involves peers in the analytical process. An investigator may convene a group of peers to review his or her audit trail and emerging findings, or the researcher may ask a peer to code independently a randomly selected set of data. The investigator compares the outcomes with his or her coding scheme. Areas of agreement and disagreement are identified and discussed. Either approach provides an opportunity for the investigator to reflect on other possible competing interpretations of the data. Peer debriefing may occur at various junctures in the analytical process.

Summary

Analysis in naturalistic inquiry has many purposes and formats. Some researchers seek to generate theory, whereas others aim to reveal and interpret human experiences. There are also many different analytical strategies, depending on the purpose of the query. Each purpose yields a different analytical strategy. Regardless of study purpose, however, the essential characteristic of the analytical process in the naturalistic tradition is that it involves an ongoing inductive and abductive thinking process that is interspersed with the activity of gathering information. Although the analytical process has well-described essential components, each form of naturalistic inquiry approaches this action process somewhat differently.

One of the most challenging aspects of engaging in naturalistic inquiry is being prepared for and managing the voluminous amount of data obtained. Even in a small-scale study, such as a life history of a single individual, a case study, or conduct of focus groups, the amount of information obtained and the analytical processes that are enacted can initially be overwhelming. The analytical process begins with the simple act of reading and reviewing, on multiple occasions, the interviews, observational notes, objects, or images collected. This step begins the thinking process that is essential to analysis in naturalistic inquiry. Through inductive and abductive reasoning, the boundaries of the study become reformulated, defined, and redefined, and initial descriptive queries are answered. Further data collection efforts are determined by the need to explore the depth and breadth of categories more fully and to answer "why" and "how" types of queries that lead to an understanding of the "whole." As data are obtained, they are coded and organized into meaningful categories. The boundaries and meanings of categories are further refined through the process of establishing relationships among categories. Queries that ask "Why?" and "How?" lead to the development of explanatory taxonomies. This step in turn leads to emergent patterns, meanings, and interpretations of how observations fit into a larger context. Existing theoretical frameworks or constructs in the literature may be brought into the analytical process to refine emerging interpretations or to serve as points of contrast. A refined and final interpretation is usually derived after the investigator exits the context of the study and begins the writing process. Gubrium eloquently summarized the analytical process as follows:

Analysis proceeds incrementally with the aim of making visible the native practice of clarification, from one domain of experience to another, structure upon structure.[22]

Throughout the analytical process, the investigator must remain flexible and open to constantly challenging his or her emerging interpretive framework.

EXERCISES

1. Return to Exercise 1 in Chapter 18, which asks you to observe a public place to determine characteristic behavior patterns. Now examine your raw data and search for categories. On the basis of the categories, code each datum and develop a descriptive taxonomy of behavior.
2. Now look at objects in the environment and engage in triangulation. How well does each source affirm your impressions? Are there any discrepancies? If so, what will you do to resolve them?
3. Develop an audit trail for your data collection and analysis activities in the previous inquiry.
4. Give your raw data set from Exercise 1 to a colleague for analysis and to establish an audit trail.

When your colleague has completed the task, compare your conclusions. Reconcile any differences by reexamining your data and your audit trails.

5. Explore some of the naturalistic analytical software to determine its strengths and limitations in coding and taxonomic development.

....

References

1. Gill L, Whyte L: A critical review of patient satisfaction. *Leadersh Health Serv* 22:8–19, 2009.
2. Creswell J, Clark VP: *Designing and conducting mixed methods research*, Los Angeles, 2011, Sage.
3. Miles MB, Huberman AM, Saldaña J: *Qualitative data analysis: a methods sourcebook*, ed 3, Los Angeles, 2014, Sage.
4. Denzin N, Lincoln Y: *Collecting and interpreting qualitative materials*, Thousand Oaks, Calif, 2008, Sage.
5. Fetterman DL: *Ethnography step by step*, Thousand Oaks, Calif, 2009, Sage, p 94.
6. Berger A: *What objects mean*, Walnut Creek, Calif, 2009, Left Coast Press.
7. *Pile sorting techniques for ethnographers*, 2011. Retrieved from Anthrostrategist: <http://anthrostrategy.com/2011/08/06/pile-sorting-techniques-for-ethnographers>.
8. Denzin NK, Lincoln YS: *Sage handbook of qualitative research*, ed 4, Thousand Oaks, Calif, 2011, Sage.
9. Northcutt N, McCoy D: *Interactive qualitative analysis*, Thousand Oaks, Calif, 2004, Sage.
10. Guest GS, MacQueen KM: *Applied thematic analysis*, Thousand Oaks, Calif, 2012, Sage.
11. Wax M: On misunderstanding verstecken: a reply to Abel. *Sociol Soc Res* 51:323–333, 1967.
12. Creswell J: *Qualitative inquiry and research design: choosing among five approaches*, ed 3, Los Angeles, 2013, Sage.
13. Gitlin LN, Luborsky M, Schemm R: Emerging concerns of older stroke patients about assistive devices in rehabilitation. *Gerontologist* 38:169–180, 1998.
14. Candlin F, Guins R: *The object reader*, London, 2009, Routledge.
15. Lofland J, Snow D, Anderson L, et al: *Analyzing social settings: a guide to qualitative observation and analysis*, ed 3, Belmont, Calif, 2005, Wadsworth.
16. DePoy E: *Inventing lameness in the Gilded Age: a study of walking sticks*, University of Maine Faculty Research Funds, in preparation.
17. Agar MH: *The professional stranger: an informal introduction to ethnography*, ed 2, San Diego, Calif, 1996, Academic Press, p 105.
18. Have PT: *Understanding qualitative research and ethnomethodology*, Thousand Oaks, Calif, 2004, Sage.
19. Corbin B, Strauss A: *Basics of qualitative research: techniques and procedures for developing grounded theory*, Thousand Oaks, Calif, 2007, Sage, p 62.
20. Glaser BG: *Theoretical sensitivity: advanced in the methodology of grounded theory*, Mill Valley, Calif, 1978, Sociology Press.
21. Ellingson L: *Engaging crystallization in qualitative research*, Los Angeles, 2008, Sage.
22. Gubrium J: *Analyzing field reality*, Newbury Park, Calif, 1988, Sage.

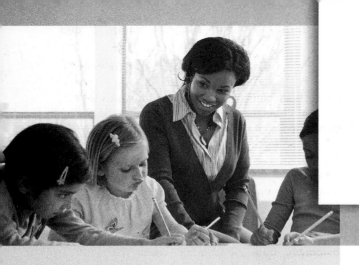

Chapter 22
Sharing Research Knowledge Before the Study

Before actually initiating an experimental-type, naturalistic, or mixed method inquiry, you most likely will have to commit your specific research ideas to writing. The document, referred to as a *proposal*, is simply a text or record that describes why and how you "propose" to carry out your research idea. A proposal details the rationale and the main thinking and action processes you intend to implement. Sections contained in the document typically include

the significance of your idea, justification for the need for your research using supportive literature, a statement as to your specific research question or query, specific hypotheses if applicable, your procedures, the analytical plan, ethical considerations, and the informed consent process. This chapter discusses the specifics of proposal preparation and the importance of sharing your research thinking and action processes before conducting the inquiry.

Reasons for Sharing Before Engagement

Preparing a document or proposal before engaging in research actions is an important aspect of the research process for several reasons. First, as we discussed in Chapter 3, for any type of research study involving human participants, you will need to submit a written proposal to a human subject board or research committee of your institution. Recall that we suggested that all studies, even when classified as evaluation, be submitted for review so that the implications for humans are scrutinized by more than just one pair of eyes. So before starting your study, institutional review board (IRB) approval should be obtained; otherwise, you are not legally and ethically permitted to implement your research plan if you are testing or otherwise involving humans.

Another important reason to prepare a proposal before starting an inquiry is to obtain financial support for the research activity. Most research, regardless of the research tradition and even if it is a pilot study, requires resources to implement. Think of the amount of time and effort that may be required of you and an interviewer, statistical consultant, or others to conduct your study. Consider the costs of materials you may need (e.g., audio or video recorder or applications on a mobile device or computer, paper, storage, computer software, specialized equipment to measure health and fitness outcomes, and so forth) or the costs associated with mailings and communications. In addition, you may want to provide a small "honorarium" to study participants as a way of thanking them for their time and effort, a common practice in research. Thus, writing a proposal to request a small or large amount of funds to support the conduct of a study may be critical. Even a small amount (e.g., $150 to $500) can help offset the costs associated with conducting a range of studies and data collection actions, such as conducting a systematic and comprehensive literature review, doing naturalistic or experimental-type meta-analysis, forming a focus group, extracting information from medical records, and testing the acceptability of a battery of standardized tests. There are numerous places to seek funding for large or small amounts, including sources internal to your department (e.g., student and faculty research funds), referred to as intramural funding programs, and external sources (e.g., federal agency, foundation, corporate), referred to as extramural funding.

Yet another important reason to write a proposal is to have a record of the specific thinking and action processes you plan to implement that you can then share with colleagues to obtain their feedback. Obtaining feedback about your research plan before implementation is an important aspect of the research process. It helps to sharpen your thinking and actions and place your efforts within the larger context of the scientific and consumer communities. Also, a documented plan can serve as your own reference or guide as you proceed with a study.

At some point in your student or professional life and involvement in the world of research, you will need to write a research proposal. Preparing a proposal is not really as intimidating as it may sound. The document can be as brief as 2 to 5 pages for an IRB submission or as lengthy as 40 or more pages when submitting a detailed research plan for consideration of funding from an external agency. Proposal writing is a technical skill. As such, proposals follow particular formats and structures that can be easily learned and applied.

Because committing your ideas to text in the form of a proposal is part of the thinking processes in research, this chapter describes the basic elements of preparing a proposal to document a study and to seek funding. Many types of proposals are written to obtain funding from external sources, such as those written to conduct a conference, purchase equipment, train students or health and human service professionals, and evaluate demonstration projects or service programs. Each type of proposal follows a different format. In this chapter, however, we discuss writing a proposal for research, whether for an experimental-type, naturalistic, or mixed method study.

A research proposal to secure funding from a particular source is referred to as a *grant*.[1,2] The process of identifying a suitable funding source and writing the proposal is referred to as *grantsmanship*.[2] A research grant will usually provide monies for salary support for the investigator and his or her team, the specific materials needed to carry out the research (e.g., equipment, supplies, communications, mailings), data analysis, and travel to professional meetings. Because obtaining money is part of the reality of being involved in research, we start by describing key aspects of grantsmanship.

Where to Seek Support for a Research Idea

Obtaining funds to support your research activity is one of the main reasons to prepare a research proposal, particularly for large-scale studies or studies requiring specialized or costly equipment or procedures. Finding a funding source for your research idea can be challenging. The funding environment for research is constantly changing, and the priorities and interests of various sources of funding are always being modified in response to advances in health care, new developments in knowledge, societal trends, and congressional activity. Therefore, finding the right *funder* for your particular research idea may take time and require knowledge of multiple sources that provide information about a wide range of funding opportunities. In this section, we outline some of the major sources of funding for health and human service research.

Where can you find a potential funding source? Your own department or institution, professional organization, student association, reference librarian, and the Internet are all worthwhile places to begin your search for support of your research idea. For example, your own department or institution may have a research fund to support pilot efforts of faculty, students, or professionals; this should be the first place you inquire. Many professional associations also provide small grants, which may range from $2000 to $50,000 or more, and predoctoral and postdoctoral research stipends. There are also special listservs and Internet-based grant-seeking programs that you can join that will help identify sources of funding based on keywords that reflect your research interests.

Funders usually post on their web pages and in newsletters what is known as a *call for proposals*, which is a notice of an opportunity to submit a proposal on a specific topic of interest to an agency or funder. Agencies publish announcements describing a problem area and inviting interested parties to propose ways to investigate all or part of the problem. These announcements vary considerably in the detail used to describe the research they would like to see submitted. The federal government tends to provide explicit descriptions of what needs to be included in grant proposals. Foundations and private companies tend to be much more general as to the format for a research proposal.

The U.S. government remains the largest source of research money available for health-related issues. It is a huge enterprise comprising an array of departments, agencies, institutes, bureaus, and centers. Although there are pockets of money for health and human service professionals throughout the federal government, two departments have a focused interest in health and human services: the Public Health Service within the Department of Health and Human Services (DHHS), which supports the National Institutes of Health (NIH), and the U.S. Department of Education. Within the Department of Education, the Office of Special Education and Rehabilitation Services (OSERS) has a variety of programs of potential interest to the health professions, as does the National Institute on Disability and Rehabilitation Research (NIDRR). We have also found that the Department of Agriculture funds research related to environmental health, nutrition, and exercise, and the Department of Defense is a source to consider for veterans' health. Funding is also available through the National Science Foundation (NSF).

Internationally, there are numerous funds that support inquiry, with eligibility for the most part depending on the countries or regions applying. The World Health Organization, Fulbright-Fogarty Awards, and other geographically specific grants are a good source for supporting collaborative research with nations outside of the United States.

Private foundations are another source of funding for health and human service research. More than 70,000 foundations in the United States offer grants to individuals, institutions, and other not-for-profit groups. The four types are independent foundations, company-sponsored foundations, operating foundations, and community foundations. Generally, only the first two types provide research support to independent investigators, although all four types offer potential funding opportunities.

Finally, corporate grants provide funding for research. Industries such as drug companies, equipment manufacturers, automobile manufacturers, insurance companies, and companies related to or concerned with public health, specific areas of health, and health care often have money available for small through large research projects. Many large corporations have funds for research projects that advance their interests. Two main interests of companies in the private sector are (1) the testing or evaluation of their own products and services and (2) research to support new innovations that can be fostered by these corporations. For example, an equipment manufacturer may want a new assistive device evaluated for its utility and acceptability, or a company may pay for a study to identify the need for new types of hearing devices.

We recommend that you examine the websites of potential funding sources to gain an understanding of the types of research questions and queries they seek to fund, to understand their values and mission,[1] and to identify the particular format they require for a proposal submission. As you search for appropriate funding sources, you may discover that your research idea is not of interest to agencies. This does not mean that your idea is without merit, but it does indicate that you will need to rethink or rework your idea to match socially and congressionally sanctioned public health concerns and values that are embraced by funding agencies. We emphasize values here to highlight the importance of addressing them in your proposal. For example, if you apply to a savings bank foundation to develop a health program, but their value is on economic development, linking your idea to economic development will be necessary. So make sure that you read the call for proposals, and all other information including the agency mission, previously funded work, publications, and materials carefully and critically to ensure a fit between the values of your research and the funder's mission.

You may find that your research idea is too advanced or "futuristic" to be of interest to funders or that although it is of great interest to your own profession, it is not considered significant from a broad public health perspective. Thus, it is necessary to cast a wide net and look for funding from a range of sources.

Consider this example. One of our students was interested in developing and examining the outcomes of a campus program for veteran students who are returning to the university after seeing combat. Because the literature suggests that public acknowledgment by students and faculty is important in increasing retention and graduation, the proposed program involves a week of seminars about veteran life and challenges on campus as well as celebrations in the evening. The variables to be investigated are campus climate and retention. The foundation to which the student is planning to apply is concerned with research and programming to promote veteran well-being, but it does not provide support for receptions, food purchase, or similar activities. If she applies to that foundation, she should omit the celebrations or seek funding for them from elsewhere and show it as leveraging other resources.

Who Reads a Proposal?

When you write a research proposal, it will be read and evaluated by a particular audience, referred to as the *reviewer*. The reviewer(s) of your proposal may be your research professor; your peers; the head of your clinical or academic department; a diverse committee of consumers, providers, and researchers who review for an institution's human subject review board; or a group of scientists or scholars from various disciplines. Therefore, you can be assured that the persons who review your proposal will come from diverse backgrounds and have various levels of exposure and knowledge of the phenomenon you seek to investigate, as well as their own professional standards as to what constitutes scientific inquiry.[2]

When you submit a proposal to your professor, department, or institution or to an external source such as a funding agency, reviewers will evaluate it using various criteria. Usually, the explicit evaluative criteria will be specified in your syllabus or in a call for proposals. For the most part, reviewers are asked to evaluate whether your research plan contributes to knowledge building, is feasible, is methodologically valid, and is worth the costs that you have budgeted. Some reviews are qualitative and you will receive written comments, whereas others are quantitative and you will receive a score. Writing a proposal is a purposeful process and, as such, must be carefully crafted to match the evaluative criteria, implicit funder values, and the background and knowledge base of the audience or reviewer. Thus, before writing down your ideas, it is important to know the nature of the review team (e.g., researchers, professionals, experts in your field, laypersons, and so forth) and the evaluative criteria that will be applied.

Suppose you need to submit a proposal to obtain funding from an agency. By going on the Internet, you identify several potential funding sources that may be appropriate or relevant to your research interest. In reading the directions for proposal development and submission on their Web pages, you learn that one agency emphasizes "innovation," whereas another agency is concerned with "dissemination" of research findings. Although your basic research idea may not change, in writing the proposal you would emphasize different aspects of your research plan on the basis of the evaluative criteria and specific interest of the target audience. •

In writing a proposal, you also need to define your key concepts carefully and articulate your ideas clearly so that they can be adequately understood by reviewers from diverse disciplines and life experiences. A concept that is core to your discipline may not be relevant to another or may be defined very differently.

> Consider the term "disability." In agencies that provide medical services, "disability" is defined as a bodily impairment that influences a major daily function for a prolonged period of time. However, in other disciplines such as contemporary disability studies, the term may refer to the social, economic, and environmentally designed barriers that impede function, having nothing to do with an embodied diagnosis.[3] Defining terms and ensuring that your definitions are consistent with the interests of the funding agency are key to success in grant seeking. •

Thus, in writing a proposal, you need to adapt to the lens of your reviewers and define and reference all key terms. In this respect, preparing a proposal is similar to sharing information in the form of a report, which we discuss in Chapter 23. That is, as in report writing, constructing a proposal is purposeful and targets a particular reader or audience, in this case the reviewer.

Writing a Research Proposal

The principles and processes involved in writing a proposal are similar to those for sharing information and reporting your study at its completion (see Chapter 23).

Basic Principles

There are five basic principles for writing a research proposal: clarity, precision, parsimony, coherence, and attention to structure. Each of these should guide

how you write, regardless of the specific purpose of the proposal.[2]

By "clarity," we mean that the proposal needs to be easily understood regardless of the reviewer. If a report is vague, verbose, or overly complex in writing style, your research ideas will not be successfully conveyed. By "precision," we mean explicating each thinking and action plan. As long as you do not exceed the page limit imposed by the funder, err on the side of detail. Consider adding tables, illustrations, and timelines, if allowable, to improve the presentation and reviewer grasp of your thinking and action. Precision also applies to appearance, grammar, and spelling. Be consistent in headings and subheadings, be vigilant in checking and correcting grammatical errors and spelling, and create a document that is easily legible. Care in form as well as content will give the reviewers the message that you are meticulous.

Parsimony is another important principle that should guide your proposal writing. Even when detailing your thinking and action, if the proposal is too lengthy or too wordy, it will be difficult or burdensome for reviewers to understand or persist in reading your work. So it is important to be "pithy" and keep your proposal to the point. A research proposal is written using simple, direct statements. It is not a place to experiment with a creative writing style or prose.

"Coherence," the fourth principle, refers to consistency among and within sections of your proposal (content and format). This element is often overlooked but critical, because you do not want to contradict yourself or omit what you may have promised to include.

For example, in a proposal to conduct research on a cognitive-behavioral approach to treating depression, if you define depression exclusively as a chemical imbalance, you would not have a rationale for your intervention. Or suppose you plan to travel by airplane to disseminate findings of your work. If you do not include a budget item for out-of-state travel, reviewers would question whether the resources that you are seeking would be sufficient to support your objectives and promises.

The fifth principle involves the need for "attention to structure," such as ensuring that all references are

BOX 22-1 *Questions to Guide Proposal Writing*

- What is your project about?
- Why is it important?
- What will you do?
- How will you do it?
- What will it cost?
- Why will it cost what it does?
- Why are you the best one to do it?

TABLE 22-1 *Common Elements of a Proposal*

Necessary Element	Information Included
Why	Title Abstract Introduction/Statement of research problem
What	Specific aims/Study objectives Literature review/Significance
How	Action plan/Methodology Reporting/Dissemination plan
When	Management of project Timeline
Who	Investigator credential
Where	Institutional qualifications Resources
Supporting material	Previous experience, publications Letters of support Formal agreements with consultants, other institutions if applicable Protection of human subjects
How much	Budget Budget justification

correctly cited, that proposal instructions are carefully followed, and, as we noted earlier, that the proposal is easy to read, with no typos, incorrect spellings, glaring grammatical errors, or inconsistent formatting. We cannot emphasize enough the critical need to follow instructions so that reviewers do not have to hunt for required information. Use techniques such as cross-referencing sections with evaluative criteria to show the reviewers that you value their time and effort.

Common Elements of a Research Proposal

As in sharing information and writing a report, writing a proposal to initiate the research process involves answering a series of questions (Box 22-1).

Although each agency or potential funding source, IRB, or department has its own format for writing a research proposal, there are common elements to such a document. Table 22-1 outlines the basic sections required for most proposals, regardless of the type of research or the research tradition. Each section of a proposal is designed to answer the core questions posed in Box 22-1, which relate to the "who, what, when, where, how, and how much" of your research idea. The basic elements of a proposal ask you to address how your research idea fits into the larger body of knowledge, as well as how you intend to use the findings or knowledge that you generate.[2]

We now examine each of these proposal elements in more detail.

Title

The title of your research study captures the main idea or theme of your proposal in a short phrase. It should not be so brief that it says nothing or so long

that a person reading your proposal has to work to determine the point of your study.

> Assume you want to conduct a study on the health conditions of elder men who are homeless and living in the shelter system. A title such as "Homeless Men" would be too brief and would not capture the main idea of your proposed research. A better title might be "Health Conditions of Older Homeless Men." •

Some agencies have specific requirements as to the length of the title. For example, a title of a research proposal submitted to the NIH must not exceed 56 typewritten spaces, including punctuation and spaces between words.

Abstract

The abstract is a brief description of each element contained in your proposal. It represents an executive summary of the study you propose. Generally, the abstract contains a statement of the purpose of your study or project, your research design, and key actions. If you are submitting your proposal to an external agency, there may be word limitations. In either case, the abstract must be clear and succinct but comprehensive. In addition to the title, the abstract is the first section of the proposal that a reviewer reads and thus provides the framework for reviewing your proposal and a first impression to the reviewer.[1] An abstract that is not clearly written, that is not comprehensive, or that has typographical, spelling, or grammatical errors can be misleading and can give the reviewer a poor impression, potentially influencing how the entire proposal is evaluated.

Because the abstract represents an executive summary of the entire project, it should actually be the last section you complete. However, keep in mind that you may write a draft abstract to guide your thinking and to send to people from whom you are requesting letters of support. For NIH grant applications, the title and abstract will be used to assign your proposal to a specific panel of reviewers. Thus, it is essential that both title and abstract reflect the core content of the proposal so that it is given to the appropriate panel.

Introduction

One way to begin your proposal is with an introductory paragraph that provides the reader with a general overview of the project's main idea and its importance. In this section, you address the questions regarding what your project is about and its merit within your field and perhaps beyond. You state the overall purpose of your study in the introduction. This section is an ideal location to link your proposal to the values and aims of the funder.

> Consider your study on the health conditions of homeless men. An opening paragraph would briefly discuss the increasing number of persons who are homeless in the United States, the types of health conditions that have been documented by previous research, and the gap in knowledge that your study will address. You might conclude with your purpose statement and its merit for knowledge development and application,[1] and then articulate how it meets the mission and values of the agency from which you are seeking funding. •

Although this introductory section is brief, it is necessary to cite data and scholarship from sources such as national studies, reports, theory, and research. Citing credible sources throughout your proposal demonstrates that you have done your homework and are familiar with the empirical work on which your study will build.

Specific Aims

"Aims" stem from a research purpose statement and concisely describe what you intend to accomplish—in other words, what will be investigated or evaluated in your research project. In addition to specifying the aims of the study, you might state hypotheses specific to each aim that you intend to test formally, if appropriate. Remember that hypotheses are only relevant when answering questions at Levels 2 and 3 in the experimental-type tradition. Of course, if relevant, you can also articulate the hunches in forms other than formal hypotheses. Box 22-2 provides an example of a specific aim and an accompanying hypothesis and a hunch for a study in which a hypothesis is not relevant.

"Aim statements" are critical building blocks of a proposal. They provide a mental template or a road map of what you plan to accomplish in the project.

BOX 22-2 *Examples of a Specific Aim and Hypothesis and Hunch Statement*

Specific aim: Test the immediate effects (up to 4 months) and long-term effects (at 6 and 12 months) of a life skills training program for men who are homeless.

Hypothesis: Homeless men who participate in the life skills program will report less depressed affect and will achieve goal attainment in specific skill areas compared with homeless men in a control group who receive no intervention or treatment.

Specific aim: To understand the reasons why some homeless men do not access shelters.

Hunch: We expect that two main reasons that men avoid shelter support are fear of theft of possessions and active substance abuse.

Rationale: Significance and Importance

Next in your proposal, you need to provide a compelling rationale for your study and discuss why it is significant and how it will address a gap in existing knowledge. Providing a brief but poignant and well-cited review of the key literature that informs your research is essential (see Chapter 6). Although having an idea that is exciting to you is a necessary starting point in conducting a research study, the idea must also have merit, must acknowledge that you are aware of previous and current work that is relevant to your area, and must be perceived as significant by the larger scholarly community and your audience, whether a human subject board, funding agency, or your professor.

You will address the "so what" question in the rationale. The "so what" question is a response that a reviewer might make after reading this section if you have not convinced the person that your idea is important and relevant to health. The "so what" response represents a fatal flaw in a research endeavor. If a reviewer cannot answer the "so what" question by reading your rationale, your work has a poor chance of being evaluated positively regardless of its methodological rigor or design validity.

The significance of your research idea must be justified with a concise critical review of other research studies that highlight the level of knowledge of the field, the need for further research and/or new theory development, and how your research addresses the gap in knowledge. Your review of previous research should demonstrate that your question or query is important but has not been satisfactorily answered. It should include only the most pertinent and current works and not a long discourse about topics only peripherally related to your project. A theoretical framework should also be clearly and explicitly linked to the variables you propose to examine when appropriate. If you are conducting a naturalistic study or a mixed method inquiry that does not contain variables, the concepts and initial queries should be articulated and justified. Remember to be succinct but inclusive in your citations. You would not want to omit the important work of one or more of your reviewers.

There are numerous ways to organize the writing of the literature review. Chronological or topical organizations are frequently used in proposal preparation. The chronological organization presents articles over a time sequence to show how knowledge has been incrementally developed, with the oldest articles first, to provide a historical perspective. Researchers using a topical organization group articles according to common themes that are relevant to the specific topic of the proposed investigation.

 In your study on the health conditions of men who are homeless, one strategy for reviewing and categorizing the related literature is to locate articles or studies that do the following:

1. Identify national and local statistics about the number of individuals who are homeless.
2. Contain demographic data about the homeless population.
3. Describe the health care needs of homeless persons.
4. Describe the problems faced by this group in accessing the health care system.
5. Discuss the strengths of previous and current work and clearly identify the gaps that you will fill in knowledge about health conditions of men who are homeless.
6. Identify the methodological challenges in sample identification and data collection and how you will address these.

Figure 22-1 presents a graphic of the literature. Each strand of literature should be carefully integrated with the others so that your literature "funnels down" to the reviewer's "Of course" statement. What we mean here is "Of course this makes sense, is well done, and will contribute to knowledge."

If you were proposing to examine reasons that men chose to avoid shelters, you might also include demographics, but you would add information to the list just given to indicate how many men who are homeless do not access shelters. You would then discuss any research proposing explanations for this choice and identify the knowledge that remains to be obtained so that these men can be safely served in their communities.

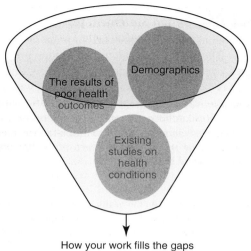

How your work fills the gaps
and builds on existing research

Figure 22-1 Funneling down to the gaps in the literature.

In reviewing the literature, it is important to consider resources outside your own field or profession and to obtain sources where the original work in an area is conducted. We find that reading in diverse fields not only enhances our knowledge but also provides a broad set of ideas that contribute to creativity and uniqueness. However, in grantsmanship, we caution you to use broad theory and research for thinking and providing a competitive proposal while also taking great care to propose a project that directly meets the funder's criteria, aims, mission, and values.

If the topic area of interest to you has not been studied or written about extensively, your review may be relatively brief. You then need to demonstrate that your topic is significant and cite the lack of research as one reason for conducting your study. A critical point to remember in writing a review of relevant literature is that the information you use and report must be from primary sources. A *primary source* is the original article or resource from which this information is reported. It is usually not appropriate to discuss a research article that is described or presented in an article by an author who did not conduct or report on the original study unless you have a reason for doing so. If you do, then indicate why you are including a secondary source in your

BOX 22-3 *Sections of Research Methodology to Present in a Proposal*

1. Overview of research design
2. Questions/queries
3. Boundary-setting procedures (description of population, sample, informants, concepts, locations, etc.)
   a. Inclusion and exclusion criteria for sample or initial rationale for informant selection
   b. Recruitment plan or plans to access the study environment
4. Action processes
   a. Procedures
   b. Materials
   c. Data collection
   d. Analytical plan
5. Human subjects (if appropriate)
   a. Assurance of confidentiality
   b. Informed consent process
6. Study rigor validity, reliability/trustworthiness, authenticity
7. Assumptions and study limitations
8. Timetable of key research activities

work. Even if you use a meta-review of literature, obtain each of the articles that you cite and critically evaluate them for yourself.

At the conclusion of reviewing relevant literature, provide a summary that reflects a synthesis and analysis of the articles. In this concluding section, you should discuss the way in which the literature you cited supports your background, significance, research question, hypotheses, and design. Also, identify the gaps in knowledge and the way in which your study or proposed program systematically contributes to knowledge building to address these gaps.

Research Plan

In this section of the research proposal, each action process is described in succinct and clear detail, including plans for bounding your study, identifying and recruiting a sample or informants, collecting information, and analyzing the data you obtain. Also, you will need to provide a justification for each action process. Box 22-3 outlines key aspects of research methodology to present in a proposal. Remember that your methodology must display coherence with the literature, your criticism of it, and your purpose—and of course your study must be "doable" with the requested and available resources.

Common mistakes made in writing this section of a proposal are an inadequate justification for why a particular action process is chosen, poor integration of ideas, lack of coherence among parts of the proposal, lack of design rigor, and lack of sufficient detail about the bounding and selecting of research study participants.

Keep in mind that there is no specific order for presenting the subsections of the research methodology discussed next. Rather, your research plan should be presented in a logical order and should reflect an integration of your ideas as well as the tradition used to conduct your study—experimental-type, naturalistic, or mixed methods.

Research Design

As discussed in Part III, the research design is the "blueprint" or plan in experimental-type design, the expression of the tradition that will be followed in a naturalistic inquiry or the rationale and plan for conducting a mixed method study. Each component of the research design must be presented and justified clearly and concisely.

One strategy is to begin this section of the proposal with a brief statement that summarizes or labels the design you intend to implement (e.g., two-group randomized experimental design, retrospective medical record review, $2 \times 2 \times 2$ factorial design, ethnography, mixed method study relying on open-ended interview followed by survey, etc.) and explain in what way the design is appropriate to address your specific research question and/or query.

Then, briefly highlight the major elements of the design. In an experimental-type inquiry, begin with your research questions and then state the independent and dependent variables, the sampling frame, sample size, selection procedures, and the number of testing occasions planned. It is important to be specific in your description. For example, when specifying the independent and dependent variables, include how each is related in the study (e.g., causal, explanatory, mediator, predictor). Box 22-4 provides an

> **BOX 22-4** *Design Statement for Experimental-Type Study*
>
> This study will describe the health conditions that present to men living in the shelter system who are aged 55 years or older. A descriptive survey design using a stratified random sample is proposed by which 100 men from 30 homeless shelters in the region will be randomly selected to complete a face-to-face interview designed to assess four areas of health: oral hygiene, mental health, physical aches and pains, and drug and alcohol use. The survey will contain demographic information, multiple-choice questions that tap knowledge of signs and symptoms of each problem, and open-ended questions that ask respondents to describe their approach to dealing with each problem.

> **BOX 22-5** *Design Statement for Naturalistic Query*
>
> This study will explore the meaning of health and wellness of men living in the shelter system who are 55 years of age or older. An ethnographic study of a large homeless shelter that houses more than 1000 men per month will be conducted. In-depth interviewing of shelter staff and residents and direct observation of daily life and shelter activities will be carried out over an 18-month period. Areas that will be explored in the interviews will be how residents participate in basic hygiene, when they seek medical care, and what it means to be in good health or feeling good. All interviews will be recorded and transcribed, and a thematic analysis will be conducted.

example of a design statement for an experimental-type study.

In a naturalistic inquiry, the same level of specificity must be provided as in experimental-type research. Specify the basic philosophical framework in which the query is based; the context in which the inquiry will proceed; the key projected data collection strategies (e.g., key informant, participant observation, object reading); and the analytical plan. Box 22-5 provides an example of a design statement for a query in a naturalistic tradition.

If using mixed methods, you may have both queries and questions, or you may be integrating only parts of your study. Indicate the purposive

This two-phase study uses a mixed method design to explore the meaning of health and wellness to men living in the shelter system who are 55 years of age or older. In Phase One, an ethnographic study of a small homeless shelter that houses more than 50 men per month will be conducted. In-depth interviewing and observation of residents will be carried out over a 12-month period. Areas that will be explored in the interviews and observations will be how residents participate in basic hygiene, when they seek medical care, and what it means to be in good health or feeling good. All interviews will be recorded, transcribed, and subjected to thematic and content analysis. Following Phase One, Phase Two, to be conducted over 18 months, will involve the development of an interview schedule testing the variables derived from the content analysis. A stratified random sample is proposed by which 100 men from 30 urban homeless shelters in the region will be randomly selected to complete a face-to-face structured interview designed to test the accuracy of the Phase One findings in a large urban population of homeless men.

nature of your proposed study, why, and how you plan to integrate methods. See Box 22-6 for an example.

Boundary Setting

This section of a proposal describes how you intend to "bound" your study. Consider outlining the following four basic points:

1. Describe the criteria that will be used to select study participants, or other units of analysis. This action process involves listing the specific criteria for inclusion and exclusion of study participants, locations, boundary-setting concepts, and so forth, and the reason or justification for each of these criteria.
2. Describe the anticipated characteristics of the study participants or units of analysis and the extent to which these are representative of the population to which you plan to generalize the study findings in an experimental-type design or the logic for selection in a naturalistic study. In discussing the sample characteristics, include any

descriptors that are supported as relevant in the literature.
3. Describe the procedures you will use for recruiting the sample, informants, or nonhuman boundaries.
4. For experimental-type proposals, discuss the sample size and the justification for its adequacy using power analysis, if appropriate. For naturalistic studies, discuss how you will enter the study environment and ensure that boundary setting is dynamic, feasible, and sufficient. For mixed methods, if you are mixing boundary-setting techniques, provide a rationale and succinct action plan.

Collecting Information This subsection should include a discussion of the procedures you will follow in collecting data and the instruments and/or techniques you will use, if applicable.

Human Subjects This subsection provides a discussion of the protection of human subjects. If they are actively participating in your study, this part of your proposal should include (1) your plans to ensure confidentiality of the information or data that you obtain from human subjects, (2) how consent from study participants will be obtained, (3) the potential benefits and risks for a subject associated with participation, and (4) the risk-to-benefit ratio (see discussion on IRBs in Chapter 3).

Design Rigor

In experimental-type proposals, you must address the validity and reliability of your design. As we have discussed, "validity" refers to whether a design and its procedures are appropriate and will yield information to answer the research question. You should explain the specific procedures you will use to ensure that your approach is the appropriate way to answer your research question. For example, if your purpose is to demonstrate causality, you might use an experimental design and discuss why the particular design you chose is most appropriate.

For experimental-type designs, you also should explain the reliability of your approach to data collection and analysis. Clearly describe the specific design features you have established that will ensure consistency of procedures in such a way that another investigator could replicate your study.

For naturalistic studies, include a discussion of your plans to ensure trustworthiness and authenticity.

If using mixed methods, assess the rigor criteria relevant to your design.

For example, suppose you are planning to use an open-ended interview approach to theorize the meaning of loss of ambulation resulting from injury to individuals who had been distance runners. You would discuss your plans for saturation, for the use of multiple analyzers, and for affirming the accuracy of your interpretations through member checking.

> You plan to make direct observations of a person's physical functioning using a standardized performance-based measure. In your research proposal, you need to discuss how you will ensure reliability and interrater agreement among the interviewers making the observations. •

You propose to both conduct open-ended interviews and rate injured runners on a standardized performance-based measure. You discuss plans for credibility, member checking, and reflexive analysis, along with activities to ensure interrater reliability.

Assumptions and Limitations

In this section of the proposal, you discuss the specific limitations of your design. Almost every study has some limitations, based either on features inherent in the design or on its application to your particular situation. Think about these limitations and how they may introduce possible sources of bias or limits in accuracy of description or interpretation. Some funders will ask you how you plan to address limitations, so you need to propose solutions as well.

> Suppose you are conducting a focus group study. A limitation of this technique is that respondents discuss their opinions with others participating in the study and thus may be swayed by social convention. This is a limitation that may have consequences for your findings. Thus, you should identify this limitation and discuss how you plan to address it. •

Timetable

It is important to outline in narrative or table format the basic actions that will be implemented and the time required. This step is essential because it provides your audience with an understanding of each necessary action and whether it is feasible to accomplish these actions within the planned time frame of the study. Also, the timetable provides a road map and schedule of the actions you will take, which will be a helpful reference as you propose your budget and, if funded, manage the research study. Figure 22-2 presents a Gantt chart format for timetable. The Gantt chart is used throughout many fields in project management and links aims, time deadlines, and accountability for project tasks in a visual image.[4]

Analytical Plan

This section involves a discussion of your analytical strategy and the statistical tests and/or qualitatively based techniques you plan to use. In your discussion, it is helpful to restate the specific aims, hunches, purposes, and/or hypotheses of your study, and then identify the analytical approaches that will be used to address each. Also, provide a brief rationale for your choice of analytical approaches, and if it is an experimental-type study or a mixed method design using statistical analysis, include the significance level that will be used to determine statistical significance.

Dissemination Plan

Sharing your research findings is one of the 10 essentials of the research process (see Chapter 2). Further, most funding sources want to be sure that their fiscal resources are used wisely and that the results of a successful project have a wide impact. From their perspective, it makes little sense to fund a project if only a few people will know about and benefit from a successful outcome. Therefore, many agencies require that you present a systematic plan to show how you will disseminate the results of your project. Two accepted ways to do this are through presentations at local, national, and international scholarly and professional meetings, and through publications in online and print journals. Also, consider other creative and innovative ways to ensure a wide distribution of your findings that target multiple

Task	Aim	Quarter 1	Quarter 2	Quarter 3	Quarter 4
Project kickoff meeting + quarterly team mtgs. + final mtg.	1/2/3	→	→	→	→
Weekly PI/PD meeting	1/2/3				→
Finalize design, design fabricate device for testing	1	→			
Strength and stability testing	1		→		
Implement weight bearing and other instrumentation	2	→			
IRB application submittal/approval	2/3		→		
Develop protocols for initial human subjects trials	2/3		→		
Monitoring system validity testing	2				→
Energy cost/biomechanics/functional ability testing	2				→
Usability testing	3			→	
Data analysis and reduction	1/2/3			→	
Phase II planning					→
Final Phase I report	1/2/3				→

Figure 22-2 The Gantt chart timetable of research to develop and test a mobility device.

audiences. These methods may include the development and distribution of instructional manuals; plans to develop webinars, workshops, or continuing education programs; blogging; locating your work on a website; disseminating your findings on sites such as ResearchGate and Digital Commons; making your raw data available to other researchers; or special ways to reach consumers as well as other professional and academic groups. We discuss this in more detail in Chapter 23.

Staffing and Management Plan

In this section, you begin to answer the question as to why you are the most appropriate person to conduct the study you are proposing in the setting and manner that you identify. Although you may have a wonderful idea, you must also assure your readership that you can accomplish the program goals efficiently, including managing the requested funds as you specify them to be spent. This section is particularly important when applying to a funding agency. You can answer this question by showing that you have a clear, logical, and efficient plan of management that will be executed by a project team of well-qualified people at an institution or context that can provide the necessary support and resources. A clear description of the organizational and management structure will answer the first part of this question. In your management plan, you will need to

discuss in detail the roles and responsibilities of key personnel, the amount of time each person will work on the project, and the time frame in which each project task will be implemented. Agencies frequently request that you organize this information in the form of a timeline or a detailed chart of major activities. The Gantt chart in Figure 22-2 is often added to a narrative to convey such information in a succinct manner.

An approach to writing this section is to visualize that you have already been funded. Think about exactly what you would have to do implement your action plan if you were to start tomorrow.[2] Whom would you need to hire? What contacts would be important? What resources would you need? Logically and rationally think through your plan before you write this section. The process may raise critical points of weakness in your research design, or it may highlight limitations in institutional resources that can be addressed before your proposal is submitted.

Investigative Team Credentials

This section also helps answer the question about your qualifications to carry out the project. Review your plan to determine the special knowledge, experience, and skills necessary to implement each step of the project. Then carefully select and describe your team and how the individual members make up a whole unit with the full complement of expertise, track record, and credentials necessary to be successful in accomplishing the goals and objectives that you propose. For example, if you are proposing a study that requires a repeated-measures design or statistical modeling techniques, make sure you have a statistician on your team with expertise in these specific analytical strategies. If your study uses naturalistic inquiry, ensure that a member of your team is an expert in qualitative methodologies and your proposed analytic applications. In writing an education research grant, make sure you are working with someone who has curriculum development knowledge and skills in evaluating educational innovation.

In writing about the credentials of the team, you should include a brief descriptive paragraph highlighting the qualifications of each member. Emphasize past experience, publications, or presentations that show expertise in the topic of the project. You may also consider a student research assistant, highlighting the mentorship and teaching aspect of your proposal if valued by the funder.

Some funders such as the National Science Foundation require you to list current and pending sources of extramural research funding, but if not requested, this information can go into your CV or biosketch. Cite funding received by you or other members of the research team for other projects, either from sources external to your institution or from sources inside your institution. Offices held in professional organizations, teaching, or consulting experiences can provide additional credibility and demonstrate that you have the necessary background to implement the research successfully.

Institutional Qualifications

Just as your team needs to be qualified, your institution or agency context needs to have the resources to assist and support you in carrying out your project. You need to include a concise description of your institution's resources and qualifications. For example, has your institution acquired a significant amount of external funding? Does it have access to comprehensive library resources or an active research office? What information and communication technology capacities are accessible for use?

Budget and Budget Justification

These sections address questions regarding the cost of your project and the reasons for the costs. You need to prepare a budget that is not inflated or wasteful and still sufficient to accomplish all your activities. Do not try to "pad" your budget by inflating costs or adding unnecessary expenses. Also, do not underestimate what it will cost you to carry out the study or educational program. The best advice is to develop a budget that accurately reflects the cost of the activities you are proposing. Most institutions have budget offices or offices of research administration that can help you as you prepare this budget.

You also are required to justify each expense. This information should be included in a budget justification section following the actual budget. In this section, describe how each item will be used, how the budget item was calculated, and why it is necessary for your study.

References

As in all scholarly work, a reference of your sources of information is required. If the agency does not specify a reference style, we recommend using the style specified by the American Psychological Association. In any case, be sure to be coherent in the presentation of references.

Appendix Material

Appendices usually include information that supplements the narrative portion of the document. Appendix materials may include the CVs of key members of the research team in the form and length requested by the funder, sample questionnaires or examples of open-ended probes, pertinent articles you have authored that relate to the study, and, most important, letters of support from consultants or from leaders in your profession. Make sure that you only put documents in the appendix that are allowed by the funder.

Special Considerations

Special considerations in preparing proposals are based on the type of research you plan to conduct.

Preparing an Experimental-Type Proposal

Within the experimental-type tradition, language and structure for presentation are standard across the basic elements of the proposal. The language used is logical, sequenced, and detailed. Because of the principle of objectivity and elimination of bias that characterize this research tradition, ideas are presented in the third person and detached from personal opinion. The experimental-type report usually has six sections in the body of the report, an abstract, and a list of references used to support the inquiry.

The abstract precedes the narrative report and serves as a summary of each section of the proposal. The reference list contains full citations of all literature identified in the proposal. Many citation formats exist. We suggest that you consider the use of a computerized program (e.g., ProCite, EndNote, Microsoft Word, RefWorks) to keep track of your literature and to format your references automatically in your style of choice. The degree of detail and precision in each section will depend on the purpose, funder guidelines, and audience for the proposal.

Preparing a Naturalistic Proposal

Because of the many epistemologically and structurally different types of naturalistic designs, we cannot assert a single proposal structure. Although some funders call specifically for naturalistic proposals, most funders still issue guidelines that require you to conform to the basic elements previously outlined. Unfortunately, this structure favors the linear approach of experimental-type research. If this situation presents itself, the proposal format, particularly the demand for details before initiating the study, can be a challenge to the naturalistic researcher. In addition, many audiences or reviewers of proposals are schooled in the tradition of experimental-type research and do not understand the naturalistic tradition or the vast differences in approaches to research design.

In writing a proposal to a linear request for proposals and most likely a reviewer audience not well informed in the naturalistic tradition, the naturalistic researcher must be sure not only to lay out the details of the action plans but also to explain clearly why a particular action will be implemented according to its appropriateness for the tradition in which the research is based. For example, the researcher might want to offer a set of "working" hunches and explain why in naturalistic research it is not appropriate to offer testable hypotheses. Or the researcher may need to specify approaches to data collection (e.g., watching, in-depth interviewing, review of documents) but must explain that the approaches used will unfold at different points in time, to be decided after the investigator is in the research environment. Again, it is important to provide a detailed justification for each action statement and why it is appropriate in a naturalistic approach. Thus, in writing the proposal, you not only have to provide an explanation of your study but also must help educate the reviewer as to how to evaluate your design within the specific tradition you are following.

Preparing a Mixed Method Proposal

In developing a proposal for a study that uses mixed methods, care must be taken to provide sufficient justification and details for each methodological component. Because a mixed method study may involve different research traditions, there is an added level of complexity to the proposal writing process. As in any proposal, the writer must strive for clarity and precision in presentation as well as completeness. Each component of the designs and how and why methods are being mixed must be carefully detailed.

Submitting the Proposal

Previously proposals were submitted by mailing a signed original and the required number of paper copies to the funding source. Several foundations, international funders, and corporate funders still request this format. However, for federal and foundation grants, the vast majority are submitted online. The majority of federal grants are submitted on www.grants.gov or www.fastlane.gov (the site for the National Science Foundation). You should familiarize yourself with the process of registering and submitting early in the process of preparing your proposal.

If you are submitting a proposal through an institution or agency setting, the institution is the applicant and must be registered with the funder. If you are submitting for an individual fellowship, you must be registered as an individual. Registration can often take up to 5 days, so register early. University and health institutional settings must have an identified representative who can sign the grant and assurances required by the funder. Working with your sponsored programs office, if you have one, will help you know who this individual is and the time needed for signatures.

We offer a word of advice regarding timing. Online proposal submission systems are not always user-friendly, so we suggest that you give yourself time to become familiar with them. Although we realize that proposals are often prepared under stringent time deadlines, try to submit before the final hours. Doing so will prevent the loss of many hours of work because you missed the deadline due to hiccups in the electronic submission system.

Summary

You now should have a basic understanding of how and why researchers share their thinking and actions before engaging in a study. One important reason to share at this early point in time is to secure financial support for your research activity. Grantsmanship is a critical component of the thinking processes in which researchers engage, and we refer you to other books that provide more comprehensive and focused discussions of grantsmanship that you may find useful.[2] Key to writing a research proposal is careful consideration of fit with the values of the funder, your purpose, and proposal format, audience, and detail. Use of technical research language specific to the tradition in which you are working and direct, clear simple statements are optimal. Readers—usually a group of the investigator's peers, that is, persons knowledgeable in the content of the research question or query—will scrutinize each statement in a proposal. Most critical in justifying the research question and/or query and proposed action plan is to provide supporting evidence that is compelling and credible. By knowing the audience (i.e., who will be reading your proposal), you can also select the approach and rationale that are most valued by that group. If you are writing for a medical audience, you might emphasize the significance of your research for quality of care; if you are writing for a health policy audience, emphasizing cost effectiveness may be more important. No matter what research tradition you are using or which proposal format you use, five principles should guide its development: clarity, precision, parsimony, coherence, and attention to structure.

EXERCISES

1. Obtain a grant proposal from a funded investigator or from your university's office of research and outline its basic structure; provide a critique of each section. Did the investigator explain the terms adequately? Did the investigator justify key aspects of the action plan? Did the investigator convince you that the proposed research question or query will significantly contribute to knowledge building?

2. Write a "mini" proposal (up to five pages) that contains the essential structure as outlined in Table 22-1. What aspects of the proposal were challenging? Show your proposal to a colleague and ask for critical feedback.

3. Go to a funder website of interest to you. Look at the guidance provided by the funder, the projects that have been funded, and the mission statement or priorities of the funding entity. What values are expressed, and what is important to the funder? How do you know? Identify the "clues" that lead you to specific values.

References

1. Gilson S, DePoy E: *Nitty gritty of proposal writing*, 2010. http://www.astos.org/our-projects#eval-practice.[ppt#282,17, Boilerplate: Resources and Institutional Setting].
2. Gitlin LN, Lyons KJ: *Successful grant writing: strategies for health and human service professionals*, ed 4, New York, 2014, Springer.
3. DePoy E, Gilson SF: *Studying disability: multiple theories and responses*, Thousand Oaks, Calif, 2011, Sage.
4. Kara H: *Research and evaluation for busy practitioners: a time-saving guide*, Chicago, 2012, Policy Press.

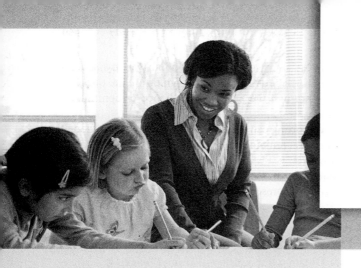

Chapter 23
Sharing Research Knowledge During and After the Study

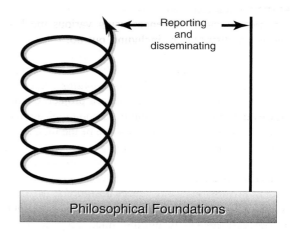

Although you may have completed the collection and analysis of information for a study, your efforts as a researcher are not quite finished until the 10th essential is accomplished. The 10th essential of research, "sharing research knowledge," involves two important action processes: purposeful reporting

and dissemination of knowledge gained from a study. Unless you report and disseminate, the full impact and benefit of your work are not realized. Unfortunately, this essential is too frequently overlooked or bypassed. Some researchers may move on to conduct another investigation without reporting and sharing results from their completed inquiry. Sometimes researchers are under a lot of pressure to continually seek funding, and thus they devote their attention to sharing before the study by developing fundable research queries and competitive grant applications.[1] However, sharing the knowledge gained from a completed study is critical to knowledge building, and thus we consider it an obligatory essential of the research process. If you do not share your results in venues that are appropriate to the audiences who can benefit, then a major purpose of your work—contributing to knowledge that informs health and human services—is left undone. Sharing knowledge from inquiry is important for study participants, other researchers, agencies who funded the study, practice settings, health organizations, policy stakeholders, or all or a combination. We further assert that it is the researcher's ethical responsibility to record the outcomes and propose the relevance of the inquiry.

By *reporting* research knowledge, we mean the preparation of a communication of all or part of an inquiry to one or more audiences. Related to the reporting function in research is dissemination. *Dissemination* is the action process of purposely sharing a research report with key stakeholders or different intended audiences using various mechanisms for distribution, including but not limited to journal outlets, news outlets, conferences, website postings, interviews, and speeches. These action processes, reporting and disseminating, usually occur at the conclusion of a research project. Often, however, there are opportunities to communicate the progress of a study and report some of the methodological challenges or preliminary findings before completing all the actions of data collection and analysis. As an example, many researchers participate in professional conferences designed to provide a venue for sharing of methods and results in order to obtain feedback to improve their projects or to share preliminary or emerging themes or other outcomes. In randomized trials, for example, it is possible to report descriptive, cross-sectional findings from the initial point of data collection, even though collection at subsequent data points has not been completed.

Think about our definition of research in Chapter 1. Do you remember the four criteria to which a study must conform; logical, understandable, confirmable, and *useful*? The last is the focus of this chapter. "Usefulness" is the one research criterion that cannot be accomplished without communicating the findings of a completed study and their meaning to others.

The detail, specificity, format, and nature of your sharing is purposeful. How you go about creating and communicating the knowledge derived from your research is purposive and driven by several factors, the most important of which are the question or query and the particular audience or community on whom you want to have an impact.

Reporting can occur in different formats, although narrative remains the primary outlet for research. However, with the spread of online and open-access journals, some are encouraging and providing a platform for presenting research findings in formats other than or complementing the written word, such as video and auditory formats that accompany a written text. Further, some schools now require their masters' and doctoral students not only to generate a written final thesis report but also to develop a 2- to 3-minute video clip synopsis of their study that is then widely distributed on the Internet. Multiple methods of dissemination not only expand the reach and use of your research, but also are methods to create full accessibility for people who acquire and learn in diverse ways.[2]

Because writing remains the primary reporting approach for experimental, naturalistic, and mixed method forms of inquiry, we focus our attention on this approach. You can extrapolate the principles to other forms of communication as well. We believe that four basic principles should inform the action process of reporting: writing, accessibility, linguistic sensitivity, and integrity of presentation.

Crafting a Report

The traditional approach to reporting is to write one or more manuscripts that report on the key findings from the inquiry. For most researchers, particular manuscripts are then submitted for consideration for publication in a peer-reviewed scholarly journal. However, there are many other outlets for sharing a report and different methods for doing so including writing for community organization's newsletter or an organization's annual report, submitting your work to proceedings of conferences at which you have presented your research, sharing results in an op-ed piece, or publishing your work on your personal site on ResearchGate or Digital Commons.

ResearchGate is designed as a social network specifically sharing scientific and scholarly work with the following mission:

We believe science should be open and transparent. This is why we've made it our mission to connect researchers and make it easy for them to share, discover, use, and distribute findings. We help researchers voice feedback and build reputation through open discussion and evaluation of each other's research.[3]

Similarly, Digital Commons is an open access and open publishing site. However, unlike ResearchGate, Digital Commons is institutionally situated, mostly in universities as part of the library.[4] Further adding to the many venues and formats are open-access online journals, blogs, and imagery. All can be used to present research findings. Mapping is another example of images that are powerful in sharing results. It is not unusual for a single inquiry to generate multiple reports in multiple formats.

As you probably have surmised by now, each type of inquiry has a distinct language or set of languages, images, and structures that organize the reporting action process. Nevertheless, all reporting, regardless of the research tradition that the report will reflect, is based on a common set of principles. These include issues related to clarity, purpose, knowledge of target audience, and citation style. We address these primarily within written format but again remind you that each principle applies to all formats.

Clarity

Writing a report serves little purpose if it is not understood.[4] Therefore, an investigator should be certain that his or her report is clear and well articulated. There are many books on writing and many ways to approach this task, which is often difficult, particularly for the new investigator. As in any professional activity, the more you do it, the more proficient you will be and the easier the task will become. It is important to recognize that writing is an important aspect of the research process; it takes time, thought, and creative energy.

Purpose

As we have stated throughout this book, multiple purposes drive the selection of research action processes. These purposes also structure the nature of

the reporting action process.[4] Consider, for example, two different purposes for writing a report: for publication in a professional journal and a written evaluation for a community organization. Researchers who write for the purpose of publishing their research in scholarly venues must conform to the style and expectations of the outlet to which the manuscript is submitted. The researcher may also consider writing an article for practitioners and thus will present results and interpretations somewhat differently. The researcher who has just completed an evaluation of a community program may need to write a report to the board of directors or the funding agency to ensure continuation of financial support. In this case, the researcher may emphasize positive programmatic outcomes and write the research report so it is consistent with the expectations of the funding agency. For the journal, a full and detailed report using the technical and professional language of the journal and readership would be warranted. However, for the agency, an executive summary with bullet points might be a better means through which to report findings. Each purpose for conducting and reporting research must be carefully considered.

Multiple Audiences

As stated earlier, being aware of the many audiences that can benefit from an inquiry is critical in order to meet the "useful" criterion in our definition of research. Audiences are diverse in their languages, the meanings they attribute to language, their priorities and what they consider to be important, their level of engagement and interest in the research process, and their values regarding credibility. Thus, along with purpose, the audiences for whom the report is prepared will determine, in large part, how the report will be structured, what information should be contained within it, how the information will be presented, and the degree of specificity that will be included. The audience may also vary with regard to their areas of expertise and knowledge of the research methodology. The important point is to identify, up front, your reason for reporting to a particular audience and to assess how that purpose can be communicated to that group. You need to communicate in a style that is consistent with the level of understanding and knowledge of the targeted reader.

As an example, suppose you have completed a participatory action research project in which individuals with intellectual impairments functioned as researchers and informants to identify recreation needs in rural communities. Careful attention to the literacy levels of multiple audiences, including those with limited literacy skills, would be warranted. To this end, the concepts of accessibility and linguistic sensitivity are important,[5] as discussed later.

Or let's say you have completed a research project examining beliefs shaping participation in cancer screenings among middle-aged Korean men and women to derive recommendations for outreach and to increase the participation of this group in preventive health practices. The challenge will be to present an understanding of the beliefs and recommendations in a linguistically appropriate and sensitive manner so that community can move forward with practices that support their health but that also are respectful of cultural traditions and preferences.

Citations

You need to be aware of several other important points as you develop reports of your research. The first is the issue of plagiarism. Most researchers who plagiarize probably do not do so purposely. To avoid this potential and devastating mistake that is often made by novice researchers, you need to be aware of the norms for citation and credit. All work produced by another person, even if not directly quoted in your work, must be cited.[6] Many different citation formats are used in health and human service research. We refer you to your publication source for the correct format and urge you to become very familiar with it. If necessary, have someone else check your work to ensure that you have properly credited other authors. It is important to note that even using your own written work verbatim that was published elsewhere is a form of plagiarism. Even in this case, you will need to express your ideas differently and then cite your previous work. Another important point to remember in reporting is that it is *not* an acceptable practice to excessively quote from other research studies in the literature review of an article for a journal. Many students of research like to review a body of literature by stringing together a series of quotes from different articles. However, the review of the literature section in a report must reflect a summation and critical analysis of the most salient aspects of existing studies. By quoting, you are simply reiterating the work of others without providing a synthesis and critical commentary.

Another common error among newcomers to formal writing is the use of citations that you have not directly read. Consider the following example.

> You read an article by an author, Dr. Smith, who cited in her review of the literature a number of other authors and their studies. You are interested in these other studies and include them in your study on the basis of your reading of Dr. Smith's article, and you cite them in your reference list. However, you have never obtained and read the original articles. In this case, you are actually using Dr. Smith's interpretations of these studies. Remember, Dr. Smith selected the most salient points from these studies that supported her particular approach. Therefore, her interpretation may be different from the intent of the original work. If you had read the articles yourself, you might have derived a different understanding. In writing a research report, it is very important to remember that only primary citations that you have read yourself are acceptable for inclusion in an article.
>
> Therefore, you have two choices. You can report Dr. Smith's interpretation of the studies she reviewed and cite her article in your reference list. For example, you may say, "According to Dr. Smith, the literature on the adequacy of home care for elders is underdeveloped." A second strategy is to retrieve the articles cited in Dr. Smith's report, read them, and report your interpretation of this body of literature. In this case, you will then cite each study you read and include it in your reference list. •

Before we leave the section on citation, we call your attention to the wonders of technology. As we noted earlier, citation formats differ according to discipline and venue. Before the advent of electronic databases and automated formatting, one major element of report preparation was formatting the reference section and citations within the text. Now, with software programs such as EndNote or RefWorks and embedded bibliographic databases in word processing programs, citing and referencing can be a snap. All you need to do is enter complete information about a source into fields in your database and select the format. The software does the rest by automatically locating citations in the text and formatting your reference or bibliography according to the style that you have chosen. Current versions of applications such as RefWorks even keep PDF copies of articles and use automated searching and citing, saving you much time while simultaneously creating a cumulative database for your references.

With these commonsense principles, let us now consider the specific reporting considerations for each tradition.

Experimental-Type Reporting

Reports of experimental-type research use a common language and follow a standard format and structure for presenting a study and its findings. The language used by the experimental-type researcher is "scientific" and technical in nature. As we noted earlier, it is logical and detached from personal opinion or beliefs. Interpretations are supported by numerical data and theory. There are typically eight major sections in an experimental-type report (Box 23-1). Although investigators sometimes deviate from this order of presentation, these sections are usually considered the essentials of a scientific report and are, for the most part, required in journals reporting this form of inquiry. As you begin to develop a report for

---

BOX 23-1 *Major Sections of an Experimental-Type Report*

1. Abstract
2. Introduction
3. Background and significance
4. Method
   • Design
   • Research question(s)
   • Population and sample
   • Instrumentation
   • Data analysis strategies
   • Procedures
5. Results
6. Discussion
7. Conclusion

---

publication in a peer-reviewed journal, be sure to first review the journal's author instructions, which will specify requirements for each of the sections discussed here. Let us examine these basic sections and the information included in each.

The title page starts the report for a peer-reviewed journal. Although each journal specifies different information and organization for this initial page, typically all ask for the authors' full names, titles, and affiliations in the order of attribution from first to last. The first author, called the primary author, takes responsibility for orchestrating all sections of the report and is ultimately responsible for accuracy, as well as being the corresponding author for questions, review recommendations, and decisions about publication. This author is typically the primary investigator of the study being reported and is responsible for the study concept and design.

In most academic environments, the last author is the senior investigator who may have mentored the research team or guided the team of authors. The first and last authorship spots on a journal article are usually coveted and considered the most important or prestigious among the authors listed. The order in which the names of the other authors are listed will depend upon each person's contributions and efforts to the study idea, design, its conduct, and the development of the report. The order of presentation of authors requires thought and is typically decided by the first author in consultation with each coauthor. It is best to make these types of decisions up front even before starting to prepare the report so there are no surprises and everyone agrees as to his/her roles and responsibilities concerning the preparation of the formal report.

Most journals will require that authors specify their role in the study and preparing the manuscript on its submission for consideration of publication. When crafting a report, whether for submission to a journal or elsewhere, the order in which authors are listed has significance. The first author is typically the one who initiated the idea for the study or manuscript, developed the study design, and had primary responsibility for writing the report and interpreting findings. Other authors may have other roles, such as working on the data analyses and data tables and critically reviewing the manuscript. To qualify for authorship, it is not enough to have collected information for a study; an author has to have participated in the manuscript preparation at some level. If an individual did not contribute to the actual writing but did collect data or was part of the study in another way, authors frequently acknowledge them in a footnote or endnote early in the manuscript.

For most journals, authors must complete a form indicating whether they have a conflict of interest with the material presented such that they or their family members would realize a financial gain from the publication of the study. This step asserts that the conduct of the study and the reported findings are free from undue bias.

This situation may sound unusual to you, but conflicts of interest are actually very common in research. Let's say you are a consultant for an assistive technology company and you have been helping them understand use rates and preferences for certain types of home technologies. You also have been working on a study that examines the benefits of some of the technologies that this company distributes. This could pose as a conflict of interest, given that positive results could directly benefit the company that retains you as a consultant. Or you may be swayed to present the most positive findings from the study that favor the consultancy work you have been doing, even when this is not your intention. In writing the report, you would have to report this potential financial arrangement and how you are managing it and the study to minimize bias. For example, you could manage the study and the reporting process by having an independent researcher review all findings and write up the results section.

As you can see, all matters concerning authorship are important, and well-considered thought must be given even to the title page. In brief summary, the four basic considerations of authorship are: who should participate as an author of a report, roles and responsibilities of each listed author, order of authorship (who should be first, second, third, and so forth), and ruling out and disclosing potential conflicts of interest for each author.

In addition to author information, the title page might also include keywords, funding acknowledgments, and possibly the word count of the narrative section. Again, requirements for this title page will vary widely from professional journal to journal, or by dissertation style or other reporting outlet. Always check the guidelines for submitting a report.

The abstract is the next section. It appears before the full report and briefly summarizes or highlights the major points in each subsequent section of the report. It includes a statement of the research purpose, brief overview of method, and summary of the major findings and implications of the study. Usually the abstract does not exceed one or two paragraphs. Professional journals usually specify the length of the abstract; some journals require brief abstracts that are no longer than 100 words, whereas others allow for up to 250 words.

The structure of the abstract will vary widely depending on the professional journal or reporting outlet. Some journals, for example, require highly structured abstracts that include subheadings such as objectives, study design, population, setting, measures, results, and conclusions. Other professional outlets require a brief paragraph that describes the study purpose, main results, and conclusions.

Following the abstract is the introduction. This section presents the problem statement, the purpose statement, and an overview of the questions that the study addresses. In this section, the researcher must show (1) how the study is embedded in and builds on a particular body of literature, and (2) the study's specific intended contribution to the discipline and professional knowledge and practice. The introduction sets the stage for the study findings and also indicates the gap in knowledge that the study is designed to address. In the introduction, it is important to be concise and use the most relevant and updated references.

For professional journals, the introduction will provide the background and significance of the study and present the problem addressed. In other types of reports, such as final reports for funding agencies, there is a separate background and significance section. The background and significance section reviews the literature and establishes the conceptual foundation for your research study. In this section, key concepts, constructs, principles, and theory addressed by the study are critically summarized. (Refer to your literature chart or concept matrix to help organize the background and significance section.) The degree of detail in presenting the literature will depend on the researcher's purpose and intended audience. For example, in a journal article, the researcher usually limits the literature review to an overview of the broad field of inquiry and then focuses on the seminal works that precede the study, whereas in a traditional doctoral dissertation, all previous work that directly or indirectly informs the research question is detailed and critically reviewed.

The method section consists of several subsections:

1. The articulation of well-structured and complete research question/s
2. A clear description of the design
3. The population and sample, including techniques used for sample selection and size
4. The measures or instrumentation, including the constructs that measured and validity and reliability of each instrument
5. The specific data analysis strategies linked to the questions answered by each
6. The procedures used to conduct the research

The degree of detail and specificity is again determined by the purpose and audience and can vary as well by the style of the professional journal. However, sufficient information must be provided in each subsection of methods so that the reader has a clear understanding of how data were collected and the specific procedures that were implemented.

The analyzed data are presented in the results section. Usually, researchers begin by presenting descriptive statistics, then proceed to a presentation of inferential and associational types of statistical analyses. A rationale for statistical analysis is presented, and the findings are usually explained. However, interpretation of the data is not usually presented in this section. Data may be presented in narrative, chart, graph, or table form. You should be aware that there are prescribed formats for presenting statistical analyses. Ary and colleagues[7] provided excellent information to guide both the preparation and the evaluation of written reports.

The discussion section may be the most creative part of the experimental-type research report. In this section the researcher summarizes the key findings and then discusses their implications, statistical significance, and meanings; poses potential alternative explanations; relates the findings to published work and theory contained in the literature review; and suggests the potential application or use of the research results. Most researchers include a statement of the limitations of the study in this section as well.

The conclusion section is a short summary that provides interpretations and application of the study findings to future research directions or health care and human service practices.

As you can see, preparing an experimental-type report follows a logical, well-accepted sequence that includes basic essential sections. The degree of detail and precision in each section depends on the purpose and audience for the report and the particular outlet. Because professional journal articles, dissertation formats, progress and final reports to funders, and other forms of research reports are diverse in formats and requirements, you must read the instructions provided for authors before and while writing the report.

Specific Reporting Requirements

There are specific reporting structures for certain types of experimental-type inquiries. Various organizations have developed helpful guidelines that establish clear, transparent standards for research reports for different types of research. For example, the American Educational Research Association provides published guidelines for reporting education research (experimental or naturalistic type) and humanities research in their publications.

The American Psychological Association (APA) publishes and regularly updates a detailed manual of the reporting style that is used by all APA and other related journals.[9] The APA manual also specifies specific reporting standards for different designs such as meta-analysis reports. Remember that these guidelines change relatively frequently, so keep up with the formatting revisions. You can do this in two ways: obtain regular updated manuals, or use the most current referencing applications discussed above. Updates to these software programs include the most recent changes to referencing styles.

Other specific guidelines include the Consolidated Health Economic Evaluation Reporting Standards (CHEERS),[10] also available online. This resource provides guidelines for cost effectiveness and other forms of economic evaluation.

Because of their importance to evidence-based practice, we now review guidelines for reporting randomized clinical trials. Although the randomized controlled trial is upheld as the most rigorous design strategy for testing predictive statements and establishing evidence for interventions, programs, or services, their reporting in professional journals has been suboptimal. To enhance the scientific utility and transparency of each thinking and action process in the randomized trial design, efforts have been made to standardize their reporting. In the 1990s, an international body of researchers engaged in clinical trials put forth the CONsolidated Standards of Reporting Trials (CONSORT) in an effort to provide standard language and structure and enhance the ability of readers to evaluate the validity of trials. The CONSORT is periodically updated, with the most recent version being March 2010.[11] CONSORT provides the tools for developing highly structured reports, all with a common template. Tools include a 25-item checklist for authors and a flowchart to depict subject process through the clinical trial.

Most medical journals that report randomized trials endorse the CONSORT and require that on submission, authors submit the CONSORT checklist indicating the page number of the manuscript that addresses each item.

The CONSORT checklist has been adopted by most medical journals, including *The Lancet* and the *Journal of the American Medical Association*, which now require written manuscript submissions that are reporting trials to use the checklist and flow diagram.[11]

Preparing Tables and Figures

Tables, charts, and figures are important parts of experimental-type research reports. They reduce complicated data by systematically organizing important findings. Different from narrative, which tells a story, tables and figures present visuals of rankings, relationships, and significance. In experimental-type reports, tables, charts, and figures are used to present data in the results section of a report.

Tables present numeric data in rows and columns, whereas charts are displays of information that may be numeric but may also be in the form of a picture or image such as a pie chart or polygon. Both tables and charts can be univariate (presenting data from one variable) or multivariate (presenting data depicting the relationships among two or more variables). Tables also can present related numeric information, most typically raw scores adjacent to computed values of a statistic and probability.

Among the most frequently used univariate charts are pie charts (depicting relative percentages), bar charts comparing frequencies, scatterplots, and curves (such as the bell curve) showing the distribution of scores on a variable.

With the increasing use of computer programs, figures and tables are simple and fun to create. Even freeware has built-in automated functions that convert numeric findings from numbers into tables. Of course, we have all seen tables and figures of the same data that visually present different pictures. Care should be taken to create figures, tables, and charts that are not misleading but are designed to clarify and highlight important findings. Your narrative about these visuals should call attention to important points and trends without repeating what is contained within the visual displays.

Consider the example of age. Suppose you have the following ages represented in your sample: 21, 25, 56, 67, 30, 32, 35, 65, 62, 32, and 25. What might you want to communicate about age? You could rank order the numbers from youngest to eldest for clarity, but you might want to make it easier for your readers to understand the age trends of your sample.

You might want to use a table to show the two extremes in your sample shown in Table 23-1. Or you might present these data in the form of a pie chart as shown in Figure 23-1. As you can see, the

TABLE 23-1 *Age Table*

Under 50 (n, %)	50 and Over (n, %)
6, 60%	4, 40%

Age of Sample

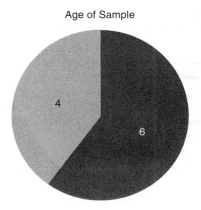

Figure 23-1 Age pie chart.

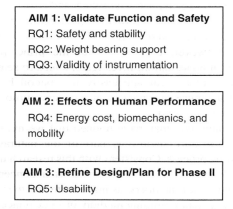

AIM 1: Validate Function and Safety
RQ1: Safety and stability
RQ2: Weight bearing support
RQ3: Validity of instrumentation

AIM 2: Effects on Human Performance
RQ4: Energy cost, biomechanics, and mobility

AIM 3: Refine Design/Plan for Phase II
RQ5: Usability

Figure 23-2 Flow chart of R & D of innovative mobility device.

pie chart is simply an image that tells a story in a clear format.

Figures are frequently used to map the study design and flow and allocation of study participations such as that required by the CONSORT checklist. Also, figures can be presented that display a conceptual model that is being tested or specific analytic outcomes such as in sensitivity analyses, interaction or moderator effects, or mediation models. Figure 23-2 presents the flow of a current research and development study for an innovative mobility device.

We now move from highly structured reporting to the diverse approaches used in sharing naturalistic research.

Preparing a Naturalistic Report

By this time, you probably expect that naturalistic reporting takes on many acceptable formats, depending on purpose, epistemology, and nature of data. Consistent with this tradition, there is no single, accepted format for preparing a final report. However, some basic commonalities among the varied designs can guide reporting in this broad tradition. Unlike experimental-type reporting, naturalistic reporting does not follow a prescribed format with clear expectations for language, nature of data, and structure. Reports tend to be rich in detail and description and draw on data in the form of narratives, images, or both to illustrate major themes and interpretations. The structure of the presentation is not standardized, and there is great variation in the format, sequencing, and nature of information[12] and approach.[13] Unless the design does not call for investigator interpretation, most naturalistic reports reflect the investigator's underlying interpretive scheme. Interpretive schemes are often presented as a "story" in which main themes and subtexts unfold as the story is told.

Consider the following examples: In your effort to develop meaningful fitness activity for youth with intellectual impairments who reside in an urban area, you review the evidence-based practice literature and find that for your population, the recommended strategies are not productive. So you plan a naturalistic study to investigate the type of activity that would be meaningful and engage these youth in physical activity. Through observation of the children and interviews with parents and teachers, you find that socialization during physical activity combined with a goal of increasing competition for the number of city blocks walked are two strategies that are meaningful and thus are likely to achieve the outcomes of voluntary participation and increasing physical activity and fitness of these youth. In preparing your report to communicate a compelling need, you keep a log of the social interactions, activities, and stories told by the youth themselves.

Now consider that you have just moved from an urban to a rural border area in northern New England to develop a similar fitness program in this area. Although there is a significant body of evidence-based practice literature and you have just documented yet another successful programmatic approach, you become aware of different geographic and place-bound factors that raise questions about the relevance of urban approaches to your population. For example, you realize that unlike the urban outdoor walking in which youth could compete on sidewalks that have easily measurable distances, walking in rural areas occurs on roadsides and trails. Moreover, snow and ice for much of the year may require the use of snowshoes or other equipment. So you decide to conduct another naturalistic inquiry to support a direction and grant application for your program. Although the stories, customs, and recommendations of families and community members are convincing, you find that in this inquiry, your photographs and video images of the youth in context "tell the story" most graphically and are most powerful in communicating the rationale for this approach, particularly in the winter months when outdoor fitness is a challenge. So you seek permission to include these visuals as data, and interpret these images for the audiences reviewing the report in your analysis.

An important aspect of reporting in naturalistic inquiry is the inclusion of a section that describes the researcher's personal biases and feelings in conducting the study. Remember that we referred to this action process as reflexivity.[14] For example, in the rural study, you realize that your own distaste for being cold has shaped some of your interpretations and recommendations. Many researchers discuss their personal perspective on conducting the study as part of the introduction to their report.

Although the report in naturalistic inquiry may be structured in many ways, it contains some of the same basic elements used in report preparation for experimental-type research. Using the language of naturalistic research, Box 23-2 provides the basic sections contained in a report. Documentation in naturalistic research may not follow the sections in the sequence as shown, but each report usually addresses these basic elements.

The introduction in naturalistic design contains the purpose for conducting the research. An investigator may include personal reasons as well as the aim related to the development and advancement of professional knowledge.

BOX 23-2 *Basic Sections of a Naturalistic Inquiry Report*

1. Introduction
2. Query
3. Epistemological foundation
4. Theoretical framework(s)
5. Research process
6. Information
7. Analysis
8. Meaning and implications

The query, epistemological foundation, and theoretical framework may appear separately or combined in one section of the report. As described in previous chapters, these thinking and action processes are integrated throughout the conduct of naturalistic research and therefore can be presented as such. However, consistent with the principle of clarity in presentation, investigators need to select a format that is clear and easily understood by the target audience and consistent with the purpose of the study and report.

By now you may have noticed that we have not listed literature review as part of the naturalistic reporting process. Consistent with this research tradition, literature may be presented as a conceptual foundation for the query, as inadequate and thus promoting a theory building method, or as evidence that supports the data or main interpretations presented by the investigator. In most reports, the literature is used to ground the research in a body of knowledge, to support the main findings, to justify the method, or to examine competing interpretations of the findings.

Reporting naturalistic research departs from experimental-type sharing in the presentation of the research process and information. Naturalistic investigators rely heavily on the narrative and, increasingly, images to report their data.[8] Quotations from informants may be woven throughout the narrative text. Visual and numeric display of information, such as taxonomic charts, photographs, and content and thematic analyses, are also used in naturalistic reporting, depending on the query, epistemological foundation, purpose, and intended audience. Let us now consider how the reports from various naturalistic designs may be structured.

Ethnography

Although there are diverse formats within the broad category of ethnography, the primary function of this approach is to identify patterns and characterize a cultural group. Therefore, the report tells a story about the underlying values, roles, beliefs, and normative practices of the culture. It is not unusual for ethnographers to begin with "method"; that is, the investigator frequently begins by reporting how he or she gained access to the study environment. The report may be developed chronologically, and literature, other sources of information, and conclusions are interspersed throughout and summarized in the end.

Harple and colleagues[15] demonstrated the use of ethnography in the complexity of the contemporary health care industry. As the basis for developing health care technology, they examined the emotional aspects of health professional work and the meaning that these devices held within the culture of the hospital for patients and staff. Throughout the report, they reminded the reader that their respect and caution not to invade patient privacy influenced their work and what they chose to observe. They also reflected why they used ethnography over other methods. Listen to what they say at the beginning of their report:

> In the complex and rapidly changing health care ecosystem, ethnographic methods are uniquely able to illuminate not just how individuals act, what motivates them, why and how they feel, but also how actors' interactions are shaped by the context. (p 129)

In contrast to experimental-type reporting, this type of statement highlights that context, not literature, served as the purpose for the method and study.

Phenomenology

Because the focus in phenomenological research is on the unique experience of one or more persons, the report is often narrative and written in the form of a story recounted to the investigator. Photographic images may be included to enhance the data. If specific points about the lived experience of the informants are made, they are fully supported with information from the informants themselves, frequently in the form of direct quotes from interviews. Because the length of phenomenological studies varies greatly, they may appear as full-length journal articles, books, or other literary styles among these formats. The reports highlight life experience and its interpretation by those who experience it, and they minimize interpretations imposed by the investigator.

The nature and purpose of phenomenological designs differ from those of ethnography, as does the reporting format. In both cases, form follows function. In ethnography, the function of the investigator is to make sense of what he or she has observed, whereas in a phenomenological study, the investigator reports how others make sense of their experience. These differences are clearly reflected in the report.

In summary, naturalistic researchers use a variety of reporting action processes to share their findings. Although there is a heavy reliance on narrative data, the naturalistic investigator has the option of using numeric and visual representations, as well as other media. All reports contain the basic sections (see Box 23-2), but the order and emphasis differ among naturalistic designs and the preferences and personal styles of the investigator, as well as the requirements of the journal or other outlet for the report.[13]

Preparing a Mixed Method Report

Because mixed method studies use diverse combinations of methods from both traditions, throughout or within only some of the ten research essentials, there are no specific guidelines for language and format.[16] Thus, the nature and structure of the report depend on the level of integration, types of designs used, purpose of the work, and audience who will receive the report. We can, however, offer two principles that may help your reporting action process. First, you should include the components of a complete research report (see Boxes 23-1 and 23-2). Regardless of its length, organization, or complexity, your report should contain a statement of purpose, review of the literature (if indicated), methodology section, presentation of findings, and conclusions. Second, because a mixed method design is not as well established as designs that are distinctly experimental type or naturalistic, it is often useful to include a sound rationale for the methodology in the report as well as the way in which each complements the other.

Accessibility

In addition to the principles for writing and presenting, there is another important reporting principle. Communicating knowledge brings with it an important obligation, that of providing knowledge in accessible formats for all groups who may benefit. *Accessible* is a term that describes the usability of a product or service. In the case of communicating research, the "product" is the research report.

In the past 30 years, three approaches to expanding information access have emerged: accommodative, universal, and interactive (recognizing the importance of considering the person in context). Accommodative strategies refer to those that adapt and customize information to meet individual condition or group-specific needs. For example, providing a screen reader to a person with low vision would be classified as an accommodation. Universal approaches (often called "universal design" or "universal access") are distinct from group-specific approaches in that they provide information in forms that all people, to the extent possible and regardless of group-specific diversity characteristics, can access without the need for adaptation. Universal access is governed by seven principles that avoid the need for retrofitting or accommodating.[18] Automated online screen readers for low-vision and blind users would be an example of universal approaches, as the strategy is designed to anticipate expansive methods of accessing information. Most recent is the interactivity of both person and environment as the major consideration for access.[17] Through this view, researchers would strive to make their work accessible through multiple formats but also see that individuals may choose their own methods. Thus, the presentation of material would be configured for "reader control." For example, the report would be structured so that it could be accessed through video, audio, print, and other preferred methods, but the investigator would realize that he/she could not provide them all. Specific tools such as automated

language translation and text to speech might be hosted or referenced with the report.

To the extent that it is possible and purposive, we believe that it is incumbent on researchers to plan communications so that they can be accessed by all who can benefit. Universal and interactive approaches to communication of information provide the framework for this goal (see later discussion on dissemination). Yet, it is also appropriate to tailor the messaging of the findings of a study to different intended audiences and to provide resources rather than trying to anticipate a format that all people prefer.

Before we leave accessibility, we highlight the role of technology in expanding access through preference instead of one approach. Although not perfect, text to speech and speech to text, as well as language translation applications such as BabelFish and Google Translate, are extremely useful for enlarging the scope of individuals and groups who can understand your report through diverse chosen approaches. For example, text to speech, speech to text or Braille, and many other developments are extending access beyond what we could have imagined even a decade ago. We can now read languages with which we are not at all familiar or even know the alphabet.

Linguistic Sensitivity

The third principle we discuss in reporting research concerns how language is used in a particular context, or linguistic sensitivity. By *linguistic sensitivity* we mean having knowledge about the target audience and the meaning of language to that group. Our point can be best illustrated by the language incidents that we discussed in Chapter 18. A third event presents yet another complication of communicating and reporting research.

At a conference on employment law and disability for attorneys and researchers, a colleague noticed that in the research presentations, the attorneys looked rather bored and that in the law presentations, the researchers expressed skepticism about claims made by the attorneys, claims that were supported only by individual and anecdotal stories about clients.

In all situations, much can be learned about communication and the meaning of words, or language. As we highlighted in Chapter 18, the Egyptian and Chinese experiences illustrate that people who speak the same language do not necessarily speak the same "meaning." The conference incident demonstrates that what is considered as credible evidence varies between and within groups. That is to say, the language of evidence that is convincing to one group or individual may not be believable or even interesting to another. Keep these stories in mind as you plan and implement the action strategies of sharing knowledge.

As suggested throughout this book, there are multiple research languages and structures. Likewise, there are multiple ways in which you may choose to present and structure the reporting and dissemination of your research. The reporting language and structure you use must be congruent with the epistemological framework of your study; it must fit the purpose for dissemination and the target audience. In all types of communication, keep in mind the important points made earlier about diversity in meaning, differing perceptions of the criterion for credibility, and universal access. Also, remember that research reporting and disseminating are analogous to telling a story. As Richardson eloquently stated over 20 years ago:

> Whenever we write science, we are telling some kind of story, or some part of a larger narrative. Some of our stories are more complex, more densely described, and offer greater opportunities as emancipatory documents; others are more abstract, more distanced from lived experience, and reinscribe existent hegemonies.[19]

Integrity of Presentation

Any type of query will yield a lot of information that the researcher will need to make sense of and synthesize. The first and primary report in a research agenda typically focuses on and communicates the outcomes of the main research query that the researcher initially posed. Following it, other reports or manuscripts may be developed that focus on subquestions or other related important study outcomes.

In any type of report, the researcher needs to present a tightly woven story, as we have indicated, that includes the statement of research problem, the essential findings, and how those findings fit within the context of a larger body of knowledge and science. In developing the report, researchers must balance the level of detail needed to provide an understanding of the query and its outcomes with page limitations imposed by the journal or venue, and the main points must be made without misrepresenting or compromising the integrity of the study. There will always be more findings from any one study than can be reported, posing a challenge in choosing what to include. Thus, the researcher has to make a decision as to what aspects of the data collected or research findings make sense to share, support the main question/query initially proposed, and do not reflect only the researcher's perspective or preferences. This task may sound straightforward, but actually in many cases it is not. For example, let's say you conducted a study of the experimental type and your findings are mixed— that is, some of the outcomes support your a priori hypotheses and others do not. Or let's say none of your findings support your initial hunches and thus the results of your study are negative. Ethically, you will need to report both. Negative findings can have as much scientific and knowledge-building value as positive outcomes. However, it can be challenging to find a publication outlet, as many journals are reluctant to publish studies that have only negative outcomes.

Thus, researchers, regardless of the tradition they are working in, confront three essential ethical challenges when reporting findings: (1) what to include and what not to include in the report and why; (2) assuring that both positive and negative findings are accurately reported; and (3) making certain that the essential components of the study are well described, balancing reporting requirements of a journal with the details needed to accurately represent the study.

Publishing Your Work

The process of publishing your work is exciting but sometimes frustrating if you are new to the process. The first step in considering publication is to ensure that your work is high quality and meets the rigorous standards for research discussed in previous chapters. However, crafting a sound report does not ensure publication. If you are attempting to publish your first piece of work, we suggest that you consult with someone who is knowledgeable about the process and possibly obtain an editor familiar with the scholarly requirements of the journal you are targeting.

It is critical to select a medium that is compatible with the design, purpose, focus, and level of development of your work. Each publication has a set of guidelines and requirements for authors that are usually available online. Scholarly and professional journals usually publish instructions for authors in selected journal issues and leave them available online throughout the year. These guidelines include the required format for writing, typing, notation style, image clarity, permissions, and submission processes. For refereed journals, after you submit your work, it is sent to several (usually three) reviewers for comment and evaluation. This process takes between 3 and 6 months. Do not be surprised if your work is rejected. Most journals have many more submissions than they can publish, with some having only a 10% acceptance rate. Rejection does not mean your work is poor. The subject matter or methods may not fit the goals of the journal, or it may be the wrong audience for your work. It is not unusual for editors to suggest alternative journals that may accept your work. If your report is accepted, most likely there will be a request for a revision from the reviewers or the editor. Few manuscripts are accepted on their first submission without minor to major revisions. After revisions and final acceptance, the work may initially be published online ahead of a print copy if there is one. Before publication (online or print version), you will receive a set of proofs for your review. These proofs are typeset pages of your work and may contain queries to you from the copy editor to clarify statements or check references or figures. Be vigilant in reviewing them to ensure that no mistakes have occurred in the typesetting process.

Celebrate your work as you see it in publication. You have met the research criterion of "usefulness"!

Sharing Your Research Through Other Methods

Dissemination in journals is not the only method for sharing your work. There are many other outlets, including presentations at professional and scholarly conferences, oral presentations in other forums, continuing and in-service education, collaborative work with colleagues, and many options for online sharing as we have discussed through the book. Communicating your work not only is useful to others, but also helps you receive constructive criticism that will advance your own thinking and conceptual development.

Summary

Disseminating your research is a major and essential part of the research process, and adequate time, consideration, and energy should be devoted to this research step. Sharing your work provides the knowledge you gained from your inquiry to others to inform practice or policy, new directions for research, and new knowledge and theory. Dissemination ultimately promotes the collective advancement of knowledge and well-informed practices in health and human services.

EXERCISES

1. Find a research article reported in a professional research journal. Also, identify a research report published in a practice-oriented newsletter for a professional association and a blog entry reporting a full study. Compare the style of writing and the basic elements of the research process in light of the intended audiences.
2. Identify a published research study using an experimental-type design, a study using a naturalistic design, and one using mixed methods. Compare the style of the work, the basic elements of the report, and particularly the presentation of data.

References

1. Gitlin LN, Lyons KJ: *Successful grant writing: strategies for health and human service professionals*, ed 4, New York, 2013, Springer.

2. Gilson SF, DePoy E: The student body. In Carey AC, Scotch RK, editors: *Disability and community*. In Altman B, Barnartt S, series editors: *Research in social science and disability*, vol 6, Bingley, UK, 2012, Emerald Publishing Group, pp 27–47.

3. ResearchGate, 2014. https://www.researchgate.net/about.

4. Babbie E: *The practice of social research*, ed 13, Belmont, Calif, 2012, Wadsworth.

5. DePoy E, Gilson SF: *Evaluation practice*, New York, 2008, Taylor and Francis.

6. Caroll J: *A handbook for deterring plagiarism in higher education*, Oxford, UK, 2013, Oxford Centre for Staff and Learning Development.

7. Ary H, Jacobs LC, Sorensen CK, et al: *Introduction to research in education*, Belmont, Calif, 2013, Wadsworth.

8. *AERA shaping research policy*, 2013. http://www.aera.net/ResearchPolicyAdvocacy/AERAShapingResearchPolicy/tabid/10297/Default.aspx.

9. Cooper H: *Reporting research in psychology: how to meet journal article reporting standards*, Washington, DC, 2011, American Psychological Association.

10. Husereau D, Drummond M, Petrou S, et al: Consolidated health economic evaluation reporting standards (CHEERS)-Explanation and elaboration: a report of the ISPOR health economic evaluations publication guidelines good reporting practices task force. *Value Health* 16:231–250, 2013.

11. *Consort transparent reporting of trials (website)*. http://www.design.ncsu.edu/cud.

12. Pink S: *Doing sensory ethnography*, Thousand Oaks, Calif, 2009, Sage.

13. Wolcott H: *Writing up qualitative research*, Thousand Oaks, Calif, 2009, Sage.

14. Denzin N, Lincoln Y: *Sage handbook of qualitative research*, Los Angeles, 2011, Sage.

15. Harple TS, Taha G, Vuckovic N, et al: Mobility of more than a device: understanding complexity in health care with ethnography. In *Ethnographic Praxis in Industry conference proceedings*, 2013, pp 129–142.

16. Tashakkori A, Teddlie C: *Sage handbook of mixed methods in social and behavioral research*, ed 2, Thousand Oaks, Calif, 2010, Sage.

17. DePoy E, Gilson SF: *Studying disability: multiple theories and responses*, Thousand Oaks, Calif, 2011, Sage.

18. Center for Universal Design, North Carolina State, 1997. http://www.ncsu.edu/ncsu/design/cud/about_ud/udprinciplestext.htm.

19. Richardson L: *Writing strategies: reaching diverse audiences*, Newbury Park, Calif, 1990, Sage, p 34.

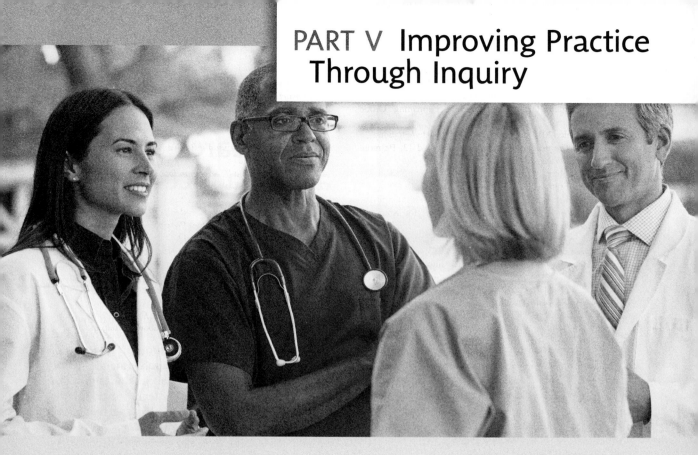

PART V Improving Practice Through Inquiry

We have finally arrived at the part of the book that answers the question, "So now that I am familiar with the thinking and action processes of both research traditions and their integration, how do I use this learning to improve my own practice and contribute to practice knowledge?" We now depart from the conceptual framework that we have used throughout the book to locate experimental-type, naturalistic, and mixed methods of research in the larger context of practice examination, efficacy, and our own practice experience. In Part V, we examine specific professional applications of what you have studied throughout the text.

As you enter Part V, congratulate yourself on your learning, and see what research can be all about in your health and human service practice.

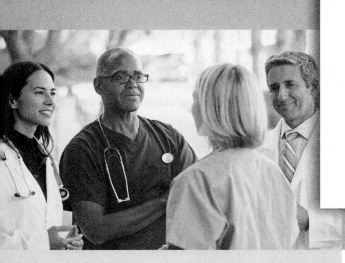

Chapter 24
Reciprocal Role of Research and Practice

You now have some level of comfort with the thinking and action processes involved in the experimental-type, naturalistic, and mixed methods research traditions. These processes serve as your working tools to develop knowledge for a health or human service practice arena. However, for us, research is not complete until it is used, and in turn that use informs the further development of new knowledge. Therefore in this chapter, we turn to the action of "application," or applying research principles to the practice arena and vice versa. In the pages that follow, four approaches that attempt to bridge the research-practice gap are discussed and illustrated: *evidence-based practice*, *translational research*, *practice-based research*, and *evaluation practice*. As you read, keep in mind that collaboration is an important part of each of these. We also see the intersection of research and practice a fertile ground for cooperation and conversely suggest that the critical relationship between research and practice can only be maximized through the collaborative efforts of professionals, clients, patients, and researchers.

Evidence-Based Practice

If you are a practicing health or human service professional, you most likely have heard of evidence-based practice. Most professional organizations highly espouse this practice as the best research and knowledge support to guide treatment and clinical. If you are not involved in a practice arena, you may be asking, "What's all the fuss about?" After all, you probably assume that all health and human service practices are based in or derived from evidence or knowledge that has been systematically obtained, rather than from hearsay, trial and error, or casual decision making. However, your assumption has not exactly been accurate. At issue are the definitions of evidence and what constitutes "adequate evidence" for informing practice decisions. Recall the debate between experimental-type and naturalistic researchers. Those espousing experimental-type approaches charged naturalistic researchers with storytelling while naturalistic investigators claimed that human experience cannot be reduced to numbers.[1,2] So as you have seen throughout this book, even within systematic research, each tradition had argued about the efficacy and value of the other, at least until mixed methods came along. And even mixed methods is not exempt from criticism, as researchers do not agree that methods from disparate philosophical foundations should find a comfortable home in a purposive framework.

Evidence-based practice is not a research method or design. Rather, it is a model of professional practice that draws heavily on and is driven by research that uses particular methodologies to assert conclusions from research literature. Major aspects of evidence-based practice propose which research methods and conclusions should underpin practice, how to organize a clinical setting to engage in this form of practice, how to teach this approach, and the barriers to its implementation.[2] However, our focus here is how evidence is defined in this approach and how evidence-based practice uses research principles to justify evidentiary-based conclusions to inform practice. We begin our discussion with a brief history, then define and provide critical comments on this contemporary practice approach.

Definitions and Models

Since early in the 20th century, policy makers, scholars, and practitioners have been debating the nature and role of research in professional practice.[3] Numerous terms have been used in these discussions to describe professional activity that in some way uses or generates knowledge based on the principles of scientific inquiry. In part, the disagreements about what constitutes science (and by extension, scientific inquiry) and how or even if science should form the foundation of professional practice have contributed to the conflict about scientifically driven practice.[3,4] Remember that research has the following properties:

1. It is theory based or theory generating.
2. It is developed according to the rigor criteria of systematic use of inductive, abductive, and deductive logic structures in all phases of thinking and action processes.
3. It involves detailing the explicit evidence and reasoning on which knowledge claims are based.

Keep these definitional elements in mind as you learn more about evidence-based practice, because they form both its strengths and its limitations. Many terms are used to discuss models of inquiry in professional practice. In general, all models posit the value of systematically derived knowledge to support professional decision making and to examine the extent to which desired outcomes have been achieved.

Public health and education were the first professional fields to emphasize the importance of systematic evaluation for practice accountability.[5] In the early 1950s, proliferation of federally supported programs resulted in the expansion of evaluation into a field of its own, with its focus on fiscal accountability.[6] Concurrently, debates emerged between those who espoused "empiricism" and those who opposed it in a "value-based" practice context.[7] As evaluation was espoused by health and human service fields, debate increased about how best and even if to conduct empirical inquiry to support practice. Discussion shifted away from polar arguments to a more expansive and complex analysis of the nature of evidence, when evidence is appropriate, and methods to generate it.[7]

The following definitions of evidence-based practice have been used in medicine,[8,9] nursing,[10] and rehabilitation[11]:

• Sackett's classic definition—The most common definition of evidence-based practice (EBP) is from Dr. David Sackett. EBP is "the conscientious, explicit and judicious use of current best evidence in making decisions about the care of the individual patient. It means integrating individual clinical expertise with the best available external clinical evidence from systematic research."[8]
• The best integration of our research evidence with clinical expertise and patients' unique values and circumstances. By best research we mean

clinically relevant research, sometimes from the basic sciences of medicine but especially from patient-centered clinical research into the accuracy and precision of diagnostic tests, the power of prognostic markers, and the efficacy and safety of therapeutic, rehabilitative, and preventive strategies.[9]

- EBP unifies research evidence with clinical expertise and encourages individualization of care through inclusion of patient preferences. The elements in the definition emphasize knowledge produced through rigorous and systematic inquiry, the experience of the clinician, and the values of the patient.[10]
- A process that begins with clinical, questions, appraisals of the evidence, application of the evidence considering the client's wishes and needs, and finishes with an evaluation of the outcomes.[11]

As you can see, each definition emphasizes the use of research evidence in the context of clinical expertise, although they all differ slightly. Two primary models have been reflected in these definitions. In one model, intervention is selected from an array of efficacious, empirically supported practices. In the second model, practitioner and client collaboratively consider best evidence to make decisions together.

In the 21st century, increasing debates about the nature of knowledge itself raise many questions about the meaning of evidence. Thus, current models of evidence-based practice are based on a broadened understanding of evidence as ranging along a continuum from anecdotal experience of providers and consumers, organizational guidelines, consensus groups or single-study review to highly structured systematic review of the literature (meta-analysis). Most prominent however is the traditional approach that remains grounded in the assumption of a "hierarchy of evidence" in which judgment about the value of knowledge is based on the methods of inquiry. The randomized controlled trial (RCT) is still considered the highest level of evidence to support intervention efficacy, and other forms of knowledge are less valued. Thus, the true-experimental design to support claims about the

efficacy of interventions remains as the methodological pinnacle of desirability, whereas other design approaches (e.g., quasi-experimental, naturalistic inquiry) tend to receive less acclaim, or they are not systematically considered in the evaluation of evidence.[2]

In general, all evidence-based practice models can be defined by their use of "best evidence" to guide practice decisions, thereby creating standard, valid interventions to the extent possible for specific conditions, diagnoses, and problem areas that are well researched.

Approaches to Identifying Evidence

As stated earlier, evidence-based practice is not a methodology, but it does label and thus use preferred methodologies for systematically reviewing evidence and linking the evidence to actual practice decisions. There are four methodological steps in applying evidence to clinical practice in this framework: reviewing the literature, rating the evidence, developing clinical guidelines, and applying or translating guidelines to a clinical case.

The key action process in this form of practice is systematically reviewing published research literature, including clinical practice guidelines, meta-analysis (both qualitative and experimental type), and Web-based searches for relevant systematically generated information. That is, key to the success of basing a clinical decision on the evidence is how investigators review the literature (see Chapter 6), including how they bound the topic or query through the selection of key terms and how they tailor the search. As in a search for any research inquiry, it is critical to know the limitations of the databases that are searched and how these boundaries shape the evidence obtained. Given the complexity and time-consuming nature of conducting a comprehensive and adequate literature review, we find that meta-search engines specifically designed for finding evidence-based practice sources are most useful. For example, PubMed provides access to Medline databases (www.ncbi.nlm.nih.gov/PubMed), Sum-Search2 (http://sumsearch.org) searches databases that contain sources for evidence-based guidelines, and TRIP "is a clinical search engine designed to allow users to quickly and easily find and use

---

BOX 24-1 *Examples of Rating Systems in Evidence-Based Practice*

"ABCD" System

A = Evidence from well-defined meta-analysis

B = Evidence from well-designed controlled trials (randomized and nonrandomized) with results that consistently support a specific action

C = Evidence from observational studies (correlational, descriptive) or controlled trials with inconsistent results

D = Evidence from expert opinion or multiple case reports

"1-2-3" System

1 = Generally consistent findings in a majority of studies

2 = Based on either a single acceptable study or a weak or inconsistent finding in multiple acceptable studies

3 = Limited scientific evidence that does not meet all criteria of acceptable studies

"I-II-III-IV" System

I = Evidence from at least one properly randomized controlled trial

II-A = Evidence from well-designed controlled trials without randomization

II-B = Evidence from well-designed cohort or case-control analytical studies

III = Evidence obtained from comparisons between times or places with or without the intervention

IV = Opinions of respected authorities based on clinical experience, descriptive studies, or reports of expert committees

---

BOX 24-2 *Sample of Clinical Guidelines Based on Rating the Evidence*

- Best to individualize music selection in accordance with patient preferences (evidence grade = B)
- Best to intervene 30 minutes before a person's peak level of agitation (evidence grade = B)
- Music intervention session should last approximately 30 minutes (evidence grade = B)
- Use of headphones may be confusing (evidence grade = D)

Modified from National Guideline Clearinghouse (www.guideline.gov), 2002.

BOX 24-3 *Applying Evidence to Practice*

- What were the results?
- How large are treatment effects?
- Are results valid?
- Will results help me in caring for my cases/clients/community?
- Can results be applied?
- Were all outcomes of clinical significance considered?
- Are treatment benefits worth the potential harms and costs?
- Are there specific characteristics of the group/persons with whom I am working that differ from the study populations so as to affect treatment outcome?
- Are the contextual differences that may change the outcomes of a treatment or intervention (e.g., geography, nationality, physical or virtual world)?

---

high-quality research evidence to support their practice and/or care" (http://www.tripdatabase.com). We have found Google Scholar (www.scholar.google.com) to be efficient in locating sources as well. And of course, university and medical center libraries have access to databases that are not publicly accessible.

After relevant research articles have been identified and retrieved, the next methodological step involves applying a systematic rating to each type of research study and form of evidence retrieved (Box 24-1). Then, on the basis of the ratings that

are derived, a series of clinical guidelines can be articulated (Box 24-2). The final step involves translating the evidence and guidelines to a particular application. In this step, the researcher must ask numerous critical questions (Box 24-3). It is particularly important to determine whether differences exist between study populations and the particular population or case to which the knowledge will be applied and whether these may diminish the treatment response or change the risk-to-benefit ratio. This translational step draws on clinical knowledge and judgment.

Limitations of Evidence-Based Practice

From our discussion thus far and what you have learned in this book, what do you see as some of the important limitations of an evidence-based practice approach?

First, as an empirically based approach borrowed principally from medicine, its application to health and human service practices can be problematic for several reasons. Health and human service professionals engage in practice to address a wide range of human problems for which knowledge through systematic inquiry is necessary. However, the knowledge required to understand human problems is not necessarily amenable to true experimentation in the form of RCTs. Other forms of knowledge may be of equal importance in understanding, for example, dynamic processes between therapist and client and how best to involve a clinical population in a disease prevention activity. Health and human service practice extends far beyond the focus on medical intervention or single treatments and the "magic bullet" medicine approach amenable to randomized design strategies.

A second significant limitation of this model of practice is that it is based on the assumption that the RCT is the primary valid design to generate knowledge that is useful in clinical practice. Although changing somewhat, measurement remains the cornerstone of evidence-based practice with true experimentation held as the gold standard.[2] This approach diminishes other forms of knowledge, particularly many of the approaches we have discussed that are feasible and practical within the daily practice context, and scholarship derived from the naturalistic tradition, participatory inquiry, or other experimental-type design strategies that can contribute different types of knowing.

A related but critical point is that evidence-based practice involves the application of nomothetically derived knowledge to idiographic concerns.[1] In this case, the issue for the evidence-based practitioner becomes how best to translate group data to the individual case. Given the growing emphasis on diversity and multicultural competence, knowledge of central tendencies through nomothetically generated research does not necessarily capture a full range of varied and unique experiences and needs and may not be appropriate to inform individual circumstance. The assertion that true-experimental design rigor and structure determine knowledge quality may be extremely limiting to the critical assessment of knowledge for use in professional practice and leads to mechanistic thinking and action. Consider this simple example. Stephen, who has a fused left hip, injured his rotator cuff. To improve his range of motion, the physical therapist, using well-supported evidence-based practice, sent him home with a large exercise ball and a regimen of prone exercises. Unfortunately, the physical therapist neglected to assess how this evidence-based strategy could be used by an individual who was not able to move his hip. Stephen, in attempting to be compliant, harmed himself when he fell off the ball.

The nature of evidence continues as an important area of debate. Because practice theories in so many health and human service professions stress use of self and the relationship between client and practitioner, students and practitioners often identify the incompatibility of logical, systematic thinking with the relational foundations of practice. Recent acceptance of faith and spirituality in professional theory and practice and the recognition that diversity is a critical consideration in any clinical relationship[12] are even more incongruent with positivist approaches to understanding human experience and human need as currently used in evidence-based practice. Thus, although we believe that different forms of evidence are credible for different professional and other stakeholder interest groups, evidence-based practice approaches discount this view and are often antithetical to the professional commitment to respect for diversity as it applies to acceptable evidence for practice process and outcome.

Although recent adaptations to the original model of evidence-based practice have added professional judgment and client values as important considerations, it is curious that the values of the professional have not been considered. Look at what Byer says about the thinking and action processes of research itself:

The story that science tells about itself is an activity pursued by human beings, [that] is objective and empirical; that it concerns itself with the facts and nothing but the facts. . . . And yet science is a human activity. This is an obvious statement but it bears repeating since part of the mythology of science is precisely that it is independent of human beings; independent of mind and intelligence. . . . How do human beings create a system of thought that produces results that are independent of human thought?[13] (p 7)

While we agree with the major limitations of current models of evidence-based practice for supporting professional practice, we do not want to "throw out the baby with the bath water." As we have said throughout this book, we encourage you to be critical thinkers and fully evaluate for which professional challenges and questions evidence-based practice is important and whether and how it may be useful in your daily professional life. This point brings us to another related issue for which evidence-based practice is extremely useful: treatment fidelity.

Treatment Fidelity

As we discussed previously, clinical trial methodology uses true-experimental design to conduct the systematic evaluation of an intervention, and to a large extent this forms the basis for evidence-based practices. Thus, if you are engaging in the establishment of evidence-based practice or using methods that have been supported by these approaches, a critical aspect of such trials is the assurance that the intervention is delivered to study participants assigned to the experimental group as it is intended and as specified by a written protocol. Attention to the integrity of implementing the intervention is referred to as *treatment fidelity.*[14,15] Actions that an investigator can take to enhance treatment fidelity include (1) creating a detailed manual of the intervention so that it can be delivered consistently, is reproducible, and is independent of interventionist style; (2) providing careful training in the intervention; (3) providing constant oversight of its delivery through direct observation of treatment sessions or review of audio or video recordings of its delivery; and (4) tracking adherence and reasons for nonparticipation.

One way to understand treatment fidelity is by a model used in psychotherapeutic intervention studies.[14,15] This model posits three components (domains) of treatment fidelity that need to be enhanced and monitored: delivery, receipt, and enactment (Table 24-1). Basically, for an intervention to be effective in meeting its intended outcomes, it must be delivered consistently, it must be received and be acceptable to participants, and finally, intervention strategies must be enacted or used. This model provides a helpful tool for thinking about the procedures that need to be considered and put into place to ensure the integrity of an intervention, particularly one that is considered evidence-based.

TABLE 24-1   *Three Domains of Treatment Fidelity*

Domain	Enhancement Strategy	Monitoring and Data Collection Strategy
Delivery	Systematic training of interventionists	Frequency of contact and intensity
	Manual of procedures	
Receipt	Use of different implementation strategies (e.g., video, hands-on instruction, role-playing)	Participant's acknowledgment of participation and receipt of intervention materials
	Evidence of receipt (e.g., knowledge test, improved understanding)	
Enactment	Identification of how and when to implement strategies	Evidence of integration, use of knowledge, skills or intervention strategies
Recording forms	Participant's feedback as to use	
	Enhanced proximal outcomes	

Practice-Based Research

Different from evidence-based practice, which applies specific types of research to guide practice, practice-based research starts with practice as its focus of inquiry. Its purpose is to use existing or "present" data (clinical notes, observations, organizational and institutional policy statements, and so on) to create knowledge that generates a complex understanding of practice from which new and creative strategies can emerge. Consider what Candy said:

> Practice-based research is an original investigation undertaken in order to gain new knowledge partly by means of practice and the outcomes of that practice. Claims of originality and contribution to knowledge may be demonstrated through creative outcomes which may include artefacts such as images, music, designs, models, digital media or other outcomes such as performances and exhibitions. Whilst the significance and context of the claims are described in words, a full understanding can only be obtained with direct reference to those outcomes.[15]

Unlike the linear sequence of evidence-based practice in which literature is selected and then applied to practice, practice-based research is embedded within the actual action processes of daily professional activity and observations of outcomes. In the United States, the Agency for Healthcare Research and Quality (AHRQ) has espoused a model of practice-based research as a network of collaboration in which professionals, clients, and other key persons engage in research to investigate, characterize, and improve the nature of practice.[15] Consider this example.

Suppose you were interested in examining the relationship between perceptions of clinical efficacy and clinical outcomes in a population of individuals with recent mild cardiovascular accidents (CVAs) who are receiving outpatient services. You decide that this inquiry is complex and that the perceptions of multiple groups interact to influence outcome. Through practice-based inquiry, a team is assembled to record and organize existing data such as verbal interchanges between clinicians and clients, client records, evaluations completed by clients of their

experience, and minutes of staff meetings. Analysis of these already "present" data sources provides a rich forum for the inquiry and for subsequent evidence-based change that emerges from analysis of daily practice.

Translation Research

The term *translation research* refers to the application of traditional "basic research findings" to clinical practice. Two primary levels have been discussed in the literature, applying laboratory research to intervention with specific individuals and then expanding the application to intervention practices in general.[14] Thus, this model is a collaboration among academic researchers and professionals who put the results of studies into practice in clinical, health care, and community settings to:

> 1) captivate, advance, and nurture a cadre of well-trained multi- and inter-disciplinary investigators and research teams; 2) create an incubator for innovative research tools and information technologies; and 3) synergize multi-disciplinary and inter-disciplinary clinical and translational research and researchers to catalyze the application of new knowledge and techniques to clinical practice at the front lines of patient care.[16]

Consider the following example. The field of advanced robotics is often conducted and contained within academic and laboratory settings. To resolve mobility barriers commonly encountered by wheelchairs, a clinician turns to a robotics laboratory in an academic setting. A specialized wheelchair that uses sensors and automated robotic navigation is fabricated. The outcomes are significant, improving community life and employment opportunities for this client. Capitalizing on this success, a team of clinicians and robotics researchers frame a development project in which they are now creating simple, commercially available robotic solutions to eliminate a variety of navigational barriers in urban communities.

Evaluation and Examined Practice

Consistent with practice-based and translational research models that bridge the research-practice gap, evaluation is moving in that direction as well. The evaluation practice model infuses everyday practice with an evaluative and systematic knowledge-generating framework. In their model of evaluation practice, DePoy and Gilson[6] defined "evaluation" as the conduct of three major thinking and action processes: problem and need clarification, *reflexive intervention*, and *outcome assessment*. All rely on the systematic thinking and action processes. Examined practice that builds on the steps of the evaluation practice model has been further elaborated as "anchoring its conceptual and praxis components on current thinking in which knowing and doing co-exist in a network of globalism, technology and post-postmodern marriage of previous disciplinary strangers." Examined practice proposes knowledge derived in the practice area as a "credible, reciprocal avenue for research evidence."[17] Although the nature of acceptable evidence is expanded in examined practice, both models contain the same essential elements. We turn to those now.

Problem and Need Clarification

Because of the complexity of defining and understanding health and social problems, methods to address and alleviate them are often unclear. As we frequently see in professional practice, why a particular approach to intervention is necessary and to what problem it responds are often omitted from the thinking and action processes of many health and human service efforts. Without a clear understanding of what problem is being addressed, and without evidence supporting the method needed to address it, we cannot fully demonstrate the value of our practices.

Clarification of the problem is critical to any professional effort because how a problem is conceptualized, who owns it, who is affected by it, and what needs to be done about it are all questions based in political-purposive and ideological arenas. Thus, the problem forms the basis from which all subsequent systematic evaluative activity takes place, and it provides the ultimate foundation for the implementation and continuation of interventions. In all arenas of practice, a clear and well-supported understanding of "problem" and "need" is essential. Without problem and need clarification, interest groups may define

problems differently and thus expect different outcomes from the same intervention.

In the models of evaluation and examined practice, a clear understanding of need must be based on credible evidence. Although we may make claims as to what type of intervention is needed to resolve problems, accountability in making informed professional decisions depends on the presence and organization of empirical evidence of need. Setting goals and objectives for intervention is derived directly from need.

Reflexive Intervention

As discussed in previous chapters, reflexivity is an important construct, defined as self-examination for the purpose of ascertaining how the researcher's perspective influences the interpretation of data. In both evaluation and examined practice, the term is expanded to denote the set of thinking and action processes that we believe should take place throughout interventions. The term "reflexive intervention" reminds us that the intervention action processes, resources, and influences are essential parts of evaluation practice and are thus subject to the same systematic scrutiny as needs assessment. Moreover, systematically examining what we do in our daily professional activity provides important data (evidence) to contribute to the knowledge base of health and human services. Thus, the objective of reflexive thinking processes in evaluation and examined practice is not limited to an individual; rather, it is applied to the sum total of the intervention and scope of influences on the process and outcome of intervention.

Reflexive intervention involves three important foci: monitoring process, resource analysis, and consideration of indirect influences on the intervention.

Monitoring (Process Assessment)

Monitoring, or *process assessment*, is the element of evaluation that examines whether and how the intervention is proceeding. Monitoring is an essential evaluation and examined practice action in which the actual implementation of an intervention is systematically studied and characterized. Monitoring processes not only examine the scope of the intervention but also scrutinize it to determine whom it affects, to assess the degree to which goals and process objectives are efficaciously reflected in the intervention, to provide feedback for revision based on empirical evidence, and to add to the evidence repository that can be subjected to clinical research.

> Here is an example. To monitor systematically funding, transportation, and elder involvement in activity, you set up a tracking system. You can determine what was done, who participated, and the frequency of participation. Without this information, you would not know what was done and could not attribute any changes in outcome to your program. •

Resource Analysis

Similar to monitoring, resource analysis occurs throughout the intervention and requires reflection. When we think of resource analysis, cost in dollars for services rendered is the resource most often examined. In evaluation and examined practice, however, resource analysis includes the full host of human and nonhuman resources used to conduct an intervention and that are related to its need and outcome.

Consideration of Influences on the Intervention

Part of the process of reflexive intervention must be a consideration of factors external to the intervention that affect both process and outcome. Without widening the scope of examination, it can be difficult to determine why change is occurring (or why it is not occurring) in the desired direction. What if you neglected to look at community influences and a local church had implemented a community program for elders serving your same population? You can see how this unplanned influence might change your expectations and attribution of outcomes.

Outcome Assessment

Outcome assessment is the action process of evaluation and examined practice that is most familiar. It answers the question, "To what extent did the desired outcomes occur?" Outcome assessment also examines the parts of an intervention and the intervention

context that relate to outcome, as well as differential outcomes resulting from other influences (e.g., intervention processes, target populations, complexity of outcome expectations). Although its aim seems obvious—to judge the value of an intervention in its achievement of goals and objectives—outcome assessment serves many other important purposes. Outcome assessment provides empirical information on which to make programmatic, policy, and resource decisions that influence and shape social and human services at multiple levels.[18]

Evaluation and examined practice models provide a systematic framework by which to develop a knowledge base of professional practice. Documenting your systematic thinking and action processes throughout every practice sequence provides credible evidence from which to support practice claims and improve practice. Thus, evaluation practice provides a systematic and "doable" link between practice and research.

Summary

In this chapter, we have discussed four models of inquiry that inform or are informed by practice. The current model of interjecting evidence into practice is the evidence-based model generated primarily from medicine. Espousal of this model outside of medical fields has led to difficulties in application, primarily because of its underlying assumptions of a hierarchy of knowledge, dismissal of all forms of research-generated knowledge except that derived from true-experimental designs, and attempt to enforce nomothetically generated knowledge on ideographic contexts. Collaborative models include practice-based research, translational research, evaluation practice, and examined practice. Each relies on collaboration and aims to improve individual outcomes and overall health and human service practice.

EXERCISES

1. Find an evidence-based literature review on a topic of interest to you and examine its use in informing your practice. Would you seek additional information to make sound practice

decisions? Why or why not? What information might you acquire beyond the research evidence presented in the literature review?

2. Identify a practice issue or problem and develop a plan for practice-based research. Then develop an evaluation or examined practice design that includes all elements of this new model.

3. Look for two articles that discuss collaborative research. Identify the roles and responsibilities of each participant and critically examine how the collaboration contributes to the knowledge that was generated by the study.

References

1. Cohen B: Design-based practice: a new perspective for social work. *Soc Work* 56:337–346, 2011.
2. Rubin A, Bellamy J: *Practitioner's guide to using evidence-based practice*, ed 2, Hoboken, NJ, 2012, Wiley.
3. McCarthy J: *Some problems of philosophy, empirically considered*, Oxford, UK, 2013, Oxford University Press.
4. Letherby G, Scott J, Williams M: *Objectivity and subjectivity in social research*, Los Angeles, 2013, Sage.
5. Brownson RC, Baker EA, Leet TL, et al: *Evidence-based public health*, ed 2, Oxford, UK, 2011, Oxford University Press.
6. DePoy E, Gilson SF: *Evaluation practice*, New York, 2008, Routledge.
7. Kincaid H, Dupré J, Wylie A: *Value-free science? Ideals and illusion*, Oxford, UK, 2007, Oxford University Press.
8. Sackett D: Evidence-based medicine—what it is and what it isn't. *BMJ* 312:71–72, 1996.
9. Strauss S, Glasziou P, Richardson S, et al: *Evidence-based medicine: how to practice and teach EBM*, ed 4, St Louis, 2011, Elsevier, p 1.
10. Stevens K: The impact of evidence-based practice in nursing and the next big ideas. *Online J Issues Nurs* 18:4, 2013.
11. Law M, MacDermid J: *Evidence-based rehabilitation: a guide to practice*, ed 3, Thorofare, NJ, 2013, Slack.
12. Seaward BL: *Health of the human spirit: spiritual dimensions for personal health*, Burlington, Mass, 2013, Jones & Bartlett.
13. Byers W: *The blind spot*, Princeton, NJ, 2011, Princeton University Press.
14. Hulley S, Cummings SR, Browner WS, et al: *Designing clinical research*, ed 4, Philadelphia, 2013, Lippincott, Williams & Wilkins.
15. Candy L: *Practice-based research (University of Technology, Sydney CCS Report: 2006-V1.0 November 20AHRO-AHRQ), Support for Primary Care Practice-Based Research Networks.* http://www.creativityandcognition.com/content/view/184/103.
16. National Institutes of Health: The NIH Common Fund. *Transl Res* September 2009. http://nihroadmap.nih.gov/clinicalresearch/overview-translational.asp.
17. DePoy E, Gilson S: *Examined practice*, Los Angeles, 2015, Sage.
18. Grinell R, Unrau Y: *Social work research and evaluation: foundations of evidence-based practice*, Oxford, UK, 2014, Oxford University Press.

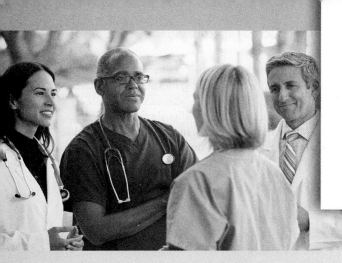

Chapter 25
Stories From the Field

Here we are at the end of our book but certainly not, we hope, at the end of your involvement in research. The beauty of research is that you learn from doing, and it is a never-ending process. At each step of the process, new, more refined, and complex queries and questions will emerge and whet your appetite.

We have introduced you to what some may believe are "heavy" philosophical topics, technical language, and logical ways of thinking and acting. These are your tools to creatively explore the challenges and questions that arise in your practices,

daily life, professional experience, or study, and in your reading of the literature. As you apply these thinking and action tools to health and human service–related issues, you will discover both the artistry and the science involved in research and its application to your professional practice.

Research, like any other human activity, has its low and high points, its tedium and thrill, its frustrations and challenges, its drastic mistakes, and its clever applications of research principles. Research is foremost a thinking process. If you think about what you are doing and reflect on what you have done, you can learn from mistakes, and you can keep refining your skill as an investigator.

In the first part of this last chapter, we give an overview of a soup-to-nuts mixed method study with you to "put it all together." Each of the 10 essentials is showcased, and integration of methods is illustrated. Then in the last part, we share some classic and some new stories from our own research to highlight the twists and turns of research and how this human activity occurs.

Soup to Nuts

We have referred throughout the book to our research on assistive technology and mobility device use. We now illustrate mixed methods research in health and human service practice with an overview of part of this research agenda. The impetus for the project we discuss next emerged from personal experience, in which a colleague who had sustained cerebellar damage wanted to participate in fitness activity but did not because of equipment barriers.

When a walker was prescribed, our colleague learned how to use it in the rehabilitation setting, but abandoned it on discharge like many others who need such devices for safe navigation. The reasons for refusal were limited functionality of the equipment for sports that she wanted to do (hiking and jogging with friends) and the stigmatizing appearance of the walker. We therefore became aware that abandonment of devices was complex in its causes and outcomes and embarked on a substantive needs assessment to meet several purposes. First, we wanted to uncover unanticipated influences on equipment use and nonuse. Second, we sought to quantify the magnitude of theorized causes that might be uncovered. Third, we anticipated writing a grant proposal to support the development of a device that would not meet with abandonment.

These purposes pointed to a mixed method inquiry in that our aims were both to develop new theory and then test it so that we would have sufficient data to rationalize a larger project. We proceeded to conduct an initial comprehensive literature review to ascertain the scope of research on the reasons that people abandon needed mobility devices. The literature documented the increasing risk of falling as one ages, particularly in the presence of mobility instability or other impairment. Thus age and previously existing mobility impairment were clearly factors that led to need and prescription. The literature on abandonment suggested that limited functionality and inconvenience were the primary causal factors in nonuse. However, further review of research on the magnitude of abandonment revealed that the theorized causes of abandonment[1] were incomplete, given the steady rate of nonuse even in the presence of efforts to convince device users that they needed walking supports to be safe. Synthesized with knowing derived from object reading studies of assistive devices,[2,3] the role of appearance and perceived stigma in abandonment of mobility equipment emerged as an important area to investigate.

Based on the literature review, a mixed method design was selected to answer the following questions:

1. What are the articulated reasons for nonuse of mobility equipment among mobility device users?
2. What is the relationship between gender of user and abandonment of mobility device? (This question was rationalized by literature that pointed to different perspectives on fashion and appearance related to gender.)

The population for the study was made up of:

1. Adults 21 years of age or older with long-term or permanent mobility impairment
2. Adults who were prescribed a walker within the past 6 months
3. Adults who were known to have abandoned the walker outside of the rehabilitation setting

A sample of convenience representing all genders and the full range of age from early adulthood through old age was identified by rehabilitation providers who were asked to recruit known "abandoners" from individuals who were receiving outpatient rehabilitation services in the local hospital.

To answer question 1, 25 individuals who consented participated in face-to face semistructured interviews. Responses were thematically analyzed and then content analyzed so that they could be coded for frequency. The most frequent reason given by respondents for abandoning devices was stigmatizing appearance. To answer question 2, we computed a chi-square that revealed no significant differences related to gender.

We then decided to conduct a follow-up study to further understand the meaning of stigma related to device appearance. The query that provided the initial entrance in to the study context was articulated as "What is the meaning of mobility device appearance to adults who been prescribed such devices?"

From the group of respondents, we recruited 10 informants. Using an open-ended, face-to-face interview strategy, informants were asked to reflect on how the use of mobility device made them feel, what it meant to them to be using a walker, and how the use of this device affected their lives. Several of the informants noted that using a walker made them feel old, one informant indicated that she did not like the way she looked when she saw her gait with the walker in the mirror, and several others said that they were embarrassed to be using this device.

Thematic analysis revealed the following categories induced from interview data about the causes for abandonment:

Lack of perceived need
Inconvenience
Inability to use
Appearance as barrier
Perception of dependency
People stare
Pitied

The device function was secondary to a majority of the informants. Thus, the material symbol, the walker, had diverse meanings to those interviewed. This knowledge guided us to write a grant proposal to conduct a large-scale needs assessment that focused on both form and function of mobility supports.

This brief overview illustrates the power of mixed method design in answering research questions using multiple methodological approaches, each complementing the other. Naturalistic thinking and action led to discovery. Experimental-type boundary setting and analysis produced an understanding of magnitude in a targeted population and provided the opportunity to test group difference.

We now move to the last part of the book, in which we share with you some of our own experiences in conducting research. We keep adding to the list because each time we engage in a project, we are met with surprises and new lessons.

Just Beginning

It was an urban anthropology class, and we were split into groups to conduct urban ethnographies on health practices by different ethnic groups in the city. The big assignment? The Chinese community. The research group? A hippie-type woman, a rock musician, and a topless go-go dancer who dressed the part day and night. The threesome entered the Chinese community, a relatively self-contained 5- by 10-block area of the inner city. As you can imagine, we were quite a sight. How would we ever be able to "enter" the world of this community and engage in passive observation and active participation in community activities? We started out by walking around and

scoping out the area. We made observations of the physical environment and spent some great times eating lunch and dinner in various restaurants.

We became Chinese restaurant experts for friends and family, but we had no breakthroughs. No Chinese family agreed to meet with us or to be interviewed. Young people were curious and asked lots of questions about us, but their parents remained removed, detached, and unavailable. We caused quite a stir in the community. We split up a couple of times to see whether one of us could gain access, but we had no luck.

Then one day we happened to pass a small building with an announcement for a Chinese Political Youth Club. The sign was posted in Chinese and English (a sign of a new acculturated generation?), and we walked directly to the address of the club. We were welcomed and engaged in long discussions of the political climate and the dilemmas confronting the community. Bingo! This was a beginning. Although our access to the community remained through the ears, eyes, and thoughts of this radical subgroup, we were able to delineate health practices and health issues as perceived by this group. This was a lesson in nonreactive research, gaining access, and the impact of key informants on the type of information and understandings that are obtained.

What Did You Expect?

One of our students was assigned to an anti-graffiti program for urban adolescents who had been convicted of defacing public property. This program was new, and so this student decided to conduct research with the adolescents to find out why they engaged in graffiti and to ask what strategies they would find helpful in reducing this behavior. So the student gave each adolescent several sheets of paper with open-ended questions. You guessed it. When she went back to her office and opened the file of paper, the teens responded with graffiti. What did she expect from giving the tools of the trade to offenders?

In Search of Significance!

Five years of intensive interviewing, data entry, data cleaning, and sophisticated statistical analyses, but where is the significance? Accepting no significance when you want to find statistically significant differences between an experimental and a control group can be difficult. Nonsignificance can be as important a finding as obtaining significant differences, but it can also present a challenge to getting the findings published.

Is Health Care Effective?

In our research class, students are required to develop a research question or query and a proposal that describes how they intend to answer the problem. Our most frustrating but popular "research question" is the one posed by many beginning students in research, "Is nursing effective?" or "Is occupational therapy effective?"

Is this question researchable? Can you explain what is wrong with the way this question is posed?

Does This Work for You?

Similar to the example just given, our social work students wanted to examine the outcome of a fund-raising effort to purchase service dogs for children in need. To examine the most efficacious strategies, they developed a questionnaire in which they asked other students what types of fund-raising strategies worked? Worked to do what? Once again, we ask if this question is researchable? Can you explain what is wrong with the way this question is posed?

A "Good" Research Subject

We established what we believed were clear, objective criteria by which to identify eligible subjects from a pool of older adults who were in rehabilitation for a stroke, a lower limb amputation, or an orthopedic deficit. The purpose of the study was to identify the initial perceptions and attitudes of older patients toward the assistive devices they received in the hospital and whether these issued devices were used at home after hospitalization.

As the recruitment process began, periodic meetings were held with therapists who were responsible for identifying potential study subjects. At one

of these initial meetings, we asked how recruitment was proceeding and if everyone understood the study criteria. Therapists relayed that all was going well, and that they were very pleased they had been able to identify the first few subjects who would "do very well" in this study. The therapists were asked what they meant by "doing well." We learned that therapists had referred patients to the study who they believed greatly valued their assistive devices and would use them at home. Therapists were systematically referring only the "good" patients and were ignoring the potential study eligibility of those patients whom they did not like or who they suspected would be noncompliant to device use.

This represented a fatal flaw in the recruitment process that would have contaminated the entire data collection effort and study results. We immediately changed the recruitment process and examined the hospital census records to determine who may have been available for study participation but systematically excluded by the therapists at this initial study phase.

A "Bad" Research Subject

In a study of family caregiving, an eligible subject enrolled in the study and was randomly assigned to receive an experimental intervention. The intervention involved in-home occupational therapy visits designed to help the caregiver modify the home environment to support caregiving efforts. This particular subject had unusual religious beliefs and social practices that upset the member of the research team providing the experimental intervention. Initially, the interventionist was unable to handle these value differences and suggested to the investigators that the subject was inappropriate for the study and should be considered ineligible. In actuality, there were no objective criteria for excluding this caregiver from the study. The caregiver fit all eligibility criteria. In addition, the individual had agreed to participate in the study and had signed an informed consent form.

It is for this very reason that criteria for subject selection are developed. Furthermore, oversight of their implementation and protection of the protocol must be maintained by the investigator. Subjective reasons for excluding individuals from study participation are a serious source of bias. In this case, the investigators worked with the interventionist to alleviate her anxiety and to proceed with the implementation of the intervention according to protocol.

Literacy Is Not Literacy

Recently, we developed a Web portal that translated higher literacy into lower literacy on tobacco-prevention websites. In testing comprehension, we went to an adult literacy center and recruited subjects who were reading at an equivalent literacy level of fourth-grade English. Given their similar literacy level, we hypothesized that they would show consistent comprehension. Their responses were highly dispersed, leading us to query what had gone wrong with the translation. We neglected to look at the numerous variables that influenced not only reading level but comprehension and found that the greatest difference in comprehension existed between immigrants and nonimmigrants. Immigrants who were well educated in another language were able not only to read the words but to comprehend complex written ideas despite the reading level in which they were presented. Dissimilarly, citizens of the United States who did not score well were not educated in written text. Thus, although they could easily comprehend oral information, they struggled with meanings of text even if they could read the words and sentences.

Native American?

Because we were interested in the ethnic background of our sample of elder women, we added an item on our survey seeking that information. We were surprised when we found that 98% of the respondents had checked "Native American." Living in Maine, and knowing that almost all persons in our sample were white, we were perplexed. So we asked our respondents why they checked Native American. One woman replied, "Well, what else would I check? I was born here, lived here all my life, and expect that I will die in America."

The Pearson, or the Moral of the Coding Story

A student was almost finished with her dissertation when a crisis occurred. She had measured two constructs: years that faculty members were teaching and their attitudes toward their jobs. She coded years in actual numbers of years teaching from 0 and then ascending. She coded attitudes, measured with interval level data from 1 to 5, with 1 denoting most positive and 5 denoting least positive. When she conducted her analysis, she calculated a Pearson r value of -0.7 and interpreted it as a strong association between years teaching and positive attitudes. She finished her conclusion section on the basis of this finding. Because the Pearson value was negative, however, the student's faculty advisor told her that she would have to rewrite the findings section. So she missed her desired graduation date. But who was correct? The student was correct. What are the morals of the story?

Code clearly. If you choose to code as this student did, be clear in your discussion of findings. And if you are a faculty advisor, read carefully, and think!

If You Can't Deliver, Don't Ask

We were embarking on a needs assessment study in which we convened a series of focus groups composed of individuals who were receiving long-term care services. We wanted to know what could be improved in the service system. When we arrived, all the focus group members were present. One by one, each spoke and clearly told us that if we could not deliver what they requested, we should not take their time by conducting another group interview.

Don't Ask If You're Not Prepared to Answer

In a randomized controlled trial to evaluate an intervention to support family caregivers, we were concerned that families assigned to the "no treatment" control group would lose interest in the study and decide to withdraw. We thus decided to conduct monthly telephone check-in calls to control group caregivers to maintain their interest in the study and enhance retention. The problem, however, was what to say to this highly stressed and emotionally vulnerable population. We learned quickly that a simple statement (e.g., "Hello, Mrs. Smith; how are you today?") elicited clinically revealing statements about the person's psychological and physical health. Some caregivers began to cry, expressed feeling extremely depressed and not knowing whom to turn to, and revealed serious health complaints and incidents of physical abuse. We were ethically bound to respond appropriately, and this quick check-in telephone call to maintain study contact turned into a meaningful clinical intervention.

No Detail Too Small

To set up a randomization scheme based on stratification by gender, a blocking scheme was developed for both men and women and provided to a research assistant to create envelopes with appropriate group assignment sheets (experimental or control). As study participants were enrolled, we noticed that the first 10 women to enter the study were assigned to control, and all four men were assigned to intervention. With the blocked randomization scheme we were using, this was not possible, so an investigation was performed.

It was discovered that the research assistant had placed only control sheets in the envelopes for women and only intervention sheets in the envelopes for men. This required official notification of the institutional review board and the data and safety monitoring board, as well as a plan of action to determine how best to preserve the original randomization scheme and manage the errors to date. The lesson learned? Even the smallest details, such as reading a person's handwriting and stuffing envelopes, can have profound methodological implications for a study.

Inductive? No Way

A colleague set out to understand disability identity and identify factors that might contribute to it. He selected informants with all types of impairment conditions, from diverse ages, and with varied times of onset from birth through injury in adulthood. He conducted open-ended interviews claiming to be engaged in naturalistic inquiry, only to be perplexed that the only informant who professed she was a member of disability culture was a former student of his in his class on disability culture!

Wow, You Got It!

Your heart starts to beat, you feel a rush; it all clicks, falls into place; you've uncovered a pattern, a finding, something really striking, and it is significant. The data are right before your eyes. The result has the potential of having an impact on how professionals practice, on how clients feel and function, and on their health and well-being! Wow, you got it! You feel great.

This is so important—you have to do it again.

References

1. Bateni H, Maki B: Assistive devices for balance and mobility: benefits, demands, and adverse consequences. *Arch Phys Med Rehabil* 86:134–145, 2005.
2. Candlin F, Guins R: *The object reader*, London, 2009, Routledge.
3. Pullin G: *Disability meets design*, Boston, 2009, MIT Press.

Glossary

Abductive reasoning Patterns and concepts that emerge from an examination of information or data, which in some cases may relate to available theories and in other cases may not.

Abstract Research report that appears before the full report and briefly summarizes or highlights the major points made in each subsequent section.

Abstraction Symbolic representation of an observable or experienced referent.

Accessible Comprehensible to the user.

Accidental sampling See Convenience sampling.

Action processes Set of actions that researchers follow to implement a design; include setting boundaries of the study, collecting and analyzing information, and reporting and disseminating study findings.

Action research Inquiry undertaken to generate knowledge to inform action.

Adequacy Satisfactory according to rigor criteria.

Analysis of covariance Statistical technique that removes the effect of the influence of another variable on the dependent or outcome variable.

Analysis of variance Parametric statistic used to ascertain the extent to which significant group differences can be inferred to the population.

Artifact review Data collection technique in which the meaning of objects in their natural context is examined.

Assent Agreement to participate in a study of subject who cannot legally consent.

Associational statistics Set of procedures designed to identify relationships between multiple variables; determines whether knowledge of one set of data allows inference or prediction of the characteristics of another set of data.

Attention factor Phenomenon in which research subjects may experience change simply from the act of participating in a research project; also known as Hawthorne effect or halo effect.

Audit trail Path of a person's thinking and action processes that enables others to follow the logic and manner in which knowledge was developed.

Axial coding Set of procedures whereby data are put back together in new ways after open coding by making connections between categories (see Chapter 18).

Bias Potential unintended or unavoidable effect on study outcomes.

Bimodal distribution Distribution in which two values occur with the same frequency.

Boundary setting One of the first action processes of research in which the investigator establishes the conceptual limits of the study, as well as the types of information and study participants that will be included.

Breakdowns Points in data collection in naturalistic inquiry in which the expectation of the researcher does not match the observation or information gathered.

Call for proposals Announcements and requests from federal foundations and other sources for investigators to submit research plans for potential funding.

Case study Detailed, in-depth description of a single unit, subject, or event.

Casuistry ethical reasoning in which every case is treated as unique.

Categories Basic analytical step used in naturalistic inquiry in which the investigator groups phenomena according to similarities and labels the groups.

Celeration line Approach to the visual analysis of data points obtained in single-subject designs; drawn across pretest and posttest data points, reflects the central tendency of the data.

Chi-square Nonparametric statistic used with nominal data to test group differences.

Cleaning data Action process whereby the investigator checks the inputted data set to ensure all data have been accurately represented.

Clinical trial Research designed to investigate treatment efficacy.

Closed-ended question Data-gathering strategy in which a question is formed and the study participant is asked to choose a response among prescribed sets of answers.

Cluster sampling Random sampling technique whereby the investigator begins with large units, or clusters, in which smaller sampling units are contained, then randomly selects elements from these clusters.

Codebook Record of variable names for each variable in experimental-type research; record of categories, codes, and line placement in naturalistic inquiry.

Coding An analytic step in which both quantitative and non-quantitative data are categorized and labeled.

Coding of categories Repeated review and examination of the narrative in naturalistic data analysis.

Cohort study Research that examines specific subpopulations as they change over time.

Concept Symbolic representations of an observable or experienced referent.

Concept matrix Two-dimensional organizational system that presents all information that the investigator reviews and evaluates.

Conceptual definition Stipulates the meaning of concepts or constructs with other concepts or constructs; also known as lexical definition.

Concurrent validity Extent to which an instrument can discriminate the absence or presence of a known standard.

Confidence interval Estimated range of values in which an unknown population parameter is likely to exist.

Confidence level The probability value associated with a confidence interval; usually represented as percentage.

Confidentiality Assurance, on the part of the investigator, that no one other than the research team can have access to a respondent's information unless those who see the data are identified to the person before participation; the information cannot be linked to a person's identity.

Confirmable One of the four basic characteristics of research (see Chapter 1); the researcher must clearly and logically identify the strategies used in a study, enabling others to follow the sequence of thoughts and actions and to derive similar outcomes and conclusions.

Confirming cases Naturalistic boundary-setting strategy in which the investigator purposely selects participants to support an emerging interpretation or theory.

Confounding variables See Intervening variables.

Consequentialism Ethical decision making model in which the outcome or consequences of action form the basis for value judgment.

Constant comparison Naturalistic data analysis technique in which each datum is compared and contrasted with previous information to fit all the pieces together inductively into a bigger puzzle.

Construct Symbolic representation of shared experience that does not have an observable or directly experienced referent.

Construct validity Fit between the constructs that are the focus of the study and the way in which these constructs are operationalized.

Content validity Degree to which an indicator seems to agree with a validated instrument measuring the same construct.

Context specific One of the central features of naturalistic inquiry; refers to the specific environment or field in which the study is conducted and information is derived.

Contextualization Placement of data into a larger perspective (see Chapter 18).

Contingency table Two-dimensional frequency distribution primarily used with categorical data.

Continuous variables Variables that take on an infinite number of values.

Control Set of action processes that directs or manipulates factors to minimize extraneous variance in order to achieve an outcome.

Control group Group in experimental-type design in which the independent variable is withheld; thus the control group represents the characteristics of the experimental group before being changed by participation in the experimental condition.

Convenience sampling Boundary-setting action process that involves the enrollment of available subjects as they enter the study until the desired sample size is reached; also known as accidental sampling, opportunistic sampling, or volunteer sampling.

Correlational analysis Method of determining relationships among variables.

Counterbalance design Variation on experimental design in which more than one intervention is tested and in which the order of participation in each intervention is manipulated.

Credibility Truthfulness and accuracy of findings in naturalistic inquiry; also referred to as truth value.

Criterion validity Correlation or relationship between a measurement of interest and another instrument or standard that has been shown to be accurate.

Critical theory Worldview that suggests both an epistemology and a social change purpose for conducting research; complex set of strategies united by commonality of sociopolitical purpose designed to know about social justice and human experience as a means to promote social change.

Critical value Numerical value that indicates how high the sample statistic must be at a given level of significance to reject the null hypothesis.

Cronbach's alpha Statistical procedure used to examine the extent to which all items in the instrument measure the same construct.

Crossover design Variation on true-experimental design in which one group is assigned to the experimental group first and to the control condition later, and then the order for the other group is reversed.

Cross-sectional studies Studies that examine a phenomenon at one point in time.

Crystallization See Triangulation.

Culture Explicit and tacit rules, symbols, and rituals that guide patterns of human behavior within a group.

Data Set of information obtained through systematic investigation; data can refer to information that is numerical or narrative; singular, datum.

Data and safety monitoring board (DSMB) An independent group of experts who (1) review and approve all study procedures; (2) provide oversight for procedures regarding the safety of human subjects and ethical research practices, including reviewing the investigator's approach to recruitment and the informed consent process; (3) determine whether and when a study should be terminated because of adverse events that can be attributed to study procedures; and (4) if interim analyses should be conducted to evaluate study outcomes and if the study should be stopped midstream because it is either overwhelming beneficial or harmful.

Database An organized set or collection of data.

Database management Set of actions necessary to develop and maintain the raw data and statistical control files that are developed in experimental-type studies.

Data reduction Procedures used to summarize raw data into more compact and interpretable forms.

Data set Set of raw numbers generated by experimental-type data collection.

Deductive reasoning Moving from a general principle to understanding a specific case.

Degrees of freedom Values that are free to vary in a statistical test.

Dependent variable Presumed effect of an independent variable.

Descriptive questions See Level 1 questions and query.

Descriptive research Research that yields descriptive knowledge of population parameters and relationships among those parameters.

Descriptive statistics Procedures used to reduce large sets of observations into more compact and interpretable forms.

Design Plan, or blueprint, that specifies and structures the action processes of collecting, analyzing, and reporting data to answer a research question or query.

Deviant case Naturalistic boundary-setting strategy in which the investigator selects participants who have experiences that deviate or are vastly different from the mainstream.

Directional hypothesis Type of hypothesis in which the direction of the effect of the independent variable on the dependent variable is clearly articulated.

Disconfirming cases Naturalistic boundary-setting strategy in which the investigator selects participants who challenge an emerging interpretation or theory.

Discrete variables Variables with a finite number of distinct values.

Dispersion Summary measure, such as range or standard deviation, that describes the distribution of observed values; also referred to as variability.

Effect size Strength of differences in the sample values that the investigator expects to find.

Embedded case study Design in which the cases are conglomerates of multiple subparts, or are subparts themselves, placed within larger contexts.

Emic perspective "Insider's" or informant's way of understanding and interpreting experience.

Endogenous research Inquiry that is conceptualized, designed, and conducted by researchers who are "insiders" of the culture, using their own epistemology and structure of relevance.

Epistemology Branch of philosophy that addresses the nature of knowledge and how one comes to know.

Equipoise Maintaining a stance of neutrality in the way in which all study procedures are explained and implemented.

Ethics Integrity of the scientific process, with specific concerns for the behavioral conduct of the investigator throughout the research process and for the ethical involvement of human subjects in research.

Ethnography Primary research approach in anthropology concerned with description and interpretation of cultural patterns of groups, as well as the understanding of the cultural meanings people use to organize and interpret their experiences.

Etic perspective Systematic understanding of phenomena developed by those who are external to a group.

Evidence-based practice A model of practice in which decisions are supported by research.

Exempt status Institutional review status in which a study protocol is exempt from formal review from either the full board or its subcommittee.

Ex post facto design One type of nonexperimental, passive observation design in which the phenomena of interest have already occurred and cannot be manipulated in any way.

Experimental group Group in experimental design that receives the experimental condition.

Experimental-type research Designs that are based in a positivist philosophical foundation and that yield numerical data for analysis.

Explanatory research Research designed to predict outcomes.

Exploratory research Studies conducted in natural settings with the explicit purpose of discovering phenomena, variables, theory, or combinations thereof.

External validity Capacity to generalize findings and develop inferences from the sample to the study population.

Extraneous variables See Intervening variables.

Extreme or deviant case Naturalistic boundary-setting technique in which the investigator selects a case that represents an extreme example of the phenomenon of interest.

Factorial design Variation on true-experimental design in which the investigator evaluates the effects of two or more independent variables (X1 and X2) or the effects of an intervention on different factors or levels of a sample or study variables.

Field notes Naturalistic recordings written by the investigator that are composed of two basic components: (1) recordings of events, observations, and occurrences and (2) recordings of the investigator's own impressions of events, personal feelings, hunches, and expectations.

Field study Research conducted in natural settings.

Flexible design One of the central characteristics of designs in naturalistic inquiry; refers to the unfolding nature of designs in which data collection decisions are based on an interactive process of simultaneously collecting and analyzing information.

Focus group design Naturalistic design that uses a small group process to facilitate data collection and analysis.

Frequency distribution Distribution of values for a given variable and the number of times each value occurs.

Full disclosure Adequacy of information provided to research participants; necessary for them to make informed decisions about the degree of their participation in a study.

Full integration Method that integrates multiple purposes and thus combines design strategies from different paradigms, enabling each to contribute knowledge to the study of a single problem to derive a more complete understanding of the phenomenon under study.

Funder Agency or organization providing financial support for research.

Gaining access Naturalistic action process of entering the context of a field study.

Grounded theory Method in naturalistic research used to generate theory, primarily employing the inductive process of constant comparison.

Guttman scale Unidimensional or cumulative scale in which the researcher develops a small number of items (four to seven) that relate to one concept and then arranges them so that endorsement of one item means an endorsement of items below it.

Halo effect See Attention factor.

Hawthorne effect See Attention factor.

Health Insurance Portability and Accountability Act (HIPAA) Legislation protecting the privacy of individuals' health information.

Heuristic design Research approach that encourages investigator to discover and methods that enable further investigation; design strategy that involves complete immersion of the investigator into the phenomenon of interest and self-reflection of the investigator's personal experiences.

Health Insurance Portability and Accountability Act (HIPAA) Federal privacy policy and ruling which mandates personal the privacy of individual health information.

History Effect of external events on study outcomes.

Holistic Philosophical approaches that view individuals as creating their own subjective realities that cannot be understood by "atomizing," or separating, experience into discrete parts.

Holistic case study Design in which the unit of analysis is seen as only one global phenomenon.

Homogeneous selection Naturalistic action process of boundary setting in which the investigator attempts to reduce variation in study participants, thereby simplifying the number of experiences, characteristics, and conceptual domains that are represented among study participants.

Human subject protection Legislated methods to reduce harm and preserve privacy of human research participants.

Hypothesis Testable statements that indicate what the researcher expects to find, based on theory and level of knowledge in the literature.

Idiographic Pertaining to uniqueness of individuals.

Inclusion and exclusion criteria Sets of criteria that determine who can and cannot participate in a study.

Independent variable Presumed cause of the dependent variable; sometimes referred to as the "predictor variable."

Inductive reasoning Human reasoning that involves a process in which general rules evolve or develop from individual cases or from observation of a phenomenon.

Inference Extent to which the samples reflect the population at both pretest and posttest times.

Inferential statistics Type of statistics used to draw conclusions about population parameters, based on findings from a sample.

Informants Participants in a research study who play an active role of informing the investigator as to the context and its cultural rules.

Informed consent Official statement developed by the researcher that informs study participants of the purpose and scope of the study.

Institutional review board (IRB) Board of experts that must be established at each institution involved in a research process to oversee the ethical conduct of research.

Integrated design Structure used to strengthen a study by selecting and combining designs and methods from both paradigms so that one complements the other to benefit the whole or contribute to an understanding of the whole.

Interactive effect Changes that occur in the dependent variable as a consequence of the combined influence or interaction of taking the pretest and participating in the experimental condition.

Interactionist Specific philosophical approach in naturalistic inquiry; assumes that human meaning evolves from the context of social interaction; human phenomena are therefore understood through interpreting the meanings in social discourse and exchange.

Internal validity Ability of the research design to answer accurately the research question.

Interpretation Analytical step in naturalistic inquiry in which the investigator examines the derived categories and themes and develops a conceptual understanding of the phenomenon.

Interquartile range Measure of variability in experimental-type research that refers to the range of scores that compose the middle 50% of subjects, or the majority responses.

Interrater reliability Test involving the comparison of two observers measuring the same event.

Interrupted time series design Quasi-experimental design involving repeated measurement of the dependent variable, both before and after the introduction of the independent variable, and no control or comparison group.

Interval numbers Numbers that share the characteristics of ordinal and nominal measures but also have the characteristic of equal spacing between categories.

Intervening variables Phenomena that have an effect on the study variables but are not necessarily the object of the study; also known as confounding variables or extraneous variables.

Interview Information-gathering action process conducted through verbal communication and occurring face-to-face or by telephone; process may be structured or unstructured and usually is conducted with one individual.

Investigator involvement One of the principal characteristics of most forms of naturalistic inquiry in which the investigator becomes fully immersed in the data collection and analytical process.

Judgmental sampling See Purposive sampling.

Kuder-Richardson formula (K-R 20) Statistical procedure used to examine the extent to which all the items in the instrument measure the same construct.

Laboratory study Research implemented in controlled environments.

"Learning the ropes" Ongoing naturalistic action process that involves negotiation and renegotiation with members of a field site or with the individual or groups of individuals who are the focus of the study.

Level 1 questions Experimental-type research questions that aim to describe phenomena; also known as descriptive questions.

Level 2 questions Experimental-type research questions that explore relationships among phenomena that have already been studied at the descriptive level; also known as relational questions.

Level 3 questions Experimental-type research questions that test concepts by manipulating one to affect the other; also known as predictive questions.

Levels of abstraction Four levels that guide theory development and testing: concept, construct, relationships, and propositions or principles.

Levels of significance Probability that defines how rare or unlikely the sample data must be before the researcher can reject the null hypothesis.

Lexical definition See Conceptual definition.

Life history Type of naturalistic inquiry concerned with eliciting life experiences and with how individuals interpret and attribute meanings to these experiences; a research approach designed to reveal the nature of the "life process traversed over time."

Likert scale Type of scale most frequently scored on a 5to 7-point range, indicating the subject's level of positive or negative response to an item.

Linguistic sensitivity Having knowledge about the target audience and the meaning of language to that group.

Literature review chart Approach to organizing a literature review in which research studies are summarized in a table format along key categories, such as type of design, measures, and outcomes.

Logical deduction Human process of reasoning that begins with an abstraction and then focuses on discrete parts of phenomena or observations.

Logical positivism Philosophical school of thought characterized by a belief in a singular, knowable reality that exists separate from individual ideas and reductionism.

Logical process One of the four criteria of research (see Chapter 1); suggests that research must be clear and conform to accepted norms of deductive, inductive, or abductive reasoning and proceed systematically and logically through the thinking and action processes.

Longitudinal study Research design in which data collection occurs at discrete points over long periods of time.

Main effects Direct effects of one variable on another.

Manipulation Action process of maneuvering the independent variable so that the effect of its presence, absence, or degree on the dependent variable can be observed.

Maximum variation Boundary-setting strategy that involves seeking individuals for study participation who are extremely different along dimensions that are the focus of the study.

Mean Average score calculated by adding the objects or items and then dividing the sum by the number of objects or items.

Measure of variability Degree of dispersion among scores.

Measurement Translation of observations into numbers.

Measures of central tendency Numerical information regarding the most typical or representative scores in a group.

Median Point in a distribution at which 50% of the cases fall above and 50% below.

Member checking Technique whereby the investigator "checks out" his or her assumptions with informants.

Memoing Particular approach to coding segments of narrative that is used in naturalistic forms of analysis; investigator indicates personal notations

as to emerging hypotheses and subsequent directions for analysis.

Meta-analysis Analysis technique of data and/or information aggregated from more than one source.

Mixing Boundary Setting Methods Using strategies from both experimental-type and naturalistic traditions to delimit the scope of a study.

Mixed-method design Combination of multiple strategies or designs that answers a series of research questions.

Mode Value that occurs most frequently in a data set.

Mortality Subject attrition, or dropping out of a study before its completion.

Multiple comparisons Statistical tests used to determine which group is greater than the others.

Multiple regression Equation based on correlational statistics in which each predictor variable is entered into the equation to determine how strongly it relates to the outcome variable and how much variation in the outcome variable can be predicted by each independent variable.

Multiple-case study Design in which more than one study on single units of analysis are conducted.

Narrative Set of words, derived from stories, interviews, written journals, and other written documents, which forms the data set in naturalistic inquiry.

Naturalistic inquiry Set of research approaches that are based in holistic-type philosophical frameworks and that use inductive and abductive forms of reasoning to derive qualitative information.

Networking See Snowball sampling.

Nominal numbers Numbers used to name attributes of a variable.

Nomothetic Referring to group characteristics.

Non-Consequentialism Ethical model which uses the inherent goodness or badness as the basis for decision making.

Nondirectional hypothesis Type of hypothesis in which the research indicates an expected effect but not the direction of that effect.

Nonequivalent control group designs Quasi-experimental designs in which there are at least two comparison groups, but subjects are not randomly assigned to these groups.

Nonexperimental designs Experimental-type designs in which the three criteria for true experimentation do not exist.

Nonparametric statistics Formulas used to test hypotheses when (1) normality of variance in the population is not assumed, (2) homogeneity of variance is not assumed, (3) data generated from measures are ordinal or nominal, and (4) sample sizes may be small.

Nonprobability sampling Sampling in which nonrandom methods are used to obtain a sample.

Nonrandom error See Systematic error.

Nonreactive methodology See Unobtrusive methodology.

Null hypothesis Hypothesis of no difference.

Object Reading Method from visual culture in which objects are analyzed for their meaning in context.

One-shot case study Pre-experimental design in which the independent variable is introduced and in which the dependent variable is then measured in only one group.

Ontology Term of philosophy that refers to a person's view or definition of reality.

Open-ended questions Form of asking questions in which the response is open and in which participants are free to formulate specific verbal responses, rather than choose among fixed response options.

Operational definition Definition that reduces the abstraction of a concept to a concrete observable form by specifying the exact procedures for measuring or observing the phenomenon.

Opportunistic sampling See Convenience sampling.

Ordinal numbers Numerical values that assign an order to a set of observations.

Panel study Similar to cohort design, except that the same set of people is studied over time.

Parametric statistics Mathematical formulas that test hypotheses based on three assumptions: (1) samples come from populations that are normally distributed, (2) there is homogeneity of variance, and (3) data generated from the measures are interval level.

Participant observation Naturalistic data collection strategy in which the researcher takes part in the context under scrutiny.

Participants Individuals who provide information in naturalistic studies.

Participatory action research Approach that directly involves study participants in each of the 10 research essentials; that is, it involves study participants that contribute to formulating the research question or query, study design, and approach to analysis.

Passive observation designs Nonexperimental designs used to investigate phenomena as they naturally occur and to ascertain the relationship between two or more variables.

Pearson product-moment correlation Statistic of association using interval level data and yielding a score between -1 and +1.

Peer debriefing Use of more than one investigator as a participant in the analytical process, followed by reflection on other possible competing interpretations of the data.

Phase I clinical trial Study of a small sample to test a new behavioral or biomedical intervention not previously evaluated.

Phase II clinical trial Study of the efficacy and safety of an intervention in a larger group of people.

Phase III clinical trial Study to evaluate comparative effectiveness and safety of an intervention in a large group of persons (several hundred to thousands).

Phenomenology Form of naturalistic inquiry used to uncover the meaning of how humans experience phenomena through the description of those experiences as they are lived by individuals.

Philosophical foundation Formal belief system guiding the research approach.

Pluralism Central characteristic of naturalistic inquiry that suggests there are multiple realities that can be identified and understood only within the natural context in which human experience and behavior occur.

Population Group of persons, elements, or both with common characteristics that are defined by the investigator.

Post hoc comparisons Statistical tests used to determine which group is greater than the others.

Posttest Observation or measurement subsequent to the completion of the experimental condition.

Practice evaluation Application of research methods to examining practice process and outcome.

Practice research Investigation of human experience in the context of health care and human service institutions, agencies, or settings.

Predictive questions See Level 3 questions.

Predictive validity Extent to which an instrument can predict or estimate the occurrence of a behavior or event.

Pre-experimental designs (experimental-type designs) Designs in which two of the three criteria necessary for true experimentation are absent.

Pretest Observation or measurement before introduction of the experimental condition.

Principles See Propositions.

Principlism A set of four rules that guide ethical decision making.

Probability sampling Sampling plans that are based on probability theory.

Probe Statement that is neutral, designed to encourage the study participant to provide additional information or elaboration.

Problem statement Statement that identifies the phenomenon to be explored and the reason(s) it needs to be examined or why it is a problem or issue.

Proposal Formal description of an intended research project.

Propositions Statements that govern a set of relationships and give them a structure; also called principles.

Prospective studies Studies that describe phenomena, search for cause-and-effect relationships, or examine change in the present or as the event unfolds over time.

Purpose statement Statement that articulates the specific purpose of or reason for conducting the research study; identifies the particular goals of the study.

Purpose statement Articulation of the reasons for conducting and using research.

Purposive sampling Deliberate selection of individuals by the researcher based on certain predefined criteria; also known as judgmental sampling.

Quasi-experimental design Experiments that have treatments, outcome measures, and experimental units but do not use random assignment to create comparison from which treatment-caused change is inferred; instead, the comparisons depend on nonequivalent groups who differ from each other in many ways other than the presence of the treatment being tested (see Chapter 8).

Query Broad statement that identifies the phenomenon or natural field of interest in naturalistic forms of inquiry.

Question Interrogative statement that a study is designed to answer. See research question.

Questionnaires Written instruments that may be administered either face-to-face, by proxy, or through the mail; may vary as to the structure of questions (closed or open) that are included.

Quota sampling Nonrandom technique in which the investigator purposively obtains a sample by selecting sample elements in the same proportion that they are represented in the population.

Random error Error that occurs by chance.

Randomization Selection or assignment of subjects based on chance.

Range Difference between the highest and lowest observed value in a collection of data.

Ratio numbers Numbers that have all the characteristics of interval numbers but also have an absolute 0 point.

Raw data file Set of numbers in a computer file that is entered from a questionnaire or other data collection instrument used in experimental-type research; its creation is the first action step in the process of preparing data for statistical analysis.

Reflexivity Process of self-examination.

Regression Statistical phenomenon in which extreme scores tend to regress or cluster around the mean (average) on repeated testing occasion.

Relational questions See Level 2 questions.

Reliability Stability of a research design.

Research Multiple, systematic strategies to generate knowledge about human behavior, human experience, and human environments in which the thought and action processes of the researcher are clearly specified so that they are (1) logical, (2) understandable, (3) confirmable, and (4) useful.

Research design Plan that specifies and structures the action processes of collecting, analyzing, and reporting data to answer a research question.

Research question Statement that guides an experimental-type investigation; must be concise and framed in such a way that systematic inquiry can be carried out; establishes the boundaries or limits as to what concepts, individuals, or phenomena will be examined.

Research topic Broad area of inquiry from which the investigator develops a more specific question or query.

Retrospective studies Describe and examine phenomena after the fact or after the phenomena have occurred.

Reviewers (review committee) Individuals who read and consider the efficacy and worth of a proposed study.

Sample Subset of the population participating or included in the study.

Sampling error Difference between the values obtained from the sample and those that actually exist in the population.

Sampling frame Listing of every element in the target population.

Saturation Point at which an investigator has obtained sufficient information from which to obtain an understanding of the phenomena.

Scales Tools for the quantitative measurement of the degree to which individuals possess a specific attribute or trait.

Secondary data analysis Analysis of a data set that has been developed in a previous study or by another investigator; usually conducted to explore specific research questions that were secondary to the primary study purpose.

Semantic differential Scaling technique in which the researcher develops a series of opposites or mutually exclusive constructs that ask the respondent to give a judgment about something along an ordered dimension, usually of 7 points.

Significance level Extent to which group differences are a function of chance.

Simple random sampling (SRS) Probability sampling technique in which a sample is randomly selected from a population.

Single-case study Design in which only one study on a single unit of analysis is conducted.

Snowball sampling Obtaining a sample through asking subjects to provide the names of others who may meet study criteria; also known as networking.

Solomon four-group design True-experimental design that combines true experimentation and posttest-only designs into one design structure.

Spearman rho Statistic of association using ordinal level data and yielding a score between -1 and +1.

Split-half technique Reliability technique in which instrument items are split in half and a correlational procedure is performed between the two halves.

Standard deviation Indicator of the average deviation of scores around the mean.

Static group comparison Pre-experimental design in which a comparison group is added to the one-shot case study design.

Statistic Number derived from a mathematical procedure as part of the analytical process in experimental-type research.

Statistical conclusion validity Power of an investigator's study to draw statistical conclusions.

Statistical power Probability of identifying a relationship that exists, or the probability of rejecting the null hypothesis when it is false or should be rejected.

Stratified random sampling Technique in which the population is divided into smaller subgroups, or strata, from which sample elements are then chosen.

Subjects Participants in experimental-type studies.

Sum of squares Descriptive statistic for interpreting variability; derived by squaring the difference between each score from the mean, which are then summed.

Survey designs Nonexperimental designs used to measure primarily characteristics of a population, typically conducted with large samples through mail questionnaires, telephone, or face-to-face interview.

Systematic error Systematic bias or an error that occurs consistently with an instrument; impacts the extent to which an instrument is valid or represents the underlying construct or concept; also known as nonrandom error.

Systematic random sampling Technique in which a sampling interval width (K) is determined based on the needed sample size, and then every Kth element is selected from a sampling frame.

Target population Group of individuals or elements from which the investigator is able to select a sample.

Taxonomic analysis Naturalistic data analysis technique in which the researcher organizes similar or related categories into larger categories and identifies differences between sets of subcategories and larger or overarching categories.

Ten essentials Ten thinking and action processes that compose any type of research that is experimental type, naturalistic, or integrated (see Chapter 2).

Test-retest reliability Reliability test in which the same test is given twice to the same subject under the same circumstances.

Theme Analytical process used in naturalistic inquiry in which the investigator identifies patterns and topics from which a theme is derived.

Theoretical sensitivity Researcher's ability to detect and give meaning to data.

Theory Set of interrelated constructs, definitions, and propositions that presents a systematic view of phenomena by specifying relations among variables, with the purpose of explaining or predicting phenomena (see Chapter 1).

Theory-based selection Approach in naturalistic inquiry wherein key informants or study participants are selected, based on their ability to illuminate the particular theoretical construct that is being explored.

Theory generating One of the primary purposes of many forms of naturalistic inquiry; use of

naturalistic approaches to link each piece of datum from which concepts, constructs, relationships, and propositions are generated or derived.

Theory testing One of the primary purposes of many forms of experimental-type research; use of experimental methodologies to test formally a set of propositions of a theory.

Thinking processes Logical thought processes of research that involve deductive, inductive, or abductive thinking; include identifying a philosophical foundation and theoretical framework, framing a question or query, substantiating the research approach, and developing a design structure.

Time series design Quasi-experimental design that involves repeated data collection over time for a single group.

Transcription Typed narrative derived from an audiotape or a video image of an interview with an individual or group; represents an action process primarily used in naturalistic inquiry as the first step in the analysis and interpretation of narrative.

Treatment fidelity Attention to the integrity of implementing an intervention.

Trend study Research examining a general population over time to see changes or trends that emerge as a consequence of time.

Triangulation Use of multiple strategies or methods as a means to strengthen the credibility of an investigator's findings related to the phenomenon under study; also known as crystallization.

True-experimental design Classic two-group design in which subjects are randomly selected and randomly assigned (R) to either an experimental or a control group condition; before the experimental condition, all subjects are pretested or observed on a dependent measure (O); in the experimental group, the independent variable or experimental condition is imposed (X), and it is withheld in the control group; subjects are then posttested or observed on the dependent variable (O) after the experimental condition.

Truth value Term used in naturalistic inquiry to refer to the accuracy of interpretation or how closely the analytical scheme reflects the natural context or focus of the investigation; also referred to as credibility.

t-Test Parametric test to ascertain the extent to which any significant differences between the means of two sample groups can be inferred from the sample to the population.

Type I error Rejecting the null hypothesis when it is true.

Type II error Failing to reject the null hypothesis when it is false.

Typical case Naturalistic boundary-setting strategy in which the investigator selects participants who are typical or representative of the particular event or experience that is the focus of the inquiry.

Understandable criteria One of the four criteria of research (see Chapter 1); refers to the requirement that a study makes sense and that all study procedures are precisely articulated.

Univariate statistics Descriptive data reduction approaches for one variable.

Unobtrusive methodology Observation and examination of documents and objects that bear on the phenomenon of interest; also known as nonreactive methodology.

Useful criteria One of the four criteria of research (see Chapter 1); refers to the requirement that a research study contributes to knowledge building.

Validity Extent to which an investigator's findings are accurate or reflect the underlying purpose of the study.

Variability See Dispersion.

Variable Concept or construct to which a numerical value is assigned; by definition, it must have more than one value, even if the investigator is interested in only one condition.

Variable label Applied to each variable in a computer file; follows certain conventions that are based on the particular statistical software used by the investigator.

Variance Descriptive statistic that reflects a measure of variability; reflects the mean or average of the sum of squares; the larger the variance, the larger the spread of scores.

Voluntary participation Informed decision to be a subject or study participant.

Volunteer sampling See Convenience sampling.

Vulnerable populations Participants in studies considered to be vulnerable or at risk; require special set of ethical procedures to ensure their protection; examples include pregnant women, fetuses, children, individuals with cognitive impairments or mental illness, and prisoners.

Index

Page numbers followed by "f" indicate figures, "t" indicate tables, and "b" indicate boxes.